*Comparative Studies and the Politics
of Modern Medical Care*

Comparative Studies and the Politics of Modern Medical Care

Edited by

THEODORE R. MARMOR, RICHARD FREEMAN, AND KIEKE G. H. OKMA

Yale University Press
New Haven and London

Set in Sabon type by Westchester Book Services

Library of Congress Control Number : 2009924986

ISBN 978-0-300-14983-8 (paperback : alk. paper)

A catalogue record for this book is available from the British Library.

This paper meets the requirements of ANSI/NISO Z39.48-1992 (Permanence of Paper).

10 9 8 7 6 5 4 3 2 1

Contents

Preface   vii

Acknowledgments   xiii

1   Comparative Policy Analysis and Health Care:
    An Introduction   1
    Theodore R. Marmor, Richard Freeman,
    and Kieke G. H. Okma

2   The United States: Risks for Americans and Lessons
    for Abroad   24
    Joseph White

3   Canada: Health Care Reform in Comparative
    Perspective   61
    Carolyn Hughes Tuohy

4   Germany: Evidence, Policy, and Politics
    in Health Care Reform   88
    Martin Pfaff

5   The Netherlands: From Polder Model
    to Modern Management   120
    Kieke G. H. Okma and Aad A. de Roo

6   The United Kingdom: Health Policy Learning in the National Health
    Service   153
    Mark Exworthy and Richard Freeman

7   Primary Care and Health Reform: Concepts, Confusions,
    and Clarifications   180
    Joseph White and Theodore R. Marmor

8   Hospital Care in the United States, Canada, Germany,
    the United Kingdom, and the Netherlands   203
    Kieke G. H. Okma and Michael B. Decter

9   Pharmaceutical Policy and Politics in OECD Countries   244
    Richard Freeman

10 Comprehensive Long-Term Care in Japan and Germany:
    Policy Learning and Cross-National Comparison   265
    John Creighton Campbell and Naoki Ikegami

11 Regulating Private Health Insurance Markets   288
    Jürgen Wasem and Stefan Greß

12 Learning from Others and Learning from Mistakes:
    Reflections on Health Policy Making   305
    Rudolf Klein

    Appendix: National Health Accounts: A Tool for International
    Comparison of Health Spending   319
    Markus Schneider

    Contributors   347

    Index   349

Preface

This book has unusual origins. It grew out of a series of ten conferences that took place in Europe and North America and, on one occasion, in Sydney, Australia, between 1995 and 2004. These gatherings, which we came to name the Four Country Conferences, explicitly articulated and addressed methodological and substantive issues of cross-national learning in health policy. Over a sustained period of time, they brought together participants working in government, health care management, and journalism as well as universities and research institutes.

The idea of a continuing and structured forum for a serious discussion of health reform cross-nationally was fueled by a deep sense of dissatisfaction about many meetings and conferences that the editors of and contributors to this book had attended earlier. Most of those meetings included experts from different countries. Most explicitly sought to learn from policy experience in other countries. However, most of such gatherings did not live up to the expectation that bringing together experts and discussing individual country experience produces a better understanding of national health policies and cross-national lesson drawing.

The model for the Four Country Conferences emerged from two meetings on international health reform experience at Ditchley House in Oxfordshire, England, in the early 1990s. The Ditchley meetings brought together policy makers, managers, and academics from a large number of countries, rich and poor, east and west. A group of attendees, including two of the three editors of this book, later became the steering committee of the Four Country

Conferences—Martin Pfaff of Germany, Michael Decter and Rudolf Klein of Great Britain, Kieke Okma of the Netherlands, and Theodore Marmor of the United States. We decided to work together and hold regular meetings, hoping to improve the quality and relevance of comparative health policy work. We came to appreciate, for instance, the benefits of creating a platform for repeated debates. We also learned the merit of organizing meetings around a semipermanent cast of participants and focusing debate on the experience of countries where comparison makes intellectual sense. This book reflects those efforts over more than a decade.

The Four Country Conferences, 1995–2004

The pairing of four countries—the Netherlands and Germany, Canada and the United States—made easier the systematic comparison of their health policy experience. Later, we added the United Kingdom, an acknowledgment of its importance as a source of health reform ideas. The initial principles of selection were few but firm: First, we selected neighboring countries with a core of shared features—cultural, economic, political, and medical—but with interesting differences. This, we hoped, would allow more disciplined debate and informed comparison, more systematic analysis and less startling anecdote than we had found in other meetings. Second, we found participants from these countries with backgrounds in government, health care management, politics, journalism, academia, and industry. Our meetings were thus multinational as well as multidisciplinary. We aimed for a considerable degree of continuity among participants in the yearly meetings to allow for the establishment of and, more important, the revision and regeneration of a body of collective understanding. This comparative format enriched our discussions in significant ways.

It allowed us to avoid the common phenomenon of the hit-and-run floating of ideas in meetings that offer no real opportunity to assess claims or distinguish facts from fiction, the faddish from the fundamental. Further, as we had found widespread confusion about the very terminology in health policy debates, we saw the need for a core of participants over time to develop a common language based on accumulated understandings. Finally, from the difficulties of finding common ground among heterogenous nations, we learned how important it is to use an explicit comparative framework for selecting the countries and topics to address.

Following the Ditchley tradition, our meetings generally lasted two days, sometimes spread out over one afternoon, one whole day, and one morning, with two evenings in between for informal meetings. Each conference began with one or two extended plenary sessions, introduced by brief keynote papers, which participants had received in advance. Plenaries were followed by an entire day of discussion in smaller working groups, each of which presented a report on its deliberations during the final plenary that returned to the main topic. What started as discussion papers for the Four Country Conferences matured into chapters of this book, as authors updated and expanded their original texts to reflect the debates of the conferences over time as well as their subsequent academic work.

This Volume

In keeping with its origins at the Four Country Conferences, this book has two purposes: first, to reflect on the challenges of cross-national comparison in health and health care, and its relationship to policy change and continuity; and second, to present papers of enduring quality to illustrate some of the features required in comparative analysis that seeks to inform policy debates. The book explores the general topic of comparative policy learning as well as specific substantial policy issues. The methodological discussions center on the use and abuse of comparative evidence in health policy developments. Among the first set of questions addressed are the following: Why countries look to others for solutions for internal policy problems, what do policy makers (and academics) know about other countries, and how do they collect and use this knowledge? What lessons can they expect to draw from experience elsewhere? What role can and should comparative analysis play in national health policy debates? What gains are there in linking national portraits of policy development with substantive analyses of topics such as drug, long-term care, and hospital care? Although the book draws on the Four Country Conference papers and debates about these topics, the chapter authors have substantially revised their original texts.

Following the introductory chapter by the editors of this volume, surveying the field of cross-national policy studies, the next five chapters explore the ambitions and realities of health care reform in specific countries. Chapter 2, by Joe White, surveys the strategies, tactics, and results of efforts in American health reform to change policy in the 1990s and beyond. Reviewing American political institutions and the contested debates about health reform, White analyzes the period following the failure of the Clinton reform and assesses to what degree American reform ideas traveled cross-nationally and warrant caution. In Chapter 3, Carolyn Tuohy uses Canadian health policy experience to illuminate the conditions under which fundamental or incremental reform takes place. Her comparative perspective illuminates all the other national accounts of reform. Chapter 4, by Martin Pfaff, describes the varied uses of evidence in German health reform, focusing specifically on the complicated politics that a former legislator so well understands. In Chapter 5, Kieke Okma and Aad de Roo portray the complex processes by which Dutch health reform efforts were introduced, partially implemented, then deflected and defeated, indirectly adjusting practices, and finally resurfacing in another disguise in 2006. Chapter 6, by Mark Exworthy and Richard Freeman, examines the United Kingdom's experience of health reform in the last decades of the twentieth century. In emphasizing policy learning—as a theme apart from health care reform—this chapter serves as a link to the more theoretically oriented second half of the book.

Chapters 7 through 11 deal with several of the most salient comparative policy topics in health care. Predicated on cross-national evidence and understanding, they are at once both abstract and practical: abstract because derived from more than one case; practical because applicable in a range of contexts. They provide introductions to both practitioners and students of health policy, both expressing and inviting useful thinking.

Joe White and Ted Marmor begin Chapter 7, for example, by discussing some of the confusions surrounding the definition of the term *primary care* and the different national understandings of this apparently simple idea. In Chapter 8, Kieke Okma and Michael Decter explore the future of the hospital in the five countries covered in the book. Chapter 9, by Richard Freeman, explores pharmaceutical policy. The author describes the tension between national industrial policies promoting research and innovation, social policies financing access to health goods and services, and economic policies concerned with controlling the growth of public spending. With a comparative perspective in Chapter 10, John Campbell and Naoki Ikegami portray the development of policy for long-term care in Japan and Germany. They emphasize the nature of the political calculations made at each stage. Chapter 11, by Jürgen Wasem and Stefan Greß, focuses on the essential features of private health insurance that require government regulation almost everywhere among rich democracies. The authors point to the substantial degree of professional consensus in the economics literature about market failure in commercial health insurance. They highlight the gap between this professional understanding and much of the policy debates about health insurance, competition, and health care reform.

In what serves as a postscript to the Four Country Conferences and as a conclusion to the book, Chapter 12 begins by questioning the meaning of the term *policy learning*. Author Rudolf Klein elaborates on the politics of the cross-border traffic in claims about policy outcomes and stresses the importance of distinguishing the process of "learning about" the experiences of other countries from that of "drawing lessons from" them. He also raises another methodological issue of great significance. What exactly are we evaluating, he asks, when we investigate the policy experiences of others? Do we evaluate stated policy as if it were in fact implemented, even though we all know it never is that simple? Do we evaluate the policy as implemented at first, sometime later, or on average? Those questions are very similar to the problems with the gold standard of biomedical research, the randomized controlled trial. Precisely because the so-called trial in social policy does not take place under tightly controlled circumstances, drawing inferences about the implemented forms of such interventions is necessarily problematic. The same applies to analyses of fiscal, professional, and regulatory policies, on both the theoretical and the practical levels.

In the Appendix, Markus Schneider presents statistical data that plays a crucial role on all international comparative efforts in health policy. His statistical data on health care expenditure in our basic set of four countries show the divergent levels and trends in expenditure. He warns that different definitions greatly complicate drawing inferences about the subject from international comparisons. His warning simply underlines the comparative point that similar terms do not necessarily refer to similar phenomena. So, for example, the concept of primary care as the first point of contact with the medical system contrasts sharply with the concept of primary care as comprehensive services by teams of nonspecialist medical providers.

In the course of the Four Country Conferences and the drafting of this book, we have acquired the usual number of intellectual and organizational debts. From the start, the steering committee directed the choice of topics, authors, and participants in the conferences. The Ministry of Health in the Netherlands supported and hosted our first and sixth conferences as did Health Canada the second and seventh. In Germany we had the financial support from not only the federal government but also the national associations of physicians and sickness funds. In the United States, we had support from Yale University, the Commonwealth Fund, and the Dutch Government for the fourth conference. And for the ninth conference in the United States we had support from Case Western Reserve University, the Commonwealth Fund, and the Dutch Government. To all these institutions we owe our thanks. In addition, we are grateful to Andrew Podger, the former head civil servant in the Australian Department of Health who attended our conferences and supported our reflection about the first four meetings in a special conference held in Sydney, Australia, in 1999.

The authors of the chapters deserve special thanks from the editors for their willingness to revise early reports and make them into chapters of a book edited by others. In the course of making a book of their chapters, we had the co-operation and help of an especially loyal set of assistants. Avi Feller was the Yale undergraduate who helped the most in the initial phase and did so with remarkable skill and welcomed cheerfulness. Camille Costelli, the assistant to editor Marmor for nearly a decade, kept track of a complex web of materials with, as all those with whom she deals acknowledge, patience and gracefulness. The summer of 2007 brought all of the work together and, for that, the assistance of Yale medical student Joe Rojas was crucial. We editors are happy to note the help we had and extend our warm thanks to all of them.

Ted Marmor, Yale University
Kieke Okma, New York University
Richard Freeman, The University of
Edinburgh

November 1, 2008

Acknowledgments

This book had its origins in a series of conferences over a decade. Each of those meetings had its own organizers, authors, and discussants, and each produced a conference report that thanked hosts and contributors. However, the authors of the following chapters deserve special thanks from the editors for their willingness to revise earlier drafts. We also want to acknowledge the help of those who assisted us in bringing this book to publication. In the course of making a book of their chapters, we had the cooperation and help of an especially loyal set of assistants. Avi Feller was the Yale undergraduate who helped the most in the initial phase and did so with remarkable skill and welcomed cheerfulness. Camille Costelli, the assistant to editor Marmor for nearly a decade, kept track of a complex web of materials with, as all those with whom she deals acknowledge, patience and gracefulness. In the summer of 2007, we brought all of the work together and, for that, the assistance of Yale medical student Joe Rojas was crucial. We editors are happy to note the help we had and extend our warm thanks to all of them.

Many others have helped in one way or another, including cordial colleagues at Yale Press. But we would be remiss if we ignored the Hanse Institute of North Germany, the site where the editors spent the fall of 2005 writing the introduction and editing the many papers that now comprise the chapters of this book. We are especially grateful to Professor Stephan Liebfried of Bremen University, a colleague of many years, who largely arranged the Hanse appointment. His welfare state unit—and its health policy participants under Professor Heinz Rothgang's leadership—provided a special bonus that fall, helpfully commenting on the work of the editors. Thanks to all from the editors and the authors whose work is published here.

Comparative Policy Analysis and Health Care
An Introduction

THEODORE R. MARMOR, RICHARD FREEMAN,
AND KIEKE G. H. OKMA

None of us can escape the "bombardment of information about what is happening in other countries" (Klein 1997). Yet in the field of health policy, which is our subject, there is a considerable imbalance between the magnitude and speed of the information flows and the capacity to learn useful lessons from them.[1] There is, moreover, a substantial gap between promise and performance in the field of comparative policy studies. Misdescription and superficiality are all too common. Unwarranted inferences, rhetorical distortion, and caricatures all show up too regularly in comparative health policy scholarship and debates. Why might that be so, and what does that suggest about more promising forms of cross-national intellectual exchange? The main purpose of this chapter is to explore the methodological questions raised by concerns about these weaknesses in international comparison in health policy. The core question is how one nation can learn from another competently in health care policy.

To address that question, this chapter first describes the political context of health and welfare state reform debates during the last three decades of the twentieth century. The first section argues that in almost all industrial democracies rising medical expenditures exacerbated fiscal concerns about the affordability of mature welfare states. Those concerns turned into increased pressure for policy change in health care and, with that, the inclination to look abroad for promising solutions of domestic problems. The second section takes up the topic of cross-national policy learning more directly, addressing some of the promises and methodological pitfalls of such work. The third section focuses on health reform debates, skeptically reviews the claims of convergence among industrialized countries, and outlines the expansive scholarship on comparative health policy. The fourth section addresses the purposes, promises, and pitfalls of comparative studies in health policy. The fifth section groups the works in categories that highlight the character, possibilities, and limits of this comparative literature. The concluding section returns to the chapter's basic theme: the real promise of comparative policy scholarship and the mixed portrait of performance to date.

The Political Context: Welfare State Debates and Health Reforms, 1970–2000

There is little doubt about the prominence of health policy on the public agenda of most, if not all, industrial democracies.[2] Canada's universal health insurance is a model of achievement for many observers, the subject of considerable intellectual scrutiny, and the destination of many policy travelers in search of illumination. Yet in the 1980s and 1990s both the national government and a majority of its provinces felt sufficiently concerned about the condition of Canadian Medicare to set up advisory commissions to chart adjustments (Okma 2002; Maioni 2008). The United States has been even more obvious about its medical care worries, with crisis commentary a fixture for decades on the national agenda. Fretting about medical care costs, quality, and access is not limited to North America. Disputes about reforming Dutch medical care have been ongoing for decades. Any review of the European experience would uncover persistent policy controversies in Germany (burdened by the fiscal pressures of unification), in the United Kingdom (with recurrent debates about the National Health Service), and in Italy and Sweden (with fiscal and unemployment pressures).[3]

The puzzle is not *whether* or *why* there is such widespread interest in health policy, but why *now*. And why has international evidence (arguments, claims, caricatures) seemed more prominent at the beginning of the twenty-first century than, say, during the fiscal strains of the mid-1970s or early 1980s? What can be usefully said, not only about the substance of the experience of different nations, but about the political processes of introducing and acting upon policy change in a national context?

There is a simple answer to these questions that, one hopes, is not simpleminded. Medical care policy came to the forefront of public agendas for one or more of the following reasons. First, the financing of personal medical care everywhere became a major financial component of the budgets of mature welfare states.[4] When fiscal strain arises, policy scrutiny (not simply incremental budgeting) is the predictable result. Second, mature welfare states, as Klein and O'Higgins (1988, esp. 219–224) argued in the late 1980s, face restricted capacity for bold fiscal expansion in new areas. This means that managing existing programs in changing economic circumstances necessarily assumes a more prominent place on the public agenda. Third, there is what might be termed the wearing out (perhaps wearing down) of the postwar consensus about the welfare state. We see the effects of more than two decades of fretfulness about the affordability, desirability, and governability of the welfare state.[5]

Beginning in earnest during the 1973–74 oil shock, with high levels of unemployment and persistent stagflation, and bolstered by the electoral victories (or advance) of parties opposed to welfare state expansion, critics assumed a bolder posture. Mass publics increasingly heard challenges to programs that had for decades seemed sacrosanct.[6] From Brian Mulroney to Margaret Thatcher, from New Zealand to the Netherlands—the message of serious problems requiring major change gained support. Accordingly, when economic strain reappears, the inner rim of programmatic protection—not just interest-group commitment, but social faith—becomes weaker and the incentives to explore transformative but not fiscally burdensome options become relatively stronger. Those factors help to explain the pattern of welfare state review—including health policy—over the last three decades of the twentieth century across the industrialized world. But even accepting this contention, there still remains the question of why these pressures gave rise to increased attention to other national experiences.[7]

Recent experience illustrates how times of policy change increase the demand for new ideas—or at least new means to old ends. Rudolf Klein once argued that "no one wants to be caught wearing yesterday's ideas" (Klein 1996). Everywhere, policy makers and analysts looked increasingly across their borders to look for the latest policy fashion. Just as some American reformers turned to Canada's example, so a number of Canadian, German, Dutch, and other intellectual entrepreneurs reviewed American, Swiss, and Swedish experience. In the 1990s, many conferences followed this pattern. Conferees were interested in getting better policy answers to the problems they faced at home. For example, participants in one such conference held in the Netherlands in the mid-1990s were explicit about their aspirations for cross-border learning: how to find a balance between "solidarity and subsidiary," how to maintain a "high quality health system in times of economic stress," even an optimistic query about "what are the optimum relations between patients, insurers, providers, and the government" (Four Country Conference 1995). Understood as simply wanting to stretch one's mind—to explore what is possible conceptually, or what others have managed to achieve—this line of thought is unexceptionable. Understood as the pursuit of the best model, absent further exploration of the political, social, and economic context required for implementation, it is wishful thinking.

Others saw the opportunity for an informational version of this intellectual stretching: quests for "exchange of policy information" of various sorts without commitment to policy importation, the "exchanging [of] views with kindred spirits," and explicit calls for intellectual stimulation. All of this is the learning that anthropologists have long extolled—understanding the range of possible options and seeing one's own circumstances more clearly by contrast.

But what about drawing policy lessons from such exercises? What are the rules of defensible conduct here, and are they followed? The truth is that, whatever the appearances, most policy debates in most countries are (and will remain) parochial affairs. They address national problems, emphasize national developments in particular domains (pensions, medical finance, transportation), and embody conflicting visions of what policies the particular country should adopt. Only occasionally are the experiences of other nations—and the lessons they embody—seriously examined.[8] When cross-national experiences are employed in such parochial struggles, their use is typically that of policy warfare, not policy understanding and careful lesson drawing. And, one must add, there are few knowledgeable critics at home of ideas about solutions abroad. In the world of American medical debate, the misuse of British and Canadian experience surely illustrates this point. The National Health Service (NHS) was from the late 1970s the specter of what "government medicine" or "socialized medicine" and "rationing" could mean. In the 1980s and 1990s, mythmaking about Canada became common in the American health reform debates (Marmor 2008).[9]

The reasons are almost too obvious to cite. Policy makers are busy with day-to-day pressures. Practical concerns incline them, if they take the time for comparative inquiry, to pay more attention to what appears to work, not to academic reasons for what is and is not transferrable and why. Policy debaters—whether politicians, policy analysts, or interest group figures—are in struggles, not seminars. Like lawyers, they seek victory, not illumination. For that purpose, compelling stories, whether well substantiated or not, are more useful than careful conclusions. Interest groups, as their label suggests, have material and symbolic stakes in policy outcomes, not reputations for intellectual precision to protect.[10] Once generated and communicated, however, health policy ideas are adopted more readily in some contexts than in others. These patterns of adoption and adaptation have to do with the machinery of government, as well as with local cultural understandings. The autonomy and authority of the governing party in Parliament in the United Kingdom, for example, as well as its position at the apex of a nationalized health service, means that "ideas can make a difference more quickly in Britain than in America" (Marmor and Plowden 1991). It may be, too, that policy ideas transfer more easily between similar types of health systems. Institutional similarity—however notional—seems to have facilitated the spread of managed competition ideas among the national health services of northern and southern Europe (Freeman 1998).

This argument must be qualified, however. Lessons from abroad often meet strong local cultural resistance. Giaimo and Manow, for example, observe that "while the market has won in international terms, the national answers to the economic pressures resulting from economic globalization demonstrate that national 'markets for ideas' have yet to be fully liberalized" (1997). Morone (1990) similarly remarks of Canada's experience with universal health insurance: "It is difficult to imagine a lesson that is more foreign to the American experience. Instead of hard conscious choices, we [the United States] have sought painless automatic solutions. Rather than explicit programmatic decisions Americans prefer hidden, implicit policies. Rather than centralize control in governmental hands, we would scatter it across many players. In short the Canadian lessons . . . are not just different—they challenge the central features of American political culture, at least as they have manifested themselves in health care policy."

It is not clear, then, whether what matters is administrative infrastructure as such or the values and assumptions it appears to embody. For it matters a lot not only how systems are configured in organizational terms but also how they are construed mentally (Freeman 1999). This understanding probably amounts to something more than ideas and values as such, pointing to the significance of ways of thinking or framing. Different national policy communities—however well networked internationally—simply see problems differently.

For all this, the field of medical care policy and management is notable for the absence of studies that set out to investigate the process of transfer or learning in any specific instance. Bennett refers to the "paucity of systematic research that can convincingly make the case that cross-national policy learning has had a determined influence on policy choice in a particular jurisdiction at a particular time" (1997). But the paucity of studies on policy learning does not apply to cross-national studies of policy origins, implementation, and change. Indeed, for that broader field of work, large and growing clusters of quite different sorts of scholarship and advocacy address medical care cross-nationally.

None of these considerations are new—or surprising. But the increased flow of cross-national claims in health policy—both in the world of academia and in politics—generates new reasons to consider the meaning of cross-national policy learning.

The Promise and Perils of Cross-National Comparative Policy Research

The presumptions of such cross-national efforts are important to explore, even briefly. One is that the outside observer can more easily highlight features of debates that are missed or underplayed by national participants. Another is that comparative commentary may bring some policy wisdom as well as illuminating asides about national debates. The common assumption is that cross-cultural observation, if accurate and alert, has some advantages. It brings a different, foreign, and arguably illuminating perspective to the debate.

A similar rationale lies behind much of the enthusiasm for contemporary comparative policy studies. Welfare state disputes—over pensions and medical care most prominently—are salient on the public agendas of all industrial democracies. There is in fact a brisk trade in panaceas for the various (real and imagined) ills of welfare states. As will become apparent in later comments on the comparative literature, however, many cross-national investigations are not factually accurate enough to offer useful illumination, let alone policy wisdom. But, properly done, studies that compare what appear to be similar topics have two potential benefits not available to the policy analyst in a single-nation inquiry.

First, examinations of how others see a problem, how options for action are set out and evaluated, how implementation is understood and undertaken—all offer learning opportunities even if the policy experiences of different polities are not easily transplantable as lessons. Second, where the context is reasonably similar, comparative work has features of a quasi-natural experiment. So, for instance, the adaptation of reference prices for pharmaceuticals in Germany and in the Netherlands—two countries with very similar institutional arrangements in health care—provides an interesting example of policy learning. The reference pricing constrains outlays in the short term. But those gains are somewhat dissipated as the actors strategically adapt to the new policy reality (Four Country Conference 2000).

Cross-national sources of information have proliferated to the extent that it has become almost impossible for a policy maker in any given country not to know something about what is going on elsewhere. But to know what, exactly? What part can and should comparative policy analysis play in these debates? Ruud Lubbers, the former Dutch prime minister, provides a striking example of trying to draw lessons from American experience, apparently without much understanding of its policy realities (Lubbers 1997). In an article for the *International Herald Tribune,* Lubbers contrasted what he called the "lean welfare state . . . with rapid job growth" of the United States with "costly social welfare system[s] with persistently high unemployment in most of Europe." He went on in the rest of the article to laud Holland's "third way," one that "tackled" the unemployment problem while "remaining within the European tradition that emphasizes quality of life rather than growth at any cost." This rather self-congratulatory theme seems odd in comparison with contemporary Dutch complaints. But the point is that the United States functions as a poorly analyzed symbol of a type of welfare state to avoid. Citing President Clinton as his source, Lubbers went on to write most of the article about the so-called Dutch miracle: a more flexible workforce, less unemployment, and a somewhat more restrained welfare state, all the result of the famous corporatist Wassenaar Agreement of 1982.

In Lubbers's article, the American example is, in fact, hardly discussed, and treated mostly as a negative symbol of what the Dutch—and other European countries—have avoided.[11] Nowhere is there any recognition that the American welfare state is quite extensive fiscally and concentrated on its older citizens, with spending levels that—when properly accounted for in tax expenditures, direct program outlays, and the like—are hardly lean. Indeed, the point of books such as Hacker's *The Divided Welfare State* (2002) is precisely to set aside this common but mistaken impression of American social policy as concentrated on the poor, miserly in its levels of benefits, and (depending on one's ideology) splendid or horrible in its social and economic results.[12]

The paradox is that the post-1970 decades witnessed the rapid expansion of public policy research, of which a significant proportion claimed to provide comparisons across countries as a base for drawing lessons. But most of those studies, in fact, consisted of mere statistical and descriptive portraitures of health systems, ignoring methodological issues of comparison. So, the argument here underlines the truism that policy making and policy research are often—if not always—pursued with little reference to each other. Nevertheless, the question remains why that truism should apply so fully in this costly area of public policy, medical care. Why are claims about system convergence so widespread in the face of persistent patterns of continuity in national models of health care?

Claims and Realities in the Health Reform Debate

The bulk of the ideological and fiscal debates about health reform took place within national borders, largely free from the spread of foreign ideas. Similar arguments that arose cross-nationally mostly represented what might be described as parallel thinking. That is to say, the common questioning of health policy reflects similarities in circumstances and problem definition. This phenomenon was evident in the common preoccupation with rising medical care costs. Figure 1.1 portrays the upward pressure of medical care expenditures in five OECD nations since the early 1970s. Even while health expenditure in each of the countries rose steadily, growth rates varied over time. Clearly, some countries, in some periods, were more successful than others in reining in health costs.

This debate about the similarities and differences in national experience intensified by the late 1980s and 1990s with the emergence of active international and supranational actors in both general welfare state disputes and, in particular, health policy. These actors include the European Union, the World Health Organization (WHO), the OECD, and the World Bank. Yet however powerful these institutions are in some areas, their role in domestic policy making within the OECD world remains indirect and limited. The European Commission, the executive branch of the European Union, has established a policy competence in public health and has become a sponsor of biomedical research.

In contrast, the European Treaty, which serves as a constitution for the European Union, leaves social policy, including health policy, firmly to the national states' competency. Yet rulings of the European Court of Justice in the 1990s have had important spillover effects on national health care policies. E.U. legislation designed originally to ensure the freedom of goods, people, capital, and services across borders no longer exempts the domain of health care (Report of Workshop on E.U. Law and National Health Policy 2004). The WHO struggles to lead health policy discussions but remains a minor actor in the funding of medical care. And the World Bank, particularly powerful in the transformation of health care in Eastern Europe, expresses some of the reform ideas found in the western industrial democracies but does not wield its influence there. Finally, OECD reports certainly affect the discussion of welfare state issues, but at one step removed from policy decision making. Yet, in spite of their limited direct role in health policy, these international

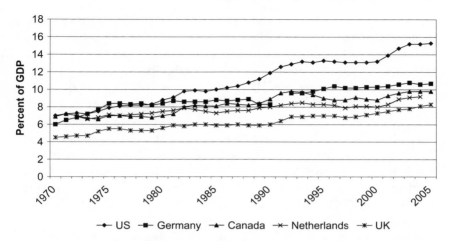

Figure 1.1 Health expenditure in the United States, Canada, Germany, the United Kingdom, and the Netherlands, 1970–2005 (share of GDP)
Source: OECD Health Data, July 7, 2007, www. OECD.org.

agencies have become platforms for debate and carriers of policy ideas across borders.

Almost everywhere, health care became relatively more expensive while public budgets were more constrained—but how much more expensive and how much more constrained have varied substantially between countries. These pressures, in turn, are mediated by different sets of actors and institutions. Debates over controlling health care expenditures took place everywhere, regardless of actual levels or growth rates of health spending. In short, the apparently common pressures on health systems are themselves uneven and indirect. And this factor is the essential source of difficulty in taking convergence as a framework for studying—or advocating—reforms in health policy. Simply put, there is as much evidence of continued difference (or divergence) in national arrangements for the finance, delivery, and regulation of health care as there is of increasing similarity. As a former official of the OECD's health policy unit claimed, "the delivery and finance of healthcare vary between nations more than any other public policy" (Poullier 1989). One does not have to agree with Poullier's conclusion to see that reducing variation has been neither the purpose nor the effect of health reform in the past decades. In medical care, as in other areas of public administration, good arguments or evidence that "one size fits all" are lacking.

To be fair, this variation is one of degree rather than of kind. At the most general level, it seems perfectly clear that some countries with roughly similar constellations of political interests, economic and political institutions, and resources develop *broadly* comparable arrangements for health care. And so, in turn, when social structures, patterns of economic organization, and expressions of political interest begin to change, health care arrangements will face pressures to change also. But what matters is what that formulation leaves unsaid. While there is value in pointing to the structural and technological context of health policy, policy makers faced not only with multiple pressures but also with myriad proposals for change, tend to choose options that are politically feasible in the short term. To them, an appeal to universal solutions seems anodyne, reductionist, or superficial. Conditions are not determining. They explain only why there should be pressure for reform but not whether change will indeed occur, let alone what shape or direction it will—or should—take.

Nonetheless, these conditions do help to explain why—if not when or where or how—cross-national trade in policy ideas should be going on and why it is increasing. Getting it right in health policy—ensuring universal access to high-quality health care without breaking the bank—makes for significant competitive advantage in the domestic political arena as well as in the international economy. Convergence in circumstances creates opportunities for learning, as well as an increased interest in applying lessons from abroad. Convergence theory, then, offers useful clues about why adaptive change might take place. It says much less, however, about the form it takes, about why one solution to a problem should be preferred over others. And for that topic, the next section addresses the purposes, promises, and pitfalls of comparative studies in health policy.

Purposes, Promises, and Perils of Comparative Inquiry in Health Policy

In this section, the emphasis is on the following three distinctions among the purposes that comparative analysis in health policy can serve: *learning about* national health arrangements and how they operate, *learning why* they take the forms they do, and *learning* policy lessons *from* those analyses. While these distinctions should be apparent to scholars of the subject, much of the comparative commentary on health care neither clarifies the different modes of comparison nor addresses the difficulties of drawing policy lessons from the experience of other countries.

First, there is the goal of learning about health policy abroad. Comparative work of this sort can illuminate and clarify national arrangements without addressing causal explanation or seeking policy transplantation. Its comparative element remains for the most part implicit: in reading (or writing) about other systems, we make sense of them by contrasting them with our own and with others we know about. The process of learning entails the appreciation of what something is by reference to what it is like or unlike. This is the gift of perspective, which may or may not bring explanatory insight or lesson drawing.

Second, there is the fundamental purpose served by comparison to generate causal explanations without necessarily seeking policy transplantation; that is, learning why policies develop as they do. Many of the historical and developmental studies of health care fall into this category. This approach uses cross-national inquiry to check on the adequacy of nation-specific accounts. Let us call that a defense against explanatory provincialism. What precedes policy making in country A includes many things—from legacies of past policy to institutional and temporal features—that *seem* decisive. How is one to know *how* decisive, as opposed to simply present? One answer is to look for similar outcomes elsewhere where some of those factors are missing or configured differently. Another is to look for a similar configuration of precedents without a comparable outcome.

Third, a still different approach is to treat cross-national experiences as quasi-experiments. The purpose is to draw lessons about why some policies seem promising and doable, or promising but impossible, or doable but not promising. All of these approaches appear in the comparative literature. With the growth of such writing came widespread optimism about the promise of lesson drawing from comparative policy analyses. But is that optimism justified?

One useful starting point to address this question is a cross-national generalization that at first sight seems misleading but upon reflection helps to clarify differences in the framing of policy problems. A 1995 article on European health reform, for example, claims that "countries everywhere are reforming their health systems" (Hunter 1995). It asserts that "what is remarkable about this global movement is that both the diagnosis of the problems and the prescription for them are virtually the same in all health care systems." These globalist claims, it turns out, were mistaken (Jacobs 1998; Marmor 1999). But the process of specifying more precisely what counts as national health care problems—whether cost control, poor quality of care, or fragmented organization of services—turns out to be quite clarifying. In this instance, the comparative approach first refutes the generalization but then helps to discipline the process of describing national health problems. So, to illustrate further, the European researcher coming to investigate Oregon's experiment in health care rationing would soon discover that it was neither restrictive in practice nor a major cost-control remedy in the 1990s (Jacobs, Marmor, and Oberlander 1999). To make this discovery is to see the issue of rationing more clearly.

Offering new perspectives on problems and making factual adjustments in national portraits are not to be treated as trivial tasks. They are what professionals might well spend a good deal of time perfecting. All too many comparative studies are, in fact, misleading caricatures rather than accurate characterizations of policies. A striking illustration is the 2000 WHO report on the ranking of the performance of health systems across the globe, which is discussed later in this chapter. While this report raised pertinent questions about what counts as good performance in health care and systems, its execution evoked sharp criticism by scholars (Williams 2001).[13] That criticism in itself should not serve as a deterrent to serious comparative scholarship. But it is a warning against superficiality.

An often-cited advantage of comparative studies is that they serve as an antidote to explanatory provincialism. An example from North American health policy provides a good illustration of how not to proceed. Some policy makers and academics in North America regard universal health insurance as incompatible with American values (Marmor 2008; Maioni 2008). They rest their case in part on the belief that the reason Canada enacted health insurance whereas the United States has not is that the two countries' values are sharply different. In short, they attribute different outcomes to different political cultures. In fact, the values of Canada and the United States, while not identical, are quite similar (Lipset 1990). Differences are there, but Canada's distribution of values is closer to that of the United States than any other modern rich democracy. Indeed, the value similarities between British Columbia and Washington State are greater than those between either of those jurisdictions and, say, an East Coast region such as New Brunswick or New Hampshire. Similar values are compatible with different outcomes, a conclusion that in turn draws one's attention to other institutional and strategic factors distinguishing Canadian from American experience with financing health care (Maioni 1998; White 1995). One can imagine many other examples of such cautionary lessons, but the important point is simply that the explanatory checks are unavailable from national histories alone.

The third purpose of comparative analysis is directly relevant to our inquiry. The desire to draw lessons from the policy experience of other nations is what has financially supported a good deal of the comparative analysis available. The international organizations have this goal as part of their rationale. The WHO, as noted, is firmly in the business of selling "best practices." The OECD regularly produces extensive, expensive, hard-to-gather statistical portraits of programs as diverse as disability and pensions, trade flows and the movement of professionals, education and health care. No one can avoid using these studies, if only because the task of collecting data and discovering "the facts" in a number of countries is so daunting. But the portraiture that emerges requires its own craft review. Does what Germany spends on spas count as public health expenditure elsewhere, or does it fall, as in the United States, under another category? Often, the same words do not mean the same things. And different words may denote similar phenomena.

For now, it is enough to restate that learning *about* the experience of other nations is a precondition for understanding *why* change takes place or for learning *from* that experience. Looking at the large and growing volume of comparative studies in health policy, we found that the majority of studies do not deliver on their claim to provide a sound base for drawing lessons from the experience of other countries. The section that follows categorizes the studies into four groups, each with its distinct purpose and applications. This grouping shows that the majority of reports and studies available (the first and second categories) provide, at best, a sound base for further analysis but hardly any ground for learning from experience abroad. The studies that are based on more solid analysis (the third and fourth groups) are less numerous, less wide in their geographical application, and more modest in their claims about policy lessons.

Comparative Health Policy Analysis: Clusters of Writing

Health policy in the OECD world is, at the same time, a matter of insistent national debate; a frequent topic of descriptive, statistical portraiture for international organizations; a sometime subject of publication in the comparative journals; and only very infrequently, in its cross-national comparative form, the object of book-length treatment. For many years, readers had to turn to Anderson's (1972) treatment of Swedish, British, and American medical care developments in the post–World War II period for acute, well-informed judgments.[14] There were many other individual country studies but few, if any, that employed a systematic, comparative method of policy analysis (Glaser 1970). In contemporary debates about Dutch health care, for instance, there appears little evidence of detailed understanding about German—or American—policy experience with health care reform in the 1990s. What is true for medical care applies just as well to other fiscally important areas of the welfare state. So, for example, American discussions of disability policy in the early 1980s drew very little from Dutch experience, though there were knowledgeable scholars in both countries who sought to have influence (Wilensky 2002).[15]

By the end of the 1980s, political scientists—particularly North American ones—had become interested in comparing relations between the medical profession, as a particular kind of interest group, and the state (Tuohy 1974; Stone 1984; Freddi and Bjorkman 1989; Wilsford 1991; Immergut 1992; Pierson 1994). By and large, their theoretical focus was on the institutions of government and the different ways in which they shape health care politics. Slowly, the field began to produce genuinely comparative political analyses of substantial industry and competence.

The years since then have witnessed a rapid expansion of cross-national health policy literature. The quality of these works varies enormously—whether measured by the standard of intellectual rigor, theoretical perspective, descriptive accuracy, or concern for systematic policy learning across borders. Roughly speaking, there are four separable but not mutually exclusive categories of such writing (Marmor and Okma 2003).

The first category includes the well-known statistical, largely descriptive documents that provide data on a number of countries assumed to constitute a coherent class. It also includes more specialized surveys that deal with public opinion, health care, and health policy (Blendon and Brodie 1997). In that way they supply much of the basic information that policy commentators explore. The OECD Health Data series has become a staple of both academic and more applied analyses alike. These studies typically provide neither behavioral hypotheses nor test explanations for why certain patterns exist. Nor do they, generally speaking, explicitly deal with the promise and pitfalls of cross-border learning. In a wider sense, the recent efforts to rank systems, countries, or institutions by means of benchmarking techniques belong to this group, too. In a much-discussed report, the WHO used its comparative data to rank the performance of national health care systems (WHO 2000).

The second category of comparative studies—by far the largest number—includes collections of international material that we label as "parallel" or "stapled" national case studies. Examples of this kind of cross-national study are the volumes by Ham, Robinson, and Benzeval (1990), the OECD (1992, 1994), Wall (1996), Altenstetter and Bjorkman (1997), Ham (1997), Raffell (1997), and Powell and Wessen (1999), as well as the Health in Transition series of booklets of the WHO European Observatory. These are usually country reports bound together, accompanied by an editorial introduction and summary conclusion. For the most part, the authors are intent on setting out how things work in whichever country they are writing about. The reports are mostly descriptive, but with some assessment of performance and the flagging of issues prompting political concern. As such, they represent a qualitative correlate of the quantitative statistical studies previously described. Done carefully, they are an invaluable resource for cross-national understanding. In many cases, they leave readers to find what is relevant and, as far as policy learning is concerned, also leave them to do the work.

The third category comprises books about a number of individual countries that employ a common framework of analysis, usually addressing a particular theme in health policy, for example, competition or privatization. That means, in principle, that comparative generalizations are possible, though not all such works actually make them.[16]

The fourth category includes cross-national studies with a fundamental theoretical orientation that take up a specific medical care theme or question as the focus of analysis.[17] One of the interesting features of this fourth category of comparative studies is that there appears a necessary trade-off between theoretical depth and the number of nations studied. The disciplined treatment of broad topics by a single author almost inevitably addresses a more limited set of countries.[18]

In this last category, Tuohy's *Accidental Logics* (1999) offers both a theoretical and an empirical analysis of policy change and continuity in three English-speaking nations. The book addresses a limited range of countries but combines theoretical sophistication with command of the relevant factual data and causal analysis in addressing the different patterns of policy change during the post–World War II years in the United Kingdom, Canada, and the United States. The likelihood of major policy changes, for Tuohy, differs according to each nation's particular "institutional mix." By that expression, she means the degree of governmental hierarchy, market forces, and professional collegiality in medical decision making and the "structural balance" between the state, medical providers, and private financial interests. Directed at understanding, Tuohy's work is of clear relevance to policy makers concerned with questions of timing for reform initiatives.

Works in this fourth category of scholarship typically use comparative methods to explore and to explain policy developments. Their practical limitations for policy makers include the relatively restricted range of countries studied and, to some degree, their considerable reliance on the theoretical perspective known as historical institutionalism. There is some irony in the fact that the most careful cross-national analyses tend to have reinforced a sense of the contingency and specificity of the way things work out at different times in different places. This kind of comparison seems to ignore (if not implicitly deny) the cross-national exchange of information and ideas in health policy that is so much a part of the very intellectual environment in which it has been produced. The most powerful studies are at the same time the most academic; the practical learning that might result from comparison is largely left implicit. Often, those books do not reach the desk of policy makers. And there is much less in them that speaks directly to the policy maker seeking to use evidence and experience from elsewhere in any straightforward way. Nonetheless, in the course of little more than a decade, the comparative analysis of health policy became a specialized field of academic inquiry, highly developed and successful in its own terms, but limited so far in its policy impact. So, we turn back to the evaluative question: How should we assess the purposes and performance of comparative policy research?

Perhaps the most important lesson we can draw from the overview of the current literature is that the development of a serious body of comparative work takes more time and effort than health policy makers are willing to spend. They sense pressure to take action and feel that they cannot wait. At the same time, policy errors based on misconceptions of the experience abroad can be costly. The eagerness of some health ministers to embrace and import policy models from the United States—such as the managed care models, the benchmark methodology, or the medical savings idea—without a proper assessment of how those ideas and models worked out in practice may lead to policies that will require repair action soon, can force politicians to reverse policies altogether, and can erode the popular support for health policy. The unwillingness of some politicians to delay action in order to study experience with similar policy elsewhere contrasts sharply with the practice of some Asian countries that have spent much time and attention before adjusting certain measures to their own national policy environments. The good news is that the 1980s and 1990s brought a large body of comparative studies. They provide a useful base for the next generation of comparative work. The statistical data are there, the materials are there, the experience in drawing portraitures of individual countries is there, and all of those are necessary conditions for the next phases of policy learning about causalities and the transfer of policy experience.

Notes

The authors wish to acknowledge that much of the work for this chapter draws upon an earlier article published by the *Journal of Comparative Policy Analysis* (Marmor, Freeman, and Okma 2005).

1. This skeptical argument is advanced, with Anglo-American examples from medical care and welfare, in Marmor and Plowden's "Rhetoric and Reality in the Interna-

tional Jet Stream" (1991). On the other hand, there is very rapid communication of scientific findings and claims, with journals and meetings regarded as the proper sites for evaluation. At present there is no journal in the political economy of medical care that has enough authority, audience, or acuteness to play the evaluative role assumed in the medical world by the *New England Journal of Medicine, Lancet, BMJ (British Medical Journal)*, or *JAMA (Journal of the American Medical Association)*.

2. Readers may be puzzled by our reluctance to treat reform as the object of commentary. This paragraph's parade of substitutes—health policy, concerns, worries, and so on—reflects discomfort with the positive marketing connotations of the term "reform." That there are pressures for change everywhere is obvious, and understanding them is this book's purpose, but the differences between change and improvement are blurred by terms like "reform" and "reforming" (Marmor 2007).

3. In the 1990s, work in English on health policy learning was for the most part concerned with a single topic, managed competition. This topic dominated reform discussion across countries between the mid-1980s and the mid-1990s. However, the focus was largely on the transatlantic relationship between the United States and the United Kingdom (Klein 1991, 1997; Marmor and Plowden 1991; Mechanic 1995; Marmor 1997; Marmor and Okma 1998; O'Neill 2000). There were complementary treatments of Western Europe (Freeman 1999), Southern Europe (Cabiedes and Guillèn 2001), and New Zealand (Jacobs and Barnett 2000).

4. Technically, this is not strictly true, of course, as is evident in the sickness fund financing of care in Germany, the Netherlands, and elsewhere. But since mandatory contributions are close cousins of taxes, budget officials must obviously treat these outlays as constraints on direct tax increases. Moreover, the precise level of acceptable cost increases is a regulatory issue of great controversy.

5. The bulk of this ideological struggle took place, of course, within national borders, free from the spread of foreign ideas. To the extent that similar arguments arose cross-nationally, as Kieke Okma has noted, these similarities mostly represented "parallel development" (Four Country Conference 1995). But there are striking contemporary examples of the explicit international transfer and highlighting of welfare state commentary. Some takes place through think-tank networks; some takes place through media campaigns on behalf of particular figures; and, of course, some takes place through academic exchanges and official meetings. The writings and activities of Charles Murray—the controversial author of *Losing Ground* (1984) and co-author of *The Bell Curve* (1994)—illustrate all three of these phenomena, as our British conferees can attest. The medium of transfer seems to have changed in the postwar period. Where the Beveridge Report would have been known to social policy elites very broadly, however much they used it, the modern form seems to be the long newspaper or magazine article and the media interview.

6. This is the argument developed in Marmor, Mashaw, and Harvey, *America's Misunderstood Welfare State* (1990), especially Ch. 3. The wider scholarly literature on the subject is the focus of the review essay by Marmor, "Understanding the Welfare State" (1993).

7. The turning to U.S. health policy experience for lessons about cost control or insurance coverage seems particularly puzzling to American scholars preoccupied with health care problems at home.

8. Some readers have suggested that this chapter is too pessimistic about the field of cross-national policy learning. And it is certainly true that some cross-national investigations have been enormously illuminating and helpful. For example, the 1964 Royal Commission on Health Services was an exemplary investigator of the experience of other countries. In the 1990s comparative policy investigations by Japanese and German analysts were important in reforming nursing homes in both countries.

9. For an elaboration of this point, see T. R. Marmor, "Patterns of Fact and Fiction in the Use of the Canadian Experience" (1994), 179–94. A particularly careful and extensive treatment of the North American experience is the review article by Evans, Barer, and Hertzman, "The 20-Year Experiment" (1991).

10. The political fight over the Clinton health plan vividly illustrates these generalizations. The number of interest groups with a stake in the Clinton plan's fate—given the nearly $1 trillion medical economy—was enormous; there were more than eight thousand registered lobbyists alone in Washington and thousands more trying to influence the outcome under some other label. The estimates of expenditures on the battle are in the hundreds of millions; one trade association, the Pharmaceutical Manufacturer's Association, spent $7 million on public relations by 1993. The most noted effort was that of the Health Insurance Association of America, which produced the infamous "Harry and Louise" advertisements. Washington was awash in interest group activities during the health care reform battle of 1993–94, but the character, impact, and meaning of those activities are far from clear.

11. A Dutch policy commentator on cross-national perspectives on the Dutch welfare state and its health system strikingly illustrates how one can oddly justify not learning much from comparative policy studies. "Comparative studies," he wrote, "are generally backward looking, so don't always provide us with the right answers for the future" (De Gier et al. 2004:113). The restrictive definition of the purpose of comparative inquiry—getting the "right answers"—limits greatly what this Dutch public servant would consider useful.

12. As Hacker rightly points out, the "share of the US economy devoted to social spending is not all that different from the corresponding portion in even the most generous of European welfare states." The sources of the spending—tax expenditures and employment-benefits especially—are what distinguish the American case. The same myth of the lean American welfare state was the object of criticism in a book published a decade earlier (Marmor, Mashaw, and Harvey 1990).

13. The 2000 WHO report seeks to rank health systems across the globe. The WHO posed good questions about how health systems work: Are they fair, responsive to patient needs, efficient? Do they provide good-quality health care? But it answered those questions without much attention to the difficulties of describing responsiveness or fairness or efficiency in some universalistic and reliable manner. What is more, the report used as partial evidence the opinions of WHO personnel to "verify" what takes place in Australia, Oman, Turkmenistan, or Canada. Moreover, while the report claims to provide data in order to improve health systems across the globe, it is hard to see how a health minister of a country ranked, say, 125th in the order has any stake to climb the ladder. Predictably, most of the uproar about the report was the battle between the countries that ranked high but not highest. Many journalists and members of Parliament

quoted the report as a critical comment on the failures of the national health system, whereas, predictably, the French minister saw the number-one ranking of his country (which in the end turned out to be based on a calculating error) as proof of effectiveness of his policy. With comparative policy studies like that, one can easily understand why some funders of research regard such studies as excuses for boondoggles. But that should not drive out the impulse for serious cross-national scholarship and learning.

14. For a retrospective appreciation of Anderson, see Freeman and Marmor's "Making Sense of Health Services Politics" (2003).

15. There is a rich scholarly disability literature, with a good deal of knowledgeable commentary on comparative policy developments. See especially Aarts and De Jong's "Able to Work?" (2003).

16. Good examples are Freddi and Bjorkman's *Controlling Medical Professionals* (1989), Ranade's *Markets and Health Care* (1998), and White's *Competing Solutions* (1995), written at the Brookings Institution to draw lessons from OECD experience for the universal health insurance debate in the United States. Sometimes journals present work of this kind: See the case studies of priority setting, for example, in the *Journal of Health Politics, Policy and Law* (2001:675–708, and 2005) for international commentary.

17. A good example of this genre is *Blood Feuds,* a book edited by Bayer and Feldman (1999) on the politics of contaminated blood in Germany, France, Japan, Canada, Denmark, and the United States. This theme is taken up in Bovens, t' Hart, and Peters's *Success and Failure in Governance* (2002), which also looks at medical professions and health care reform.

18. For instance, Pierson (1994) compares retrenchment politics in Reagan's America and Thatcher's England; Immergut (1992) compares the disputes over national health insurance in France, Switzerland, and Sweden in the early part of the twentieth century; and Maioni (1998) compares the different paths to national health insurance taken in Canada and the United States. Moran (1999) assesses the political economy of health care in Britain, Germany, and the United States; Freeman (2000), the politics of health care in five European countries.

References

Aarts, L., and P. De Jong. 2003. *Able to work? How policies help disabled people in 20 OECD countries.* Paris: OECD.

Altenstetter, C., and J. W. Bjorkman, eds. 1997. *Health policy reform, national variations and globalization.* Basingstoke, UK: Macmillan.

Anderson, O. 1972. *Health care: Can there be equity? The United States, Sweden and England.* New York: John Wiley.

Bayer, R., and E. Feldman. 1999. *Blood feuds: AIDS, blood and the politics of the medical disaster.* Oxford: Oxford University Press.

Bennett, C. J. 1997. Understanding ripple effects: The cross-national adoption of policy instruments for bureaucratic accountability. *Governance* 10 (3): 213–33.

Blendon, R. J., and M. Brodie. 1997. Public opinion and health policy. In *Health politics and policy,* ed. T. J. Litman and L. S. Robins. Albany, NY: Delmar.

Bovens, M., P. t' Hart, and B. G. Peters, eds. 2002. *Success and failure in governance: A comparative analysis of European states.* Cheltenham: Edward Elgar.

Cabiedes, L., and A. M. Guillèn. 2001. Adopting and adapting managed competition: Health care reform in Southern Europe. *Social Science and Medicine* 52 (8): 1205–17.

De Gier, E., A. De Swaan, and M. Ooijens. 2004. *Dutch welfare reform in an expanding Europe: The neighbours' view.* Amsterdam: Het Spinhuis.

Evans, R. G., M. L. Barer, and C. Hertzman. 1991. The 20-year experiment: Accounting for, explaining, and evaluating health care cost containment in Canada and the United States. *American Review of Public Health* 12:481–518.

Four Country Conference on Health Care Reforms and Health Care Policies in the United States, Canada, Germany, and the Netherlands. 1995. Conference Report. Amsterdam, February 23–25.

Four Country Conference: Pharmaceutical policies in the US, Canada, Germany, and the Netherlands. 2000. Conference Report. Amsterdam, July 13–15.

Freddi, G., and J. W. Bjorkman, eds. 1989. *Controlling medical professionals: The comparative politics of health governance.* London: Sage.

Freeman, R. 1998. Competition in context: The politics of health care reform in Europe. *International Journal for Quality in Health Care* 10 (5): 395–401.

Freeman, R. 1999. *Policy transfer in the health sector.* European Forum conference paper WS/35. Florence: European University Institute.

Freeman, R. 2000. *The politics of health in Europe.* Manchester, UK: Manchester University Press.

Freeman, R., and T. Marmor. 2003. Making sense of health services politics through cross-national comparison. *Journal of Health Services Research and Policy* 8 (3): 180–82.

Giaimo, S., and P. Manow. 1997. Institutions and ideas into politics: Health care reform in Britain and Germany. In *Health policy reform, national variations and globalization,* ed. C. Altenstetter and J. W. Bjorkman. Basingstoke, UK: Macmillan.

Glaser, William A. 1970. *Paying the doctor; systems of remuneration and their effects.* Baltimore: Johns Hopkins University Press.

Hacker, J. 2002. *The divided welfare state: The battle over public and private benefits in the United States.* New York: Cambridge University Press.

Ham, C., ed. 1997. *Health care reform: Learning from international experience.* Buckingham, UK: Open University Press.

Ham, C., R. Robinson, and M. Benzeval, eds. 1990. *Health check: Healthcare reforms in an international context.* London: King's Fund Institute.

Hunter, D. 1995. A new focus for dialogue. *European Health Reform: The Bulletin of the European Network and Database,* no. 1 (March).

Immergut, E. M. 1992. *Health politics interests and institutions in Western Europe.* Cambridge: Cambridge University Press.

Jacobs, A. 1998. Seeing difference: Market health reform in Europe. *Journal of Health Politics, Policy and Law* 23 (1): 1–33.

Jacobs, K., and P. Barnett. 2000. Policy transfer and policy learning: A study of the 1991 New Zealand Health Services Taskforce. *Governance* 13 (2): 229–57.

Jacobs, L., T. M. Marmor, and J. Oberlander. 1999. The Oregon Health Plan and the political paradox of rationing: What advocates and critics have claimed and what Oregon did. *Journal of Health Politics, Policy and Law* 24 (1): 161–80.

Journal of Health Politics, Policy and Law. 2001. Special issue: Comparative health care policy, ed. Mark Peterson, 26 (4).

Journal of Health Politics, Policy and Law. 2005. Special issue: Legacies and latitude in European health policy, ed. Mark Schlesinger, special eds. Adam Oliver and Elias Mossialos, 30 (1–2).

Klein, R. 1991. Risks and benefits of comparative studies: Notes from another shore. *Milbank Quarterly* 69 (2): 275–91.

Klein, R. 1996. *Commentary at the Four Country Conference: Health Care Reform.* Montebello, Canada, May 16–18.

Klein, R. 1997. Learning from others: Shall the last be the first? *Journal of Health Politics, Policy and Law* 22 (5): 1267–78.

Klein, R., and M. O'Higgins. 1988. Defusing the crisis of the welfare state: A new interpretation. In *Social security: Beyond the rhetoric of crisis,* ed. T. R. Marmor and J. Mashaw. Princeton, NJ: Princeton University Press.

Lipset, S. M. 1990. *Continental divide: The values and institutions of the United States and Canada.* New York: Routledge.

Lubbers, R. 1997. In seeking a third way, the Dutch model is worth a look. *International Herald Tribune,* September 9.

Maioni, A. 1998. *Parting at the crossroads: The emergence of health insurance in the United States and Canada.* Princeton, NJ: Princeton University Press.

Maioni, A. 2008. Health care politics and policy in Canada. In *Health care in crisis: The drive for health reforms in Canada and the United States.* Woodrow Wilson International Center for Scholars, Washington, DC: 14–25.

Marmor, T. R. 1993. Understanding the welfare state: crisis, critics, and countercritics. *Critical Review* 7 (4): 461–77.

Marmor, T. R. 1994. *Understanding health care reform.* New Haven: Yale University Press.

Marmor, T. R. 1997. Global health policy reform: Misleading mythology or learning opportunity. In *Health policy reform, national variations, and globalization,* ed. C. Altenstetter and J. W. Bjorkman. Basingstoke, UK: Macmillan.

Marmor, T. R. 1999. The rage for reform: Sense and nonsense in health policy. *In Health reform: Public success, private failure,* ed. D. Drache and T. Sullivan. London: Routledge.

Marmor, T. R. 2007. *Fads, fallacies and foolishness in medical care management and policy.* Singapore: World Scientific Publishing Co.

Marmor, T. R. 2008. American health care policy and politics: The promise and perils of reform. In *Health care in crisis: The drive for health reform in Canada and the United States.* Woodrow Wilson International Center for Scholars, Washington, DC.: 14–25.

Marmor, T. R., J. Mashaw, and P. Harvey. 1990. *America's misunderstood welfare state: Persistent myths, enduring realities.* New York: Basic Books.

Marmor, T. R., and K. G. H. Okma. 1998. Cautionary lessons from the West: What (not) to learn from other countries' experiences in the financing and delivery of health care. In *The state of social welfare: International studies on social insurance and retirement, employment, family policy and health care,* ed. P. Flora, P. R. De Jong, J. Le Grand, and J. Y. Kim. Aldershot, UK: Ashgate.

Marmor, T. R., and K. G. H. Okma. 2003. Review essay: Health care systems in transition. *Journal of Health Politics, Policy and Law* 28 (4): 747–55.

Marmor, T. R., R. Freeman, and K. G. H. Okma. 2005. Comparative perspectives and policy learning in the world of health care. *Journal of Comparative Policy Analysis* 7 (4): 331–348.

Marmor, T. R., and W. Plowden. 1991. Rhetoric and reality in the international jet stream: The export to Britain from America of questionable ideas. *Journal of Health Politics, Policy and Law* 16 (4): 807–12.

Mechanic, D. 1995. The Americanization of the British National Health Service. *Health Affairs* 14 (2): 51–67.

Moran, M. 1999. *Governing the health care state.* Manchester, UK: Manchester University Press.

Morone, J. A. 1990. American political culture and the search for lessons from abroad. *Journal of Health Politics, Policy and Law* 15 (1): 129–43.

OECD. *See* Organisation for Economic Co-operation and Development.

Okma, K. G. H. 2002. What is the best public-private mix for Canada's health care? Paper. Montreal Institute for Research of Public Policy.

O'Neill, F. 2000. Health: The "Internal Market" and reform of the National Health Service. In *Policy transfer and British social policy,* ed. D. Dolowitz. Buckingham, UK: Open University Press.

Organisation for Economic Co-operation and Development. 1992. *The reform of health care: A comparative analysis of seven OECD countries.* Health Reform Studies no. 2. Paris: OECD.

Organisation for Economic Co-operation and Development. 1994. *The reform of health care: A review of seventeen OECD countries.* Health Reform Studies no. 5. Paris: OECD.

Organisation for Economic Co-operation and Development. 2003. *Health at a glance: OECD indicators 2003.* Paris: OECD.

Pierson, P. 1994. *Dismantling the welfare state?: Reagan, Thatcher and the politics of retrenchment.* Cambridge: Cambridge University Press.

Poullier, J. P. 1989. Managing health in the 1990s: A European overview. *Health Service Journal* 6 (April 27).

Powell, F., and A. Wessen. 1999. *Health care systems in transition.* Thousand Oaks, CA: Sage.

Raffell, M. W., ed. 1997. *Health care and reform in industrialized countries.* University Park: Pennsylvania State University Press.

Ranade, W., ed. 1998. *Markets and health care: A comparative analysis.* Harlow, UK: Longman.

Report of Workshop on EU Law and National Health Policy. 2004. The Hague: Ministry of Health, Welfare and Sports.

Stone, D. 1984. *The disabled state*. Philadelphia: Temple University Press.

Tuohy, C. 1974. The political attitudes of Ontario physicians: A skill group perspective. Ph.D. diss., Yale University.

Tuohy, C. 1999. *Accidental logics*. Oxford: Oxford University Press.

Wall, A., ed. 1996. *Health care systems in liberal democracies*. London: Routledge.

White, J. 1995. *Competing solutions: American health care proposals and international experiences*. Washington, DC: Brookings Institution.

Wilensky, H. L. 2002. *Rich democracies: Political economy, public policy, and performance*. Berkeley: University of California Press.

Williams, A. 2001. Science or marketing at WHO? A commentary on "World Health Report 2000." *Health Economics* 10 (2): 93–100.

Wilsford, D. 1991. *Doctors and the state: The politics of health care in France and the United States*. Durham, NC: Duke University Press.

World Health Organization. 2000. *The world health report 2000: Health systems; Improving performance*. Geneva: WHO.

The United States
Risks for Americans and Lessons for Abroad

JOSEPH WHITE

Comparative health policy commentators who discuss the United States have had the unenviable job of reporting on a system that is much less equal and much less adequate than the health care system in any of the other four countries discussed in this volume—even though it is also much more expensive.[1]

However, we do have some comparative advantages that may make our participation worthwhile for the others. One is that American experience can serve as a cautionary tale. It is easy to look at any human organization and see problems. It is sometimes harder to see successes because what organizations accomplish may be taken for granted. For example, in the study of public management, civil service protections may be seen as impediments to innovation, and their function as a barrier to corruption and nepotism forgotten because success causes those problems to fade from memory. Looking at third world countries that lack honest civil services might give reformers in the United States pause. Similarly, comparing their arrangements to those of the United States may be useful to Canadians, the Dutch, Germans, or the British as a reminder of the problems they left behind when they accepted the challenges of governing systems that, for all their flaws, insure all citizens and greatly limit the opportunities to pursue material self-interest within medical delivery and health care finance.[2] We can remind the other participants what they have to lose.

The American health care system provides some citizens with excellent high-tech medicine. But the basic statistics about access, cost, and quality do not look good compared to the other members of the Four Country group, or to most other advanced industrial nations:

- The number of Americans without health insurance of any sort is only available by estimates from surveys, because there is no coherent record of who has what insurance. That figure, however, is widely agreed to be at least forty-five million individuals as of 2005.[3]
- At an estimated 16 percent of the gross domestic product (GDP) in 2004, American health care costs are far higher than in any other country. The Organisation for Economic Cooperation and Development (OECD) median was 8.7 percent of GDP; Germany was at 10.9 percent, Canada 9.9 percent, the Netherlands 9.2 percent, and United Kingdom 8.3 percent (Shea et al. 2007).
- At a minimum, the evidence that the United States receives higher quality in return for its higher spending is scant. For example, if we look at life expectancy at age forty, in the year 2000 the United States ranked eighteen out of twenty-one higher-income nations.[4]

These results occur in a system of health care finance and delivery that is uniquely complex:

- The United States has a form of government-provided social insurance for the elderly (age sixty-five and over) and disabled (defined by approval of federal disability benefits), called Medicare. It covers hospital and medically necessary physician services, and as of 2006, a pharmaceutical benefit.[5]
- Most individuals receive insurance through their workplace. Unlike in other countries with occupationally based health insurance, the American system is voluntary on the part of the employers. The employers normally pay more than the 50 percent of the premium that is common in sickness fund systems. But they also have to purchase the insurance on the market, or work out their own "networks" of providers while "self-insuring." Hence employers are more or less on their own, trying to find affordable benefits for their employees. Because costs are very high, the employee share is a fixed-dollar amount and not adjusted for income, and also employers often require much larger employee contributions to cover dependents than the employee alone, some employees do not accept the

insurance even at the subsidized price, or pay for themselves but not their dependents.

- A large range of private for-profit and nonprofit insurers offer a much wider range of policies on the health insurance market. These policies differ not only in premiums but in the benefits covered, cost sharing, administrative rules, and the health care providers whose services can be reimbursed by the coverage.

- Over forty million Americans are covered by a special program for the poor, called Medicaid. Medicaid's benefits are available mainly to low-income children and their mothers; low-income elderly (for benefits not covered by Medicare); and the disabled. Medicaid is administered by the states with oversight by the federal government, which in all cases pays more than half the costs. In spite of this subsidy, states fail to enroll a large portion of the individuals (mainly children) who are eligible for benefits.

- American health care providers, whether or not officially categorized "not-for-profit" must pursue revenue from a wide variety of sources in a highly entrepreneurial manner. In particular, the giant academic medical centers—combinations of teaching hospitals and medical schools—will have revenues from philanthropy, the huge federal government medical research enterprise, other research funders such as state governments and pharmaceutical companies, payments for hospital services and for the physicians staff's services, and in some cases direct government subsidies.

- Fairly easy access to capital and weak regulation allow providers to combine, fragment, and recombine in a kaleidoscope of organizational forms.

The complexity of American arrangements produces a second advantage of American experience for analysts, if not for citizens. The United States provides evidence about a far wider range of health care delivery and finance approaches than can be derived from any two other countries. Medicare provides an approximation of the international standard: compulsory contributions and membership, contributions related to ability to pay, and a very large pool of beneficiaries. Medicaid is an example of means-tested insurance with government sponsors. The Department of Veterans Affairs medical system is essentially a version of the British National Health Service (NHS), though restricted to one population group. Then there is the whole alphabet soup of American private insurance and health care delivery organizations. America's private insurance world not only is diverse at any given time but changes over time. The balance among different arrangements—for example, the extent of health maintenance organization (HMO) enrollment or of self-insurance—shifts regularly, and even the set of arrangements described by a term, such as HMO, changes over time.

The very diversity of American arrangements makes it impossible to explain them at reasonable length. Yet developments over time do show some patterns for policy makers and scholars in other countries to consider. Conversely, the uniqueness of these patterns may be more obvious to a participant in comparative studies than to scholars whose focus is limited to the United States.

When I wrote the first draft of this chapter, as a report on American "reforms" for the 1996 meeting of the Four Country Conference at Chateau Montebello in Canada, I was most aware of how American experience could reveal the downside risks of "reform" in other countries. In making revisions for this book with the benefit of a decade of hindsight, I still see our experience as a cautionary tale. Yet I am more impressed than before by the other side of the American story—the way it offers evidence far beyond the experience from practice not only in Canada, Germany, and the Netherlands but in all other rich democracies. Much of this experience has to do with how market competition really works.

Therefore, this chapter begins by discussing the international health policy agenda in the mid-1990s. I identify American intellectual trends at the time and how they related to international discourse. Next I raise some doubts about how accurately the discourse in the United States and abroad represented practice. Then the chapter will review what happened in the United States between 1996 and 2005. For a short time, "market" approaches seemed to many analysts to be improving the rationality and performance of American health care. Yet that pattern soon reversed, and even when there were savings, they did not work in the way the rhetoric of the time suggested.

The Health Care Policy Agenda in 1996

When the Four Country group gathered in 1996, a stated theme for the conference was "managing change." Such a theme obscured the purpose of change. Imprecision was acceptable, however, because the answer was obvious: in 1996 *change* meant, for all governments, better control of health care costs that were supposedly "unaffordable."

This "unaffordability" seemed then and now to deserve some comment. There were two standard concerns about the effects of health care costs, depending on how health care was financed. In Germany and the Netherlands, which (until 2006; see Chapter 5) largely funded health care through contributions levied as percentages of wages (up to a capped wage ceiling), the economic concern was that health care payments increase the cost of hiring, so ostensibly depress employment.[6] In Canada, where funding comes from provincial and federal general revenues, the argument was that public deficits decrease national savings and so depress economic growth. The United States had versions of both arguments: that government programs raised deficits and so reduced national savings, and that employers with high health care costs were at a competitive disadvantage.

The most striking thing about those arguments is that health care policy makers are not supposed to have the expertise to challenge them. The need for spending restraint is taken as a given on the grounds that providing health care is less important than economic growth. Yet the underlying economic arguments were and are not compelling.

In the United States, for instance, the Congressional Budget Office (CBO), in estimating the effects of enacting the policies within the congressional Republicans' 1995 budget plan, concluded that significant cuts in Medicare, much more severe reductions in Medicaid (including elimination of the entitlement to nursing care) and cutting a host of other programs by more than a quarter, would lead to the GDP being half of one percent larger in 2002 (CBO 1995). That is not a lot of gain for the pain.[7]

Arguments about the employment effects of payroll taxes are questionable in at least three ways. First, any effect on employment from the payroll charges must be compared to the possible positive effects on employment from directing resources to the relatively labor-intensive field of medical services.[8] Second, reductions in this burden could hardly make a difference for competition between, say, employers in Holland and Germany and those in low-wage countries such as Indonesia. The wage differential between the developing economies and the rich democracies vastly exceeds the few percentage points that, at maximum, could be saved from reducing health benefits. Third, if all rich democracies with sickness fund systems were to reduce payroll contributions, none would benefit vis a vis the others. The result would only be a "race to the bottom" which would result in no economy benefiting but the poor who suffer from less health care losing.[9]

Aside from the macroeconomic arguments, belief that costs were excessive was encouraged by examples of "waste" or "inefficiency." Economists can find examples in any system—even Britain's, which in 1996 may have had waste, but surely could have spent more money to good advantage (as the Blair government concluded in the late 1990s). Public health advocates always feel hospitals get too much money. Bureaucrats always know of specific hospitals that spend money badly or groups of physicians who exploit the system. Even individuals whose incomes depend on higher spending still might agree that other peoples' incomes were "unaffordable."

Yet the ability to identify, in retrospect, some unnecessary care, is very different from an ability to prevent that "waste" with policy changes. Medical diagnosis is often a process of elimination, so sensible measures as part of a pattern of investigation will seem "wasteful" as responses to the actual condition. Eliminating "waste" then may reduce diagnostic accuracy. When "managing change" implicitly means "changing the system to make it more efficient," it really requires choosing which errors to risk in conditions of uncertainty.

Nevertheless, the combination of general concern about costs and broad interest in saving by eliminating "unnecessary" spending had the effect, in 1996, of increasing international interest in health policies within the United States, which, according to many commentators, offered models for savings from reduction of unnecessary care.

MAKING CARE MORE APPROPRIATE AND THE "MANAGED CARE" HYPE

There is a standard menu of measures to eliminate inappropriate services. I call this approach "managing treatment," and it is what most people seem to think they mean by "managing care" (for a more extensive discussion, see White 1999). One is to improve knowledge about effectiveness of treatment. Another is to alter payment systems so providers (especially physicians) have incentives to provide more cost-effective treatment. A third is to create institutions to review or pre-approve treatment decisions. A fourth is to devise alternative delivery systems (ranging from chronic care teams to the ideal prepaid group practice) that can do more than physicians can (for example, remind people to take their medicine) while improving physician practice. Where there is compelling evidence as to what will work best and be most cost-effective, of course it would be preferable to change practice in that direction.

Versions of all these approaches were being implemented within the United States private insurance sector in 1996. The question I considered then, and will review here, is how those measures worked. At the time, they appeared to be being oversold. They were oversold in part because all payers, whether they are employers or public officials, are attracted to promises of blameless cost control. "Managing care" defined as giving people the right treatment in the right place at the right time (and no more) promised that patients would get what they needed—no painful "rationing"—while providers would have no legitimate gripe about any lost income.

The health services research community also promoted the idea, because knowledge of the most efficient treatments was precisely what the American health services research community was selling to its political and business clients. Supporters of the then-new Agency for Health Care Policy and Research (later renamed the Agency for Health Research and Quality) claimed that its work would yield major improvements in cost and quality—thereby implicitly promising great benefits from "managing care" according to such research.[10] The case for health services research and the case for "managed care" were very easily conflated.

Perhaps the dominant incentives for promoting "managed care" in the United States, however, involved the macropolitics of health policy. Politicians were attacted to the idea that costs could be managed by competing insurance plans—so provide a "free-market" form of cost control in place of "big government" measures. In theory the plans would compete to control costs by managing care. President Clinton had adopted this concept of "managed competition," in part, in his failed effort to create universal health insurance in the United States (White 1995). At the time of the 1996 conference, Congressional Republicans were making such an approach the rationale for turning Medicare and Medicaid over to private insurance companies. The rationale was that measures such as the development of treatment guidelines or outcome measures could create quality-based competition to improve cost control while preserving quality. "Choice" among insurance plans would enable enrollees to use the threat of "exit" to force plans to attain high quality at low prices.

Support for this approach crossed party lines in part because of distaste for alternatives. Other countries at that time mostly focused on controlling system capacity, fixed operating budgets for hospitals, and limits on prices for other services and pharmaceuticals. Fee restrictions were "price controls" and so pretty much anathema to many American economists.[11] Capacity controls, many analysts argued, imposed excessive limits on care, as symbolized by the waiting lists in the United Kingdom. Even Americans who endorsed national health insurance wrote about the "painful prescription" for cost control in the NHS (Aaron and Schwartz 1984). American opponents of universal health insurance greatly overstated the effects of these restrictions (especially in nations other than the United Kingdom), but they did exist. Germany, for example, appeared to have much less capacity for bone marrow transplantation in the early 1990s than many comparable countries and ranked low on appropriate use of that technique (U.S. General Accounting Office [GAO] 1994).

Another alternative for cost control is to give patients price incentives to consume less. This requires some sort of user charges to patients or other cost sharing between patients and insurers. Cost sharing was (and is) highly controversial in Canada (where it is essentially prohibited by the 1984 Canada Health Act), and only plays a modest role in either Germany or the Netherlands. Nevertheless, it tends to have supporters in all countries (such as economists and physicians, for very different reasons). In the United States, the influential health economist Joseph Newhouse had led the Rand Experiment, which he basically interpreted as favoring cost sharing (though others could differ; see Newhouse 1993; Rice and Morrison 1994). American right-wing think tanks took this approach to an extreme with proposals for medical savings accounts (MSAs).[12] In spite of the extensive interest on the part of conservatives and economists, however, increased cost-sharing was obviously unpopular with the voters.

A third cost-saving alternative is to devolve care decisions to some entity that lives within a fixed budget. Such budgets were already imposed on hospitals in several countries, but there were also attempts to expand their scope beyond the hospital. One example was British General Practitioner (GP) "fundholding"; another was the push in Canada to decentralize authority over both hospital and other services to local or regional "community" authorities.[13]

President Clinton had essentially proposed a combination of managed competition with a global budget and back-up price regulation. The Dutch had come up with a similar idea in their Dekker Plan of 1987. Though accepted by the legislature, it disappeared during the process of implementation but resurfaced in 2006 in a somewhat different form (see Chapter 5). President Clinton's version didn't solve the political challenges of cost control and was rejected by Congress. Next, in 1995, President Clinton vetoed the Republican Medicare proposals. Yet in 1996 there was still substantial talk in the United States about saving from competition among insurers that would manage care. Insurers, encouraged by employers, were moving employees into versions of managed care, and analysts who had previously criticized the idea jumped on the bandwagon for care management by *private* actors. Brookings Institution economists Henry Aaron and Robert D. Reischauer (1995), proclaimed the need to transform Medicare into a system in which "all Medicare beneficiaries ultimately would receive a predetermined amount to be applied for the purchase of a health plan providing defined services." They argued this was necessary because "Medicare is rapidly becoming the last refuge of unregulated fee-for-service care in the United States." They also felt it was appropriate to restrict choice for Medicare beneficiaries because, as a matter of principle, "Medicare beneficiaries should have a degree of choice among health plans similar to that enjoyed by the rest of the population" (Aaron and Reischauer 1995).

None of this advocacy recognized the practical difficulties with the managed competition and care theory. The basic problems were that sufficient evidence to govern care through guidelines did not exist, and the risk-adjustment methods needed to ensure competition on value rather than risk-manipulation also had not been found. The latter difficulty, especially, was evident to the Dutch participants in the Four-Country meetings. Nor had all American analysts endorsed the reliance on management and less choice. In a report for the Kaiser Family Foundation, Marilyn Moon and Stephen Zuckerman (1995) compared Medicare with private insurance. They found that cost per capita for Medicare insured grew more slowly than private insurance from 1984 to 1993, in essence the period when Medicare tightened its payment controls. Even in 1993, when the growth of costs in private insurance began to slow down, expenditure for Medicare insured grew by only 0.3 percent more than for private insured for a set of comparable services.[14] In line with these data, Moon and Karen Davis (1995) advocated a combination of less fundamental reforms to Medicare. In the context of an American elite debate that reflexively presumes that the Brookings Institution is "liberal," the positions of Aaron and Reischauer clearly defined Moon and Davis as left wing.

While "managed competition" seemed to be the winning horse in the rhetorical race, as of 1996 it had not won the analytical race. To pass review by the CBO, Republican proposals for spending cuts in Medicare had to include "backup," regulatory, payment controls—precisely because the case for savings from managed care was not convincing.[15] Medicaid cuts, in the Republican 1995 proposals, depended on eliminating the entitlement to benefits—which is not exactly a sophisticated policy innovation.

Nevertheless, by 1996 the growth of private sector health care costs in the United States had slowed down dramatically compared to the pre-1993 period. Advocates of "managed care" claimed that was due to their method's efficiency. The evident question was whether they were correct, and I was skeptical.

There were alternative explanations for the lower growth. Some providers (particularly the pharmaceutical industry) had held back price increases in an attempt to deflect the pressure to pass the Clinton legislation until the threat was gone—not quite a savings from "managed care." Shifting from less restrictive to more restrictive systems of delivery could provide one-time savings of perhaps 5 to 10 percent, but more restrictive systems do not necessarily slow down expenditure growth. Some of the trend was caused by erosion of insurance coverage. Five percent fewer Americans had private health insurance in 1995 than in 1989 and that probably had some depressing effect on the volume of health care.

Another alternative explanation was the possibility that the United States had applied more of the cost restraints familiar in other countries, rather than actually shifting to more appropriate treatments. While there were little reliable data as to how the private "managed care" plans were saving money, available evidence suggested it was not by actually managing care but mainly by winning discounts on fees. If lower prices were the main cost-control device, one had to wonder whether that was so different from traditional regulatory methods. In addition, academic advocates of managed care and competition argued that the greatest benefits would be achieved by driving some doctors and hospitals out of business—in short, by reducing capacity. While (political) critics of traditional health care cost-control methods talked about the rationing created by capacity controls, Alain Enthoven (1990, 1993) had long argued that the market would face fewer obstacles than the government does in the necessary task of closing unneeded facilities. Perhaps, but constriction of supply was still more like the international standard than like "managing care."

AMERICAN TRENDS AND THE INTERNATIONAL DISCOURSE

Hence international observers should not have assumed the United States was actually saving money by "managing care." If actual American cost controls differed from the rhetoric, that fact might not make it such an exception after all. In the Netherlands, for example, cost sharing had met much resistance and competition was not operating in the manner originally contemplated by the Dekker Commission, Plan Simons, or any other blueprint. Yet regulation of fees had become much stricter. In Germany, rather than creating plans and leaving the dirty work of cost control to the plan managers, the government held physicians directly accountable for pharmaceutical costs—and that seemed to be working a lot better than the previous, admittedly half-hearted, efforts to restrain costs through cost sharing, at least on the short term. In Canada, governments were limiting fees and slashing hospital capacity while emitting a fog of rhetoric about "decentralization" and "community control."

In addition to attending to the risks of "reform," therefore, the question was what mechanisms of "competition" or "devolution" really added to the old-fashioned cost-control methods—namely fee regulation, budgets, and capacity limits. Devolution schemes, whether to "bring local government close to the people" or to create "efficient, competing plans," have obvious political attractions. It is easy to see why health ministries or policy analysts will be attracted to schemes that proclaim somebody else will allocate resources more efficiently—and get the blame. But aside from packaging and blame avoidance, what are the real advantages of these strategies? And what are their special costs?

The most obvious political cost of the managed care approach involves the difficulty of getting the public to accept restrictions on choice of provider. That might have been a slightly less severe challenge in countries such as France and Australia than in Canada, Germany, the United Kingdom, or the Netherlands. In the former countries, unlike the latter, high cost sharing already restricted access by poorer citizens to some segment of caregivers.[16] But the poorer citizens are not the most powerful interests in any country, and restrictions on access to health care create political difficulties everywhere. In the United States, beneficiaries were accepting restrictions in order to reduce their cost sharing (HMOs generally having much less cost sharing than traditional indemnity plans) and because employers promoted restrictions while labor was weak. In Canada, Germany, and the Netherlands, there was no reason for voters to accept the restrictions of "managed care."

But two consequences of the newer cost-control strategies were especially evident from an American perspective—perhaps because they are aspects of the U.S. system anyway, only exacerbated by competition. One was the overhead that accompanies the proliferation of organizations involved in health care or the administration of cost sharing. The other, evident in America but also in Britain, was the difficulty of maintaining adequacy and some equity of supply in a world of devolution and, especially, competition (White 1995).

In the United States the new adequacy-and-equity concern in the mid-1990s focused in particular on academic medical centers, with their relatively large proportion of impoverished patients and their special costs of training.[17] They are to a large extent the caregiver of last resort in a system with great inequality of insurance. Those hospitals disproportionately admit the uninsured, who are treated by trainee physicians. Insured patients are more likely, for relatively uncomplicated conditions, to attend the more pleasant suburban hospitals.

In Canada, Germany, and the Netherlands—systems with virtually everyone insured and with low cost sharing—the academic medical centers did not seem to play the same safety-net role, so their viability was not so significant for equity. But in countries such as Australia and France, where cost sharing is more significant, academic medical centers did seem to be more basic to system equity.[18] The lesson for analysts from Germany, the Netherlands, and Canada was that imposing price constraints on their citizens, either directly through cost sharing or indirectly through some form of managed competition, would likely make their academic medical centers more important for equity, so that their viability could become a crucial issue. In particular, the combination of price constraints on beneficiaries and a shift of resources from hospitals to so-called "community care," might reduce equity of access. In short, while other countries looked to American experience for new methods of health care cost control, there was reason to be concerned about the equity of access. Policy makers in other countries, it seemed, should consider two questions:

- How much inequality is possible without threatening adequacy of care for the least fortunate citizens within your system?
- What are the key institutions of a "safety net" to ensure the adequacy of care for all citizens in the context of efforts to control costs?

The View from 2007

The short answer to those questions is that policy makers in Canada, Germany, and the Netherlands (at least until 2006; see Chapter 5) have been unwilling to impose significant cost sharing or to break up insurance pools. Cost control through cutting hospital capacity and limiting payments to providers did produce some significant concerns about access and quality in Canada, but the pain was spread pretty widely. Measures that would directly threaten equity remained unpopular (Tuohy 2002). After the turn of the millennium, Canadian policy makers chose to "reinvest" in health care. This approach was made easier by significant federal government surpluses and rationalized with language about primary care and outcomes measurement, which presumably made the health policy community feel better about the spending (Wong 2005).[19]

Yet what about the substance of this analysis? What really was going on in the United States in 1996, and what happened thereafter?

COST AND ACCESS TRENDS

Table 2.1 provides data on Medicare enrollment and cost per enrollee inside and outside Medicare as well as insurance premiums paid by large employers for their workers.[20] In general, small employers and individuals face higher premiums, so the table slightly understates total growth.

Annual premium amounts can differ from costs as the relationship between premium income and actual costs—the "medical loss ratio"—is not constant. Health insurance tends to follow an "underwriting cycle" in which periods of higher profits are followed by greater price competition among insurers (reducing the spread between premiums and medical costs). Next, higher "medical losses" lead to less price competition and a higher spread between premiums and costs.[21] One of the unusual developments of the 1990s and

Table 2.1 Health care costs per capita, United States, 1991–2003 (annual growth rates; negative growth in parentheses)

	GDP per capita (%)	Non-Medicare health care services (%)	Large employer premiums (%)	Medicare per enrollee (%)
1991–1993	3.3	6.2	10.1	
1994–1997	4.4	2.4	2.4	
1998–2000	4.6	6.7	5.0	0.3
2001–2003	2.8	9.0	13.3	7.2
(1990–1995)	(3.7)	(4.5)	(7.4)	(8.7)
(1995–1997)	(4.8)	(2.6)	(1.3)	(6.5)

Sources: Author's calculations are from individual year figures in the following sources: "All Services" and GDP for 1994–2003 are from Bradley C. Strunk and Paul B. Ginsburg, "Tracking Health Care Costs: Trends Run Downward in 2003," *Health Affairs,* Web Exclusives (January–June 2004): Exhibit 1, W4-356. "All Services" and GDP for 1991–1993 are from Strunk and Ginsburg, "Tracking Health Care Costs: Trends Stabilize But Remain High in 2002," *Health Affairs,* Web Exclusives (January–June 2003): Exhibit 1, W3-268. Insurance Premiums for 1991–2000 are from Christopher Hogan, Paul B. Ginsburg, and Jon R. Gabel, "Tracking Health Care Costs: Inflation Returns," *Health Affairs* 19 (6): Exhibit 3, 220. Insurance Premiums for 2001–2003 are from Strunk and Ginsberg, "Tracking Health Care Costs," W3-272). "Medicare per Enrollee" is from *2005 Annual Report of the Boards of Trustees of the Federal Hospital Insurance and Federal Supplementary Medical Insurance Trust Funds* (Washington, DC: Centers for Medicare and Medicaid Services, March 23, 2005), Table V.B1, 151.

Note on Sources: The underlying data source for health care costs per capita is the Milliman USA Health Cost Index. The index is "designed to reflect the claims trends experienced by private insurers for a typical policy" (Strunk and Ginsberg, "Tracking Health Care Costs," W3-267). Medicare spending is removed from this calculation; however, the procedure does not remove spending by Medicaid and for uninsured patients, so it will not perfectly mirror trends for spending paid by private health insurance. The underlying sources for premiums are only reporting premiums for larger employers. Therefore, they will understate overall premium trends, since large employers tend to face somewhat smaller increases (and premiums) than do small employers or individuals. Different surveys generated this data for 1991–1998, 1998–2000, and 2001–2003. Details are available in the *Health Affairs* articles. Please note also that these calculations are based on percentage figures published in the listed tables; calculations from raw data could presumably result in slightly different figures.

early 2000s was that both phases of the "cycle" were longer than usual: insurers accepted much lower margins for longer than in the past, and after they changed their mind, insisted on higher margins for longer.

Table 2.1 also shows that, in the early 1990s, costs per capita were growing much faster than per-capita GDP in the private sector and in Medicare. Thus, at the time of the battle over President Clinton's national health insurance proposals in the early 1990s, experts expected costs to soon hit 14 percent of GDP and rise to 18 percent by the end of the decade (White 1995, 239–40). Yet at the time, the trend in the private sector was dramatically reversing as the growth of costs and premiums slowed down significantly through 1997, so that national health expenditures declined as a share of the economy.[22] Meanwhile, Medicare costs burgeoned, as political stalemate prevented any agreement on new cost-control measures.

Around 1997, however, both trends reversed again. From 1998–2000 the costs in the private sector accelerated. Insurance companies did not catch on immediately—premiums lagged the trend, though they still grew more quickly than from 1994 to 1997. Meanwhile, the warring factions within American government finally agreed on a compromise set of savings measures for Medicare, in the Balanced Budget Act of 1997 (BBA-97). The savings of that act almost entirely depended on stronger versions of traditional controls. The BBA-97 strengthened controls over payments for inpatient care and physician services. It also extended to areas that had been relatively uncontrolled, such as nursing homes, physical therapy, and home health care. In short, the savings followed the recommendations of Moon and Davis, not Aaron and Reischauer (Moon, Gage, and Evans 1997; O' Sullivan et al. 1997).

In addition, the federal government initiated a crackdown on "fraud and abuse" in Medicare. Legislation such as the BBA-97 and the 1996 Health Insurance Portability and Accountability Act increased financing for investigation and prosecution (within both the Federal Bureau of Investigation [FBI] and the U.S. Attorneys' offices). Further, the use of laws with harsh civil penalties (for example, the Federal False Claims Act) and particularly visible prosecutions of large providers (the University of Pennsylvania health system and the giant Columbia/HCA for-profit hospital chain) simply scared the wits out of health care managers. In response, "DRG creep," with hospitals classifying more and more admissions as complex and costly under the prospective payment system for inpatient care, suddenly stopped in 1997. Some health care providers that provided suspiciously high rates of services per beneficiary disappeared when caps were put on per-capita payments. And Medicare cost increases suddenly slowed dramatically. Total Medicare spending even shrunk slightly between federal fiscal years 1998 and 1999 (CBO 1999, 2001).

Providers screamed with the pain caused by this Medicare cost constraint, and there was great political pressure for "givebacks." Meanwhile, the federal budget deficit had turned into surplus so the government had money to give—and the new administration in 2001 did not seem to be too interested in Medicare cost control anyway.[23] Hence Medicare returned to a pattern of rapid increase in 2001 to 2003. Yet costs in the private sector increased even more quickly, and as the insurance companies scrambled to get to the other side of the underwriting cycle (and stay there), premiums rose even more quickly.

By 2003, therefore, America's health care was back to the cost crisis of 1993. As a share of the economy, national health expenditures rose from 13.2 percent in 1998 to 15.3 percent in 2003 and were projected to rise to 18.7 percent by 2014 (Heffler et al. 2005).[24] Still, Republican control of the federal government kept national health insurance far from the political agenda.

In short, the "market" or "managed care" had a short-lived success in cost control. But Medicare then caught up; over the full period from 1990 to 2003, costs rose at very similar rates for both Medicare and private insurance.[25] Those data give no reason to believe that market competition can improve on the performance of even a weak version of the international norm; and Medicare, for example, which has little ability to limit capital spending, offers at best a weak version of cost-control methods in other countries.

In 1996, managed care and competition among hospitals threatened access to care, largely by putting the safety net provided by academic medical centers at risk. Yet effects on access were much more complicated than that dynamic. At first, the combination of rapid economic growth and significant cost controls made health insurance more affordable for employers. As a result, employment-based coverage reversed its decline and, between 1994 and 2000, rose from 64.4 percent of the population to 66.8 percent. Meanwhile, coverage for the needy through the Medicaid program declined from 12.7 percent of the population in 1994 to 10.5 percent in 1999, both because of the good economy (which reduced need) and "welfare reform" that reduced participation in Medicaid. Hence the private sector extended its role in insuring Americans.

However, both trends subsequently reversed. By 2003 only 63 percent of Americans had health insurance through employment. Meanwhile, governments in the late 1990s responded to favorable budget conditions by expanding Medicaid eligibility. When the economy then turned sour, Medicaid enrollments grew to 12.8 percent of the population; by 2003 they were higher than in 1994 (Fronstin 2004, 5). By March 2003, nearly forty-five million Americans—about 17.7 percent of the population below the age of sixty-five (so ineligible for Medicare)—were without health insurance. Hence when both governments and employers were doing well financially they tended to maintain or expand coverage, whereas they reduced or at best maintained coverage when they did worse. The net effect was a decline in private coverage and an expansion of public coverage. It appears to be easier, though not easy, to reduce private than public coverage.[26]

Both the private and the public sectors' cost controls threatened particularly negative effects on major teaching hospitals. They appeared to be at a disadvantage in contracting with private insurers, and they were hit by the antifraud campaign within Medicare. To make matters worse, many of them had made unwise investments during the 1990s. By 1999, many were in the red (Medicare Payment Advisory Commission [MedPAC] 2001, 69–71). Yet increased subsidies from the federal (Medicare and Medicaid) Disproportionate Share Hospital (DSH) programs (Zuckerman et al. 2001) gave some teaching hospitals distinctly higher operating margins from Medicare than from private payers (MedPAC 2003). Increased federal research spending also helped to offset the fiscal pressures on the academic medical centers.

Reduced income caused by the spread of "managed care" was associated with physicians providing less charity care (Center for Studying Health System Change [HSChange] 1999). Shrinking inpatient capacity (in almost all markets) and facility closures (in many) decreased access to emergency departments (EDs); ambulance diversions from one ED to another became common by 2001. Local and federal government sought to address these issues with a mix of measures. They expanded community health centers and reorganized dispatching systems for ambulance services. Hospital managers expanded emergency departments in the hope of catching more patients (Brewster and Felland 2004; Felland, Felt-Lisk and McHugh 2004; Kellerman 2004; Melnick et al. 2004).

The basic pattern, then, was that the market did threaten the "safety net," but that political decisions kept it—mostly—intact. By 2003 more Americans were uninsured than in 1993, a larger proportion of Americans were uninsured, and more Americans were dependent on government "safety-net" programs such as Medicaid, community health centers, and subsidies to academic medical centers.

THE REAL WORLD OF "MANAGED CARE"

Subsequent developments confirmed earlier suspicions about the causes of "savings" from "managed care." There were some savings as traditional HMOs reduced hospitalizations, and physicians and insurers copied that behavior. But most of the savings appear to have been from negotiating to drive down prices. As one evaluation expressed the situation as of 1997, "Health plans, in early attempts at cost control, used fairly crude measures, including leveraging aggregated purchasing power to negotiate price discounts with providers. They turned their attention next to the potential for shifting service delivery from inpatient to outpatient settings. Concurrently, they pursued strategies for reducing service demand. 'Now we're at the stage where cost savings ultimately will come from managing care better,' one analyst contended" (HSChange 1997, 2). In other words, they weren't quite "managing care" yet.

Later analyses also emphasized the dynamic of price negotiation. James D. Robinson reported on the travails of the Aetna and US Healthcare insurance companies. They each gained market share quickly, merged in 1996, and the combination grew to include twenty-one million covered lives. As Robinson explained, Aetna, "sought to move as much enrollment as possible into the fully insured HMO, counting on aggressive provider discounts to control medical costs . . . The Aetna US Healthcare managed care strategy relied above all else on massive scale, on millions in enrollment and billions in revenue to pressure physicians and hospitals to participate at low payment rates; cover the administrative overhead of utilization management, dilute adverse selection from weak underwriting; and spur continuous rounds of lower costs, lower premiums, and further growth" (Robinson 2004a, 45). Instead of size creating profits, however, the combined company had large losses. The top management team was dumped, and the company survived only by entirely reconfiguring its business. By 2003 Aetna had only thirteen million enrollees and only 3.3 million in its HMO lines.

Aetna's strategy, and the similar strategies of many other insurers, failed because providers revolted, "consolidating their local markets and demanding rate increases, litigating over delays in payment and denials in authorization, and, in some instances, simply walking away from HMO networks" (Robinson 2004a, 45). In other words, "managed care" mostly meant the exercise of market power to drive down prices, and it failed when the providers developed sufficient power to resist.

As mentioned in the introduction to this chapter, the United States is so large that it provides a variety of experiences. California was different because of the massive presence of Kaiser Permanente, the prototypical group/staff model HMO, which really *did* "manage care" through a distinct practice culture and internal management. Yet a similar pattern of market power effects occurred there, only with different players.

Attempting to follow Kaiser's example, physicians in much of the state formed into large multispecialty groups (similar to the Permanente group of

Kaiser), and contracted with HMOs to take on risk through capitated payment for patients (Casalino 2001; Robinson 2001). By the late 1990s, there were sixteen million people in HMOs in California, receiving care through 250 medical groups. "Then . . . came the crash" (Robinson 2001, 82). California's physician groups, seeking to expand their market share, had "accepted low rates because they wanted to attract patients from competing organizations." The trouble was they could not control costs outside their organizations very well. "The limits of leverage against health plans stem from the simple fact that health care is local, and even the largest medical groups never built anything approaching monopoly power in any particular submarket" (Robinson 2001, 91).

Why did physician groups (and Aetna, and everybody else) have to compete by price discounting rather than by managing care to make it more appropriate? Truly managing care, namely, managing treatments, requires building and managing complex organizations (if it is possible at all).[27] Markets not only don't make that happen, but the pursuit of market power may have made it more difficult. "The race to become large enough so that the other side must contract with you," Casalino reported, "has resulted in organizations growing at rates that HMO and group leaders acknowledge have sometimes been unmanageable and to sizes that many believe may be larger than is warranted for economies of scale" (2001, 103). Consolidation also had negative effects on culture and work incentives in bringing together "physicians who did not know or appreciate each other, who shared no common vision or culture, and who treated fewer patients per day than when self-employed" (Robinson 2001, 89). He observed that instead of creating integrated care, "amalgamation can transfer inside the organization the diversity and disunity formerly coexisting under the principle that good fences make good neighbors." Especially in more loosely structured groups, there could be fights over internal divisions of resources, with specialists threatening to withdraw en masse in order to "extort greater shares of the overall budget" (Robinson 2001, 92).

Nor did groups in a market system have incentives to compete on quality. In a real market where patients have choice about where to buy medical services but nobody has devised a plausible risk-adjustment mechanism, the threat of adverse selection meant that "we do not see billboards advertising that HMO A or Medical Group B provides outstanding care of diabetic patients . . . capitated organizations with a reputation for high quality may suffer a double financial hit: a loss on their investment in quality, and a loss from attracting sicker-than-average patients." Some groups actually "did institute disease management and other quality improvement programs during the 1990s, but as the financial disincentives became clearer, and as the groups struggled with the financial crisis of the late 1990s, these efforts [were] scaled back" (Casalino 2001, 104–5).

By 2004 John Iglehart, founding editor of *Health Affairs*, could conclude: "Lingering visions of the ideal health maintenance organization (HMO) still color policymakers' perceptions about the less organized provinces of the health system. It is still fashionable to argue that the object of policy should be to nurture competition for consumers' allegiance between high-performance health plans. In fact, though, relatively few such plans exist. Evidently, a rare and fortuitous combination of circumstances is needed to incubate the kind of large multispecialty groups on which true HMOs are built" (2004a, 35). These circumstances and time had allowed the development of Kaiser Permanente, in certain large markets, at certain times. But Kaiser's model had large management costs and could not show big enough cost advantages to triumph over other kinds of "managed care" in the 1990s. As a result, in 2004 only twelve versions of the ideal HMO remained in the country, serving 7.6 million enrollees. A decade before there had been ninety-eight, serving 11.8 million enrollees (Schoenbaum 2004).

There are real lessons here for non-Americans, even if Americans haven't learned them. First, developing integrated provision of medical care is extremely difficult for reasons that have nothing to do with our finance system: It seems to require extremely complex organizations that combine very different cultures and face immense management tasks. Such organizations *can* be created but may require special circumstances: In the United States, historically, physicians tended to self-select into the Permanente medical group. Second, in America's system of competing insurers with shifting risk pools, either employers or the workers themselves may shift enrollees from plan to plan. This shifting gives health care providers little reason to seek quality by improving the appropriateness of treatment, especially for patients with chronic conditions for whom less expensive maintenance treatments early *might* save money on expensive hospitalizations later. In the American context, the point is that traditional fee-for-service Medicare is a more logical platform for systems of disease management than a set of atomized plans with shifting membership could be (Short, Mays, and Mittler 2003). For foreigners, the lesson would be that if you want to "manage" care, it makes little sense to give that function to insurance carriers and yet let enrollees move among carriers.

The course of events in the United States also highlights the difference between managing treatments and selective contracting (White 1999). The distinction is in part reflected in standard classifications of health plans. These include HMOs, which supposedly have tighter networks of providers and extensive care-management routines; preferred provider organizations (PPOs), which mainly work through selecting providers who accept prices that the insurer can live with; and point-of-service (POS) plans, in which enrollees essentially have a choice between using a kind of HMO network (with its restrictions) or going to other providers but paying substantially higher cost sharing. These options show that the selectivity of contracting and the intensity of management of treatment are distinct dimensions of cost-control effort.

The three approaches competed with each other, and PPOs won. By 1993, there were more Americans in PPOs than in HMOs. During the 1990s enrollment in all three forms grew at the expense of nonselective, "unmanaged" indemnity insurance, with PPOs maintaining an edge. By 1999 there was very little old-fashioned indemnity insurance left (outside of Medicare). At that point, PPO coverage expanded drastically at the expense of the other forms. By 2002, PPOs enrolled 112 million Americans, more than twice the number in HMOs (Hurley, Strunk, and White 2004).

Why did PPOs win out in the marketplace over more tightly managed systems? First, more tightly managed care is less than popular with patients. While the "managed care backlash" had few and insignificant legislative victories, employers apparently decided that their employees wanted fewer restrictions. But employers might not have shifted to PPOs if they had faced greater price differences between HMO and PPO plans. HMOs interfered more in patient care, but administering such interference also caused costs. Hence, by the early 2000s, in most markets, there was little difference in costs between the two forms (Hurley, Strunk, and White 2004; Schoenbaum 2004). That factor enabled PPOs' marketing advantages to dominate decisions.

The PPO approach, precisely because it is defined by contracting rather than management, makes it easier for insurers to create provider networks. Insurers can customize plans to employers' preferences, for example, by offloading costs to employees (through cost sharing) or by fitting a network to where the employees live. The traditional group- or staff-model HMO was oriented against cost sharing and limited geographically by its clinic structures. The organizer of a PPO plan could even rent out its network to an employer that chose to self-insure—and lots of employers, in part because of regulatory requirements for health insurance, preferred to self-insure (Hurley, Strunk, and White 2004).

If all employers had been required to offer the same basic coverage, these marketing advantages would not have mattered. In the every-employer-for-itself world of the American health care market, however, the ability to customize products to fit a given employer's particular employee distribution

and financial condition in a given year became the real function of health insurers. When employers are the true purchasers, then the effective consumers,
in Robinson's words, "differ widely in their preferences and willingness to
pay for particular products," (1999, 8) and health plans gain business by offering a variety of networks and terms. In the traditional model of HMO, the
prepaid group practice such as Kaiser Permanente, there is only one plan and
little ability to customize.

But, while PPOs could beat HMOs within the U.S. market, they could not
control costs as well as Medicare. There is no reason to believe a similar selective contracting approach would control costs better than the current systems in other countries. As the analysts at the Center for Studying Health
System Change (not a big-government group) noted about legislation that
presumed PPOs could lower Medicare expenditure: "Almost certainly, PPOs
cannot get sustainable discounts from physicians or hospitals that approxi-
mate rates paid by Medicare, as even the tightest HMO networks rarely approach Medicare's administered prices. In that respect, Medicare is the
'mother of all PPOs' because it enjoys superior discounts over virtually all
private payers. That the PPO will not be able to achieve the low administrative costs of traditional Medicare is a point conceded even by proponents of
PPOs" (Hurley, Strunk, and White 2004, 67).

MARKET POWER AND PURSUIT OF SELF-INTEREST

Thus the beliefs of market participants and underlying factors of supply
and demand shaped the ups and downs of America's privately funded medical
care.

Four relevant sets of actors fueled the movement into HMOs and PPOs, the
discounting activities, and the pursuit of market shares that dominated behavior in the mid-1990s. First and foremost, entrepreneurs and managers of
insurance companies believed these approaches were how insurers should do
business. Robinson's (2004a) account of Aetna's tribulations neatly illustrates
the dynamic of belief followed by disillusion. Second, providers had to be
willing to sign selective contracts at discounted rates. In a way, the move to
selective contracting was a self-fulfilling prophecy: Because they were told
"managed care" was the wave of the future, providers figured they had to get
ahead of the wave "to ensure they did not lose patients or revenue as beneficiaries moved into managed care" (Grossman, Strunk, and Hurley 2002, 3).[28]
Third, employers' belief in the money-saving capacity of the new plans
emerged from desperation. They needed to try something, and when selective
contracting worked for a while, employers pushed their luck, shopping for

even better deals. Finally, investors believed they would get high returns from providing the capital to build and expand these networks. This belief was another temporarily self-fulfilling prophecy. As a group of Wall Street analysts told a Center for Studying Health System Change gathering in 1997, for-profit HMOs grew due to "access to capital; good balance sheets with large amounts of cash; highly valued stock that they can use as cash to make acquisitions and grow; highly sophisticated marketing and operating abilities; and innovative product development that responds to consumer interests and demands while controlling costs." The catch was, the last part was not true: They had the capital and cash based on highly valued stock, but "much of this industry" was "not profitable now" (Center for Studying Health System Change [HSChange] 1997, 1). Investors provided the money because of the perceived prospect of profits, not actual profits. Still, the story fed on itself as "some plans intentionally under-priced to gain market share . . . With the industry in its growth phase, publicly offered plans were valued based on a multiple of members and so had additional incentives to price to increase enrollment. The heavy capitalization of these plans provided a cushion for losses arising from such pricing" (Grossman and Ginsburg 2004, 97).

In short, investors who believed the story supported insurers, and it worked as long as providers believed it too. The story was so widely believed that too many people "jumped into the business" (HSChange 1998b, 1), creating even more pressure on providers to accept discount premiums and on plans to "sacrifice premium increases in exchange for entering new markets and growing their enrollments" (HSChange 1998a, 1). But the story collapsed when providers stopped playing their part in it.

A combination of provider disgust and desperation, provider consolidation (to increase market power), and provider exit changed providers' willingness to accept and play their role in the story. By 2001, the center's Wall Street analysts were agreeing that hospitals, by consolidating, had gained dominant power in many areas, and where that had not happened, insurers were propping up the weaker hospitals with better rates in order to prevent consolidation. Both plans and providers had switched to emphasizing higher prices in order to restore profitability, mainly because the "self-induced pain" of the era in which both sides believed in market share above all had been "phenomenal" (HSChange 2001, 3).

As hospital managers abandoned the strategy of lowering prices in order to increase market share, while continuing their efforts to consolidate systems in order to increase market share and raise prices, they became more willing to confront the health plans. In a widely noticed showdown, the St.

Joseph's hospital system in Orange County refused to contract with PacifiCare, and won. "St. Joseph was able to retain most, but not all, of its patients as they switched enrollment from PacifiCare to other health plans, which sent a powerful message to both sides about the consequence of contract showdowns" (HSChange 2003a, 3). Showdowns had similar results around the country, as enrollees who had a choice within their employer plans switched to follow their preferences, and employers chose to accommodate employees' preference for wider networks. By 2003 the hospitals in most markets clearly had the upper hand over the insurers and were using their market power to extract large payment increases (HSChange 2003b, 2). As a result of these developments, a new story had come to dominate—and in essence coordinate—market behavior. Managers of health plans "accepted their weaker position relative to providers" (White, Hurley, and Strunk 2004, 1) and pursued profitability by keeping charges to insured and employers high through "pricing discipline" (HSChange 2004).

Meanwhile, the insurers in turn had consolidated to match the providers. There were half as many health plans in 2004 as in 1996 (HSChange 2004). Blue Cross and Blue Shield systems used their advantages in contracting (market power as the biggest customer) to grow from sixty-five million covered lives in 1994 to ninety-one million in 2004 (Iglehart 2004b). Much of the remaining private enrollment was in the hands of Aetna, UnitedHealth Group, and CIGNA (Robinson 2004b). One might wonder, then, why this consolidation did not allow the insurers to resist providers' demands for increased payments.

The simple answer is that there were two concentrated parts of the market and one fragmented part. The insurers had to choose between a full-pitched battle with the providers or exploiting their own market power vis-à-vis the employers. Raising premiums to employers was a lot easier.

Although physicians were able to increase their fees from the mid-1990s, they could not consolidate and gain market power across specialities in the same way as hospitals (in part due to the internal challenges of integration previously described). Some sought higher income by participating in clinical trials sponsored by drug companies (for a very critical assessment, see Kassirer 2004). But medical specialists found ways to increase their market power without integrating with primary care providers (PCPs). By the late 1990s, Californian specialists realized they had "incentives to form single-specialty groups both to gain negotiating leverage with health plans and to profit from imaging and surgical services without having to share governance and revenues with PCPs in a multi-specialty group." Larger specialty groups could also attract the capital needed to purchase imaging and other equipment. Hence participation in multispecialty groups began to weaken, while single-specialty groups became more popular (Casalino, Pham, and Bazzoli 2004, 83).

In some markets, cardiac and orthopedic specialists consolidated to a point where they could consider challenging hospitals. Those services receive particularly favorable payment rates from both Medicare and private insurers, and are often profit centers for American general hospitals. Creating specialized surgical hospitals could transfer those profits to entrepreneurs and the physicians, at the expense of the established hospitals. By 2002 physicians and for-profit specialty hospital companies had created forty-eight small hospitals with substantial physician ownership. The United States has never had strong controls on capital investment, but in some states even the weak certificate-of-need (CON) programs slowed down this corporatization.[29] It occurred faster where physicians had leverage due to consolidation or relative physician shortage (Devers, Brewster, and Ginsburg 2003; Pham et al. 2004). In response to concerns about the effect of these developments on general hospitals (Devers, Brewster, and Ginsburg 2003; Hackbarth 2005), the 2003 Medicare legislation placed a moratorium on Medicare contracting with new specialty hospitals owned by physicians, and Congress's Medicare Payment Advisory Commission advised that the moratorium be continued through 2006 (Hackbarth 2005).

Hence market forces were encouraging developments away from "integrated" care led by PCPs and toward disintegration of hospitals in the interest of specialists. The consolidation of specialists to purchase equipment and even create specialty hospitals was possible, however, only *because governments allowed it to happen.* In most countries, entrepreneurs would not be able to raise capital, build a facility, and then expect the dominant public insurers or sickness funds to send their enrollees to the facility. Here is another example where policy makers outside of the United States can look to the United States and realize what they are doing right.

The specialty hospital story also points to one other aspect of market dynamics that contradicts the theory of markets' advantages. It is true that market pressures can put some supply out of business. But that does not mean it will eliminate the right supply. As we saw earlier, contraction of services had some negative aspects, such as reduced access to emergency services. Meanwhile, hospitals competed to increase supply of profitable services, such as cardiac or obstetric care. In short, the market did not rationalize supply; it just redirected supply toward the most profitable services.

As all the old stories about how the market would save American health care were disproved, American health policy elites on the conservative wing developed a new one. The new term was "consumer-driven health care."

Consumers would have "high-deductible health plan products tied to spending accounts, funded by employers. Once the consumer has exhausted the spending account, there is a gap in coverage . . . where the consumer must pay for all care before the high-deductible policy kicks in and provides coverage." These spending accounts, known as health savings accounts (HSAs), would have very favorable tax treatment. So how is this different from just having high cost sharing in the form of a deductible? It would be different because consumers would receive "information that supports cost-efficient decision making" (Trude and Conwell 2004, 1).

This chapter is not the place for an extensive review of the HSA concept.[30] Yet it seems worthwhile to note that "consumer direction" in health care is, first of all, rhetoric. A more accurate label would be "consumer constraining," since the point of high deductibles is precisely to create price constraints to inhibit consumption. Beyond the rhetoric, the idea faces a series of practical difficulties.

First, if consumers were to "take charge" of their health care (or health) they would need a great deal of information and the ability to process that information. The latter may never exist; the former is not exactly in high supply. The U.S. Government Accountability Office, the GAO, for example, found that plans offered to federal employees provided standard information about healthy behavior, but little about the quality and cost of providers (GAO 2006a, 17–18). Rosenthal and colleagues (2005, 1592) observed that most "first generation consumer-directed health plans . . . do not make available alternative measures of quality and longitudinal cost-efficiency in enough detail to help consumers discern high-value health care options; financial incentives for consumers are weak and insensitive to differences in value among the selections that consumers make; and none of the plans made cost-sharing adjustments to preserve freedom of choice for low-income consumers." In other words, "consumer-directed" health plans (CDHPs) have been no more "consumer directed" than most "managed care" plans actually manage care. CDHP is mainly a relabeling of high-deductible insurance, a very old-fashioned cost-control idea.

Even the level of cost sharing in many plans is not evidently higher than in common private insurance. Remler and Glied (2005, 1070) pointed out that with funds in an HSA available to pay for part of the deductible, and with the deductible replacing cost sharing above its maximum amount (for example, co-payments for prescription drugs), "many HSA/high-deductible arrangements would actually reduce cost-sharing for many groups. In particular, the group responsible for half of all medical spending would see no change or a decline in cost sharing at the margin and on average." Hence these plans are not necessarily more *consumer-constraining* than the alternatives. Just as the hype about HMOs enabled both supporters and critics to ignore differences between actual plans and the ideal of a tightly managed group or staff system, the sound and fury about high-deductible approaches conceals the reality as well as the variation among plans.

Enrollment in HSAs has been a moving target. It began slowly. In 2002 employers "doubted the approach would slow the growth of their health care costs" (Trude and Conwell 2004, 2).[31] By 2005, the Center for Health System Change reported that, in the twelve markets it monitored, CDHPs were being offered, "but enrollment to date is limited." The analysts added that, "few of the consumer-driven products available today offer information to help patients differentiate effectively between types of services or choose providers that deliver the best combination of price and quality" (Lesser, Ginsburg, and Felland 2005, 1, 3). By 2006 there were still only about three million enrollees in CDHPs.[32] By 2008, enrollment in CDHPs may have been accelerating; one survey reported that 13 percent of enrollees in firms with fewer than 1000 workers were in CDHPs, although the figure was only 5 percent of enrollees in larger firms (Claxton et al. 2008). Some observers suggested that growth in enrollment among employees of smaller firms might have resulted from those firms offering CDHPs as a " 'last ditch' effort to preserve some type of health insurance for employees;" alternatively, some smaller professional firms might be offering CDHPs with HSAs because they would be attractive as tax-favored savings vehicles for "highly compensated professionals" (Christianson, Ginsburg, and Draper 2008: 1365). In either case, the notion that informed consumers would shop for quality did not appear relevant. Although some data showed savings for some employers, effects are difficult to estimate because of favorable selection (Buntin et al. 2006, w521–23). A study of enrollment within a large employer plan in 2005 showed that the workers who chose the CDHP were younger and on average had lower previous medical spending than those who chose other plans (Barry et al. 2008). If employers contribute to the accompanying savings accounts, their net savings appear to be small (Gabel, Pickreign, and Whitmore 2006).

What can one make of all this? First, developments in markets are ragged and uneven. Second, as costs rise then coverage with reduced benefits does become more attractive to payers, which should be no surprise. Third, aggregate results may mask multiple causes. Fourth, doubts that CDHPs would be venues for informed purchasing, and fears that they would provide opportunities for adverse selection, appear to be legitimate. Last but not least, the promotion and adoption of "consumer-directed" insurance seems to be another example of the dangers of believing hype and stories either within American health care markets or the American health care policy community.

Conclusion: American Health Care a Decade Later

American health care performance over the decade after the 1996 Four Country Conference could have been a lot worse. After all, costs only increased by about 2 percent of GDP over the decade. There is even one advanced industrial country (Switzerland) that did a worse job of cost control (OECD 2004). In some respects, American performance was quite superior to what had happened in the decades before 1996.

One hopes that aspirations in other countries are a bit higher than this result. Yet America's experience with markets in health care still has lessons either for American policy analysts or for those who are considering reforms in other countries.

First, it is never a good idea to try to predict what will happen in a market. People pursue their interests in all sorts of ways that might only look obvious in retrospect. They also may be contracting in multiple directions, so it is very hard to predict behavior from looking at just one set of contracts.

Second, market power is very, very important. It is dynamic but not in simple ways. It depends not only on measurable aspects of supply and demand (for example, how many hospital beds) but also on the beliefs of people who are negotiating with each other. Political scientists and poker players know that negotiation involves bluff, threats, even attempts to make the other think you might not behave rationally. In a corporatist system such as Germany's, with negotiations between the sickness fund physicians and the sickness funds, expectations about what government might do also shape the bargaining. As a system is "reformed" to be more "competitive," the psychological side of bargaining becomes less predictable.

Third, because market power depends in part on beliefs, the dynamic of a market—at least initially—can be shaped by shared beliefs, or in Deborah Stone's (1999) terms, stories. In essence, the "managed care is coming and providers had better get into networks" story dominated the mid-1990s. Eventually, providers got fed up with the story, adopted consolidation strategies to break free, tested their power, and found they had some. Insurers had to abandon the story if they wanted to stay in business. Both market participants and health policy elites adopted a new story, about managed care's failures.

Sometimes stories are based more on reality, sometimes less; but they coordinate behavior (for a while) whether logically true or not. They originate as much in disciplinary biases as in reality. Thus health services researchers promote the idea that managing care can save money, public health professionals promote the idea that the "medical model" is inappropriate and inefficient, and the American health policy community in general keeps dreaming up stories about competition. Other health care systems use stories from other sources, such as the "we don't want to be like the Americans" story (particularly potent in Canada). Hence another lesson is that policy makers should be skeptical of *whatever* story is common within their own system at the time.

Fourth, markets do not create institutions. Incentives do not create institutions. Building institutions requires power, skill, personnel, luck, and time. It is silly to expect "market forces" to create integrated, high-quality multispecialty medical organizations. If anything, that kind of institution building may be easier in a system that is under less pressure for immediate results and has more hierarchical power. The ironic example, in the United States, is the Veterans Health Administration program (Oliver 2007).

Fifth, the absence of capital controls in the United States highlights how important they are in other countries. Much of what happened within the United States depended on decisions by investors who flocked to for-profit HMOs and other businesses, and then rushed away from them as they failed; or by drug companies that offered new income sources for physicians through clinical trials; or by the capital sources that allowed some hospitals to expand or specialty hospitals to be created. Capitalism means capital has power. Government management of a system means restrictions on the free flow of capital.

Sixth, how institutions work depend on other institutions. Sometimes we can only see the limits when they are removed. Consider, for example, the theory that in health care, supply creates its own demand. Hence, costs can be reduced by limiting capacity. This is a basic method of cost control outside the United States. Yet, in the United States, we saw that reducing hospital capacity allowed hospital managers to raise their prices. This dynamic does not happen in other countries because hospital managers are not allowed to set their own prices in the first place. The effectiveness of capacity restrictions depends on limits on providers' ability to raise prices.

Finally, American experience illustrates how the case for "competition" runs up against all sorts of self-interest problems and practical contradictions. For example, the theory of managed competition assumes employees will shift among health plans according to cost and quality. Yet if enrollees can shift, plan managers have little incentive to invest in prevention for the long term. In order for it to be rational to invest in enrollees' health over the long run, enrollees have to be *unable* to switch. Hence it should be no surprise that in the American market, plan managers eventually decided that the key to running their business was to manage their risks, not care. American insurers are in the business of carving up risk to maximize profits (Robinson 2004b). They might also pursue health care values—their managers would not mind keeping their enrollees healthy—but only if a way can be found to do that while serving the basic value of maximizing profits. Creating conditions where economic self-interest serves health care values turns out to be quite difficult.

There is little doubt that health policy analysts will continue to generate theories about how "competition" could solve problems of cost and quality and even access. I am sure there will be more attempts in the United States, and they will be promoted overseas, just like "managed competition." It is hoped that this chapter will remind readers to be cautious about believing those stories and to try to learn from what American actors, pursuing their economic interests, actually do—not the stories they tell.

Notes

1. This chapter is an extensively revised and extended version of the paper "Risks and Benefits of Health Care System Reform: An American Overview," which I presented at the second Four Country Conference on Health Care Reform, Chateau Montebello, Canada, in 1996. In revising I have tried to preserve the perceptions of the time, the emphasis on how American experience might be useful to observers in other countries, and the way that my own perceptions of U.S. experience were shaped by my own comparative work and participation in the Four Country Conferences. Yet I have added substantial material, some of which has been reported for an American audience, from an American perspective, in "Markets and Medical Care: The United States, 1993–2005," *The Milbank Quarterly* 85(3), September 2007, pp. 395–448. Readers interested in a much more extensive discussion of United States developments during that time period will find it in the Milbank Quarterly article. I would like to thank Alan B. Cohen for his insightful and helpful comments on the penultimate draft of this chapter.

2. As Aaron Wildavasky argued, policy making is not a process of problem "solution" in the sense that problems are eliminated, but of problem "succession": initiatives ameliorate some problems only to make others more visible. See Wildavsky (1979), especially chapters 2 and 3.

3. See Fronstin (2004) for data as of 2004.

4. The data is from OECD (2004). The comparison nations are those OECD nations with per-capita incomes over $20,000 per year in 2000. I am using life expectancy at age forty to control for the social ills that result, for example, in the United States having particularly bad infant mortality statistics, or high homicide rates among young males.

5. The cost sharing is also quite high. However, Medicare remains a far more secure source of insurance than is available to other Americans.

6. This cap is similar to the way the portion of payroll subject to Social Security taxes in the United States is limited.

7. For a good overview of the issues in translating changes in the federal government's budget position into economic growth, see CBO (1993).

8. A later and thorough analysis in Germany (Advisory Council for Concerted Action in Health Care 1998) concluded that diversion of resources to health care might actually increase employment. In subsequent Four Country Conferences, I could not see that this suggestion had any effect on German policy elites.

9. I have not mentioned the favorite argument of many economists, namely that health benefit costs are deducted from wages so do not increase total compensation. If this is true, insurance contributions would have no effect on employment. This is evidently not believed by any policy-maker who makes the argument about employment burden, so the practical reasons not to expect much benefit from reducing the "burden" appear more compelling to me.

10. This identification of a profession's interests with promising political trends, of course, did not make health services researchers any different from the traditional medical research community, when it has an opportunity to seek spending increases. It is worth pointing out that the content of the exchanges in any international conference depend on who is there. For better or worse, the American contingent in the Four Country group has been weighted against true-believers in managed care. I'd like to believe this was beneficial for participants from other countries.

11. Prominent exceptions include William Hsiao and others who helped design Medicare's fee schedule in the late 1980s.

12. In the case of MSAs, later redefined as Health Savings Accounts (HSAs), advocates try to frame cost sharing more attractively by calling it "ownership" and by providing a tax subsidy for whatever savings a person may manage.

13. Jonathan Lomas provided a fascinating account of how such "community" decision making actually worked at the 1996 conference.

14. This growth in relative Medicare spending occurred because costs in home health care especially were rocketing upward, and that service is far more important for the elderly and disabled than for other populations.

15. The plan proposed to give Medicare enrollees incentives to enroll in competing health plans but to make that option voluntary. So a portion of enrollees would remain in traditional, fee-for-service Medicare. If competition did not generate low enough premiums to match the savings targets, fees would be slashed within the remaining fee-for-service system so as to meet the target. Hence private insurers were protected against the possibility that they might not control costs by imposing the pain on providers who served the remaining public plan.

16. The high cost-sharing was restrictive only for a poor minority in France, since most had supplemental insurance through *mutuelles*. The French subsequently created compulsory and heavily subsidized supplemental insurance for the poor.

17. I say "new" concern because the most important equity-and-adequacy concern was then, and is now, the fact that so many Americans do not have health insurance at all. But that was nothing new.

18. See the discussion in White (1995).

19. The Blair government in the United Kingdom chose to implement large spending increases as well, but I am not emphasizing that because the United Kingdom is not part of the Four Country group.

20. Medicare calculations will be closer to exact than the other figures. Large-employer premiums are based on surveys. Actual costs per individual involve a wide range of measures, estimates, and adjustments. Even the Medicare figure is not ideal, as not all Medicare enrollees have the full coverage of both Part A and Part B of the program. But the data in this table should be roughly right and were the best I could find.

21. That pattern describes the market dynamic. There has also been a regulatory pattern, in which state regulators observe the retained earnings of the nonprofit health insurers (Blue Cross/Blue Shield) growing and allow smaller rate increases; then when margins shrink the regulators loosen up. Where market competition has not been too heated, the regulatory dimension may have been more important over the years.

22. From 13.4 percent in 1993 to 13.2 percent in 1998. See Heffler et al. (2005, W5–75).

23. The cynical interpretation, to which I subscribe, is that the Bush administration was so interested in privatizing Medicare that its policy makers did not want the program to control costs more successfully than private insurers did. At a minimum, there is no doubt that they wished to raise Medicare's costs for enrollees who chose private plans within Medicare, in order to attract enrollees to those plans, as they did in the eventual Medicare Prescription Drug, Improvement and Modernization Act of 2003.

24. The first column of Table 2.1 also shows that the economy grew more quickly from 1994 to 2000 than before or after. Since economic growth determines the denominator of the health expenses to GDP ratio, the relative successes of the Clinton presidency are another reason why health care's "burden" on the overall economy grew much more slowly in those years.

25. Over the long run from 1970–2001, Medicare costs per enrollee grew at 9.6 percent per year, while private sector costs grew by 11 percent per year. In addition, Medicare beneficiaries on average appear to be "generally more satisfied with their health care than are privately insured people under age sixty-five" (Boccuti and Moon 2003a, 235). For discussion of some methodological issues, see Boccuti and Moon (2003b).

26. There were many proposals to reduce insurance, particularly Medicaid, at state and federal levels, but many fewer were enacted than proposed. For a discussion on this topic, see Hoadley, Cunningham, and McHugh (2004).

27. Truly managing care also requires information about treatment appropriateness that does not exist, but a history of developments in health services research is beyond the scope of this chapter.

28. The quote refers to movement into Medicare's set of "managed care" options, and the competition between the two approaches played out more directly in that context. Within Medicare, private plan enrollment grew from 1993–97 because, as costs grew more slowly in the private sector, plans could attract enrollees with extra benefits and still make a profit. But when the plans lost market power while Medicare cracked down with more regulation and the antifraud campaign, the private insurers found they could not compete nearly so well with the traditional program. After growing to nearly

18% of enrollment by 1999, managed care fell to 13% of Medicare enrollees by the end of 2003 (Review 2004: 48). For good accounts, see Gold (2001); Grossman, Strunk, and Hurley (2002); White (2003, 251–53).

29. More than half of the specialty hospitals were in four states that did not have CON programs (Hackbarth 2005, 3). We might guess that CON processes were effective in this case because the established players in a local market objected to the interloper. CON processes usually have been weak because if the issue was whether an existing hospital could expand facilities, the existing producer interests could not agree to restrict each other. In this case, the existing providers could unite against new entrants, and apparently did. It is an exception that proves the rule about weak capital investment regulation in the United States.

30. A good overview of the origins and arguments is Jost (2007). On quality effects see Buntin et al. (2006). For early evidence see the special issue of *Health Services Research* (August 2004), including Gauthier and Clancy (2004); Lo Sasso et al. (2004); Bertko (2004); and Davis (2004). For evaluation within the closest thing to an "ideal" context of choice and an employer that seeks to provide information, see GAO (2006b).

31. Employers also worried that healthy employees would get extra benefits from the employer's savings account contribution, raising the expense for those employees more than any savings from less healthy employees, and that the information available to employees would not in fact be so useful.

32. The survey for Gabel, Pickreign, and Whitmore (2006) estimates 2.7 million enrollees; the source for Buntin et al. (2006) yields an estimate of 3.1 million.

References

Aaron, H. J., and R. D. Reischauer. 1995. The Medicare reform debate: What is the next step? *Health Affairs* 14 (4): 8–30.

Aaron, H. J., and W. B. Schwartz. 1984. *The painful prescription: Rationing hospital care*. Washington, DC: Brookings Institution.

Advisory Council for Concerted Action in Health Care. 1998. *The health care system in Germany: Cost factor and branch of the future*. Vol. 2, *Progress and growth markets, finance and remuneration*. Bonn: Advisory Council for the Concerted Action.

Barry, C. L., M. L. Cullen, D. Galusha, M. D. Slade, and S. H. Busch. 2008. Who chooses a consumer-directed health plan? *Health Affairs* 27 (6): 1671–9.

Bertko, J. 2004. Commentary: Looking at the effects of consumer-centric health plans on expenditures and utilization. *Health Services Research* 39 (4, pt. 2): 1211–18.

Boccuti, C., and M. Moon. 2003a. Comparing Medicare and private insurers: Growth rates in spending over three decades. *Health Affairs* 22 (2): 230–37.

Boccuti, C., and M. Moon. 2003b. Data concerns in out-of-pocket spending comparisons between Medicare and private insurance. *Urban Institute Health Policy Online*, no. 4. http://www.urban.org/url.cfm?ID=900615.

Brewster, L., and L. E. Felland. 2004. Emergency department diversions: Hospital and community strategies alleviate the crisis. *Center for Studying Health System Change Issue Brief*, no. 78 (March).

Buntin, M. B., C. Damberg, A. Haviland, K. Kapur, N. Lurie, R. McDevitt, and M. S. Marquis. 2006. Consumer-directed health care: Early evidence about cost and quality. *Health Affairs,* Web Exclusive (October 24): W516–30.

Casalino, L. 2001. Canaries in a coal mine: California physician groups and competition. *Health Affairs* 20 (4): 97–108.

Casalino, L., H. Pham, and G. Bazzoli. 2004. Growth of single-specialty medical groups. *Health Affairs* 23 (2): 82–89.

CBO. *See* U.S. Congress, Congressional Budget Office.

Center for Studying Health System Change. 1997. Patients, profits, and health system change: A Wall Street perspective. *Issue Brief,* no. 9 (May).

Center for Studying Health System Change. 1998a. Managed care woes: Industry trends and conflicts. *Issue Brief,* no. 13 (May).

Center for Studying Health System Change. 1998b. Wall Street comes to Washington: Analysts' perspectives on health system change. *Issue Brief,* no. 17 (December).

Center for Studying Health System Change. 1999. Managed care cost pressures threaten access for the uninsured. *Issue Brief,* no. 19.

Center for Studying Health System Change. 2001. Wall Street comes to Washington: Market watchers and policy analysts evaluate the health care system. *Issue Brief,* no. 43 (September).

Center for Studying Health System Change. 2003a. HMOs alive and well in Orange County. *Community Report,* no. 9 (Summer 2003).

Center for Studying Health System Change. 2003b. Wall Street comes to Washington: Where is health care headed? *Issue Brief,* no. 67 (August).

Center for Studying Health System Change. 2004. Wall Street comes to Washington. *Issue Brief,* no. 87 (August).

Christianson, J. B., P. B. Ginsburg and D. Draper. 2008. The transition from managed care to consumerism: A community-level status report. *Health Affairs* 27 (5): 1362–70.

Claxton, G., J. R. Gabel, B. DiJulio, J. Pickreign, H. Whitmore, B. Finder, M. Jarlenski and S. Hawkins. 2008. Health benefits in 2008: Premiums moderately higher, while enrollment in consumer-directed plans rises in small firms. *Health Affairs* 27 web supplement (24 Sept): w492-w502.

Davis, K. 2004. Consumer-directed health care: Will it improve health system performance? *Health Services Research* 39 (4, pt. 2): 1219–33.

Devers, K. J., L. R. Brewster, and P. B. Ginsburg. 2003. Specialty hospitals: Focused factories or cream skimmers? *Center for Studying Health System Change Issue Brief,* no. 62 (April).

Enthoven, A. 1990. What can europeans learn from Americans? In *Organisation for Economic Cooperation and Development, Health Care Systems in Transition.* Paris: OECD: 57–71.

Enthoven, A. 1993. The history and principles of managed competition. *Health Affairs* (Supplement): 24–48.

Felland, L. E., S. Felt-Lisk, and M. McHugh. 2004. Health care access for low-income people: Significant safety-net gaps remain. *Center for Studying Health System Change Issue Brief,* no. 84 (June).

Fronstin, P. 2004. Sources of health insurance and characteristics of the uninsured: Analysis of the March 2004 current population survey. *EBRI Issue Brief*, no. 276 (December).

Gabel, J., J. Pickreign, and H. Whitmore. 2006. Behind the slow enrollment growth of employer-based consumer-directed health plans. *Center for Studying Health System Change Issue Brief*, no. 107 (December).

GAO. *See* U.S. General Accounting Office.

Gauthier, A. K., and C. Clancy. 2004. Consumer-driven health care: Beyond rhetoric with research and experience. *Health Services Research* 39 (4, pt. 2): 1049–54.

Gold, M. 2001. Medicare+choice: An interim report card. *Health Affairs* 20 (4): 120–38.

Grossman, J., B.C. Strunk, and R. E. Hurley. 2002. Reversal of fortune: Medicare+choice collides with market forces. *Center for Studying Health System Change Issue Brief*, no. 52 (May).

Grossman, J. M., and P. B. Ginsburg. 2004. As the health insurance underwriting cycle turns: What next? *Health Affairs* 23 (6): 91–102.

Hackbarth, G. M. 2005. Physician-owned specialty hospitals. Statement before the Subcommittee on Health, House Committee on Ways and Means, 110th Cong., 1st sess., March 8, 2005.

Heffler, S., S. Smith, S. Keehan, C. Borger, M. K. Clemens, and C. Truffer. 2005. US health spending projections for 2004–2014. *Health Affairs*, Web Exclusive (February 23): W5–74–85.

Hoadley, J. F., P. Cunningham, and M. McHugh. 2004. Popular Medicaid programs do battle with state budget pressures: Perspectives from twelve states. *Health Affairs* 23 (2): 143–54.

HSChange. *See* Center for Studying Health System Change.

Hurley, R. E., B. C. Strunk, and J. S. White. 2004. The puzzling popularity of the PPO. *Health Affairs* 23 (2): 56–68.

Iglehart, J. 2004a. Physician practice: Next steps. *Health Affairs* 23 (6): 35–36.

Iglehart, J. 2004b. The challenges facing private health insurance. *Health Affairs* 23 (6): 9–10.

Jost, T. S. 2007. *Health care at risk: A critique of the consumer-driven movement.* Durham, NC: Duke University Press.

Kassirer, J.P. 2004. *On the take: How medicine's complicity with big business can endanger your health.* New York: Oxford University Press.

Kellerman, A. L. 2004. Emergency care in California: No emergency? *Health Affairs*, Web Exclusive (March 24): W4–149–51.

Lesser, C., P. B. Ginsburg, and L. E. Felland. 2005. Initial findings from HSC's 2005 site visits: Stage set for growing health care cost and access problems. *Center for Studying Health System Change Issue Brief*, no. 97 (August).

Lo Sasso, A. T., T. Rice, J. R. Gabel, and H. Whitmore. 2004. Tales from the new frontier: Pioneers' experiences with consumer-driven health care. *Health Services Research* 39 (4, pt. 2): 1071–89.

Medicare Payment Advisory Commission. 2001. *Report to the Congress: Medicare payment policy* (March).

Medicare Payment Advisory Commission. 2003. Agenda item: Hospital margins and their uses. Commission Public Meeting, October 9. http://www.medpac.gov/search/searchframes.cfm.

MedPAC. *See* Medicare Payment Advisory Commission.

Melnick, G. A., A. C. Nawathe, A. Bamezai, and L. Green. 2004. Emergency department capacity and access in California, 1990–2001: An economic analysis. *Health Affairs*, Web Exclusive (March 24): W4–136–42.

Moon, M., B. Gage, and A. Evans. 1997. An examination of key Medicare provisions in the Balanced Budget Act of 1997. *Commonwealth Fund Papers* (September).

Moon, M. and K. Davis. 1995. Preserving and strengthening medicare. *Health Affairs* 14(4): 31–46.

Moon, M. and S. Zuckerman. 1995. *Are private insurers really controlling spending better than medicare?* Kaiser Family Foundation, Menlo Park CA.

Newhouse, J. P. 1993. *Free for all? Lessons from the RAND Health Insurance Experiment.* Cambridge, MA: Harvard University Press.

OECD. *See* Organisation for Economic Co-operation and Development.

Oliver, A. 2007. The Veterans Health Administration: An American success story? *Milbank Quarterly* 85 (1): 5–35.

Organisation for Economic Co-operation and Development. 2004. *OECD health data 2004.* Paris: OECD.

O'Sullivan, J., C. Franco, B. Fuchs, B. Lyke, R. Price, and K. Swendiman. 1997. Medicare provisions in the Balanced Budget Act of 1997. *CRS Report for Congress* 97–802 EPW. U.S. Congress, Congressional Research Service, Washington, DC.

Pham, H. H., K. J. Devers, J. H. May, and R. Berenson. 2004. Financial pressures spur physician entrepreneurialism. *Health Affairs* 23 (2): 70–81.

Remler, D. K., and S. A. Glied. 2005. How much more cost sharing will health savings accounts bring? *Health Affairs* 25 (4): 1070–78.

Review of the assumptions and methods of the Medicare trustees' financial projections. 2004. 2004 Technical Review Panel on the Medicare Trustees Report. Washington, DC: Centers for Medicare and Medicaid Services.

Rice, T., and K. R. Morrison. 1994. Patient cost-sharing for medical services: A review of the literature and implications for health care reform. *Medical Care Review* 51 (3): 235–87.

Robinson, J. C. 1999. The future of managed care organization. *Health Affairs* 18 (2): 7–24.

Robinson, J. C. 2001. Physician organization in California: Crisis and opportunity. *Health Affairs* 20 (4): 81–96.

Robinson, J. C. 2004a. From managed care to consumer health insurance: The fall and rise of Aetna. *Health Affairs* 23 (2): 43–55.

Robinson, J. C. 2004b. Consolidation and the transformation of competition in health insurance. *Health Affairs* 23 (6): 11–24.

Rosenthal, M., C. Hsuan and A. Milstein. 2005. A report card on the freshman class of consumer-directed health plans. *Health Affairs* 24 (6): 1592–1600.

Rosenthal, M., and R. G. Frank. 2006. What is the empirical basis for paying for quality in health care? *Medical Care Research and Review* 63 (2): 135–57.

Schoenbaum, S. C. 2004. Physicians and pre-paid group practices. *Health Affairs*, Web Exclusive (February 4): W4–76–78.

Shea, K.K., A. L. Holmgren, R. Osborn and C. Schoen. 2007. Health system performance in selected nations: A chartpack. *The Commonwealth Fund, New York* (May).

Short, A., G. Mays, and J. Mittler. 2003. Disease management: A leap of faith to lower-cost, higher-quality health care. *Center for Studying Health System Change Issue Brief*, no. 69 (October).

Stone, D. 1999. Managed care and the second great transformation. *Journal of Health Politics, Policy and Law* 24 (5): 1213–18.

Trude, S., and L. Conwell. 2004. Rhetoric vs. reality: Employer views on consumer-driven health care. *Center for Studying Health System Change Issue Brief*, no. 86 (July).

Tuohy, C. H. 2002. The costs of constraint and prospects for health care reform in Canada. *Health Affairs* 21 (3): 32–46.

U.S. Congress, Congressional Budget Office. 1993. *The economic and budget outlook: Fiscal years 1994–1998.* Washington, DC: CBO.

U.S. Congress, Congressional Budget Office. 1995. *CBO Memorandum: The economic and budget outlook: December 1995 update.* Washington, DC: CBO.

U.S. Congress, Congressional Budget Office. 1999. The impact of the Balanced Budget Act on the Medicare fee-for-service program: Testimony of Dan L. Crippen, Director, Congressional Budget Office. September 15. Washington, DC: CBO.

U.S. Congress, Congressional Budget Office. 2001. *The budget and economic outlook: Fiscal years 2002–2011.* Washington, DC: CBO.

U.S. General Accounting Office. 1994. *Bone marrow transplantation: International comparisons of availability and appropriateness of use.* GAO/PEMD-94–10. Washington, DC: GAO.

U.S. Government Accountability Office. 2006a. *Federal employees health benefits program: First-year experience with high-deductible health plans and health savings accounts.* GAO-06–271 (January). Washington, DC: Government Accountability Office.

U.S. Government Accountability Office. 2006b. Consumer directed health plans: Early enrollee experiences with health savings accounts and eligible health plans. GAO-06–798 (August). Washington, DC: Government Accountability Office.

White, J. 1995. *Competing solutions: American health care proposals and international experience.* Washington, DC: Brookings Institution.

White, J. 1999. Targets and systems of health care cost control. *Journal of Health Politics, Policy and Law* 24 (4): 653–96.

White, J. 2003. *False alarm: Why the greatest threat to Social Security and Medicare is the campaign to "save" them.* Rev. ed. Baltimore: Johns Hopkins University Press.

White, Justin, R. E. Hurley, and B.C. Strunk. 2004. Getting along or going along? Health plan-provider contract showdowns subside. *Center for Studying Health System Change Issue Brief* no. 9 (January).

Wildavsky, A. 1979. *Speaking truth to power: The art and craft of policy analysis.* Boston: Little, Brown and Company.

Wong, J. 2005. Re-casting Canadian federalism: Health care financing in the new century. In *Reforming Health Social Security: Proceedings of an International Seminar.* Human Development Sector Unit, East Asia and the Pacific Region, The World Bank, Working Paper Series No. 2005-4 (June 2005), pp. 112–34.

Zuckerman, S., G. Bazzoli, A. Davidoff, and A. LoSasso. 2001. How did safety-net hospitals cope in the 1990s? *Health Affairs* 20 (4): 159–68.

Canada
Health Care Reform in Comparative Perspective

CAROLYN HUGHES TUOHY

It is a sobering task to revise this chapter on the Canadian health system written in 1996, especially given the history of the period from 1996 to 2008. This chapter was originally presented as a paper at a time that, history now shows to have marked the depths of an unprecedented trough in public spending on health care in Canada—the effects of which were then only beginning to be felt. Between 1992 and 1996, real per-capita public health care spending declined by about 8 percent. These fiscal changes were part of broad governmental agendas, at both federal and provincial levels, of deficit cutting and subsequent reinvestment. In 1993, combined federal and provincial deficits in Canada peaked at over $65 billion. Throughout this period, program spending had to compete not only with deficit reduction but also with tax cuts at both levels of government.

In the late 1990s, as deficits began to be brought under control, the first priority for program spending in all provinces was health care, and in 1998 per-capita health spending began a rapid climb that extended to 2006 and promises to continue (Figure 3.1).[1] These dramatic fiscal swings had two major effects—one fiscal, the other political. First, the trough in public spending on health care yielded a fiscal savings of about $30 billion collectively for Canadian governments from 1992 to 2000, as compared to what would have been spent if expenditures had steadily increased to 2000. Second, the

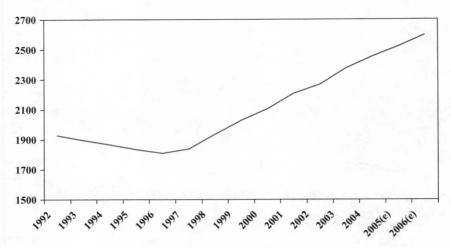

Figure 3.1 Per-capita public health care spending, Canada, 1992–2006 (constant 1997$)
Source: Conference Board of Canada (Ottawa: Conference Board of Canada)

political impact on the health system was to shake public confidence and destabilize the various accommodations upon which the system rested. Notably, in the early years of the twenty-first century, the issue of waiting times for health services rocketed to prominence on the political agenda.[2] The very fundamentals of the system were called into question (although they did not change) in a way that would have surprised the observer of the system in the mid-1990s.

This chapter is in three sections. The first briefly sets out the theoretical framework for thinking about the dynamics of change in the health care arena. The second reviews the organizational and financial structures of Canadian health care in the 1970–1995 period and addresses in particular the themes of the 1996 Four Country Conference: managing change, consumer choice, and resource allocation. The third section assesses the system in the mid-2000s and notes what remains constant and what has changed between 1996 and 2008.

A Framework for Thinking about the Dynamics of Change in the Health Policy Arena

The frameworks for governing the production and consumption of health care services vary across nations (and over time) along two key dimensions, which I term "institutional mix" and "structural balance."[3] By "institutional mix," I mean the mix of *hierarchy, market,* and *collegiality* (peer control) in the design of decision-making structures. By "structural balance," I refer to the balance of influence across three categories of actors: *state actors, health care providers,* and *private financial interests.*

These two dimensions of decision-making systems are related but not identical. A heavy weight for hierarchical, market, and collegial instruments may enhance the influence of state actors, private financial interests, and professionals, respectively. But this influence is not a one-to-one correspondence. The state may avail itself of both exchange-oriented and collegially oriented instruments to realize its policy goals; private financial interests may take the form of vertically and horizontally integrated firms and may invest in professional practices; and health care professionals may compete in markets or assume positions of authority within hierarchies. It is the intersection of these two dimensions that defines the essential character of decision-making systems.

The institutional mix establishes a logic of decision making that shapes the expectations of participants and the ways in which they will respond, rationally, to challenge. (In particular, it determines the types and flows of information upon which decisions are made.) Different institutional mixes also have different implications for the creation or erosion of trust and "social capital," and different symbolic connotations. The structural balance determines the nature of the *interests* that will be brought to bear in decision making, and in particular the way in which the interests of recipients and potential recipients of health care services are mediated. (Who, in other words, has the "consumer's proxy?")

Changes may occur within institutional or structural categories. Hierarchies may become more or less decentralized, for example, or markets more or less concentrated. Certain types of state actors, health care providers, or private financial interests may gain or lose influence. But such shifts are less radical and less definitive of the character of the system than are changes in the mix of hierarchy, collegiality, and market instruments and in the balance across state, provider, and private financial actors.

The institutional mix and structural balance of health care systems is a product of two factors: (1) public policies that establish the institutional and structural parameters of the system, and (2) the behavior of actors that can cause shift in the parameters over time. Major policy initiatives altering the fundamental institutional mix and structural balance in health care decision-making systems are episodic and rare. Such initiatives have required an extraordinary mobilization of political authority and will, on the scale of the Labour majority government at the end of the Second World War in Britain, the Democratic landslide in the 1964 presidential and congressional elections in the United States, or the era of "cooperative federalism" in the 1960s in Canada. Accordingly, in the terms of Kingdon (1995) such "windows of opportunity" have depended upon factors largely external to the health care arena.

These episodes of policy change establish the framework that shapes the behavior of the actors within the decision-making system. But that behavior in turn feeds back upon the framework itself. In some cases, such as the "corporatist" British National Health Service (NHS), the effect of this feedback has been to reinforce the status quo. In other cases, such as the more market-oriented and employer-based American system, it has created a dynamic of volatile change. These feedback effects are channeled by the logic of the system.

Within this framework, the next section sets out the argument, originally presented in 1996, that the institutional mix and structural balances of the Canadian system, seen in comparative perspective, had been remarkably stable since the full establishment of Canadian Medicare in the early 1970s. The final section will consider whether this argument still holds.

An Overview of the Canadian Health Care System,
1970–1995
PROVIDER-STATE ACCOMMODATIONS IN A SINGLE-PAYER SYSTEM

In the 1970–1995 period, Canada's institutional mix of hierarchical, market-oriented, and collegial instruments and the structural balance of influence across state actors, health care providers, and private financial interests appeared remarkably stable. Other nations, such as the United States and Britain, underwent more significant shifts on at least one of these dimensions. In the former, market forces generated not only an explosive growth of complex contracting arrangements but also the rise of very large private vertically or horizontally integrated hierarchies. In the process, the influence of the medical profession within the delivery system eroded while that of private financial interests increased (Starr 1982; White, Salmon, and Feinglass 1994). (There was, nonetheless, great variation in the role of physicians within the wide variety of organizational forms that came to characterize the American system.) In Britain, major policy changes tempered the hierarchical nature of the NHS through the introduction of market-type mechanisms within the publicly funded system. The various actors appeared, however, to adjust to these changes in ways that mitigated their effect on the overall institutional and structural characteristics of the system.

In Canada, however, the balance of hierarchy, collegiality, and market in the decision-making system in the mid-1990s remained much as it was in the 1970s and 1980s when the federal hospital and medical insurance plans were introduced, although provincial governments were experimenting with various forms of decentralization within the state hierarchy. Similarly, despite a marginal shift in the public and private shares of total health expenditure in favor of the latter (from 73.2 percent public in 1971 to 71.8 percent in 1994), the balance of influence between state actors and private financial interests also changed little.[4] And while state actors asserted their roles more strongly than in the past, the basic terms of the accommodations between the medical profession and the state that shaped Canadian Medicare remained, with one notable exception to be discussed shortly, essentially the same.

Canadian Medicare bears the marks of its birth in the 1960s. In an era in which the indemnity model of financing medical care had become well established, and in which buoyant economic growth was encouraging an expansion of governmental social spending, the plan adopted essentially involved the government underwriting of the existing delivery system.[5] Federal legislation (the Canada Health Act [CHA] of 1984) requires that in order to qualify for federal financial contributions, provincial programs must conform to the five principles of universality, comprehensiveness, accessibility, portability, and public administration. The resulting provincial programs centralized the financing of medical and hospital services in the provincial governments (with federal contributions), while leaving the decentralized delivery system in place.

Hence, from its inception, Canadian Medicare had a type of "internal market" in the limited form of a "purchaser/provider split." Hospital and medical providers are organized independently from the provincial government "purchaser," and consumers have free choice of provider, at least at the level of primary care. This "internal market" is however, far from the competitive ideal type: It is essentially made up of monopsonist-monopoly relationships with provincial governments in the role of monopsonist. Money "followed the patient" in the largely fee-for-service physician services sector but not in the hospital sector, where both capital and operating expenditures in the hospital sector are centrally controlled by provincial governments. The provinces generally did not develop a sophisticated purchasing function: they funded hospitals on a historical global-budget basis; and central control in the physician services sector related almost entirely to medical remuneration, beginning with centrally negotiated prices. Almost the last vestige of the individual physician's discretion over the price of service disappeared in 1984, with the passage of federal legislation providing for fiscal penalties to any province allowing "extra billing" (billing beyond the amount covered by the government plan) for medical and hospital services. But physicians continued to have broad discretion over the location of their practices, the inputs to their practices, and the volume and mix of services they delivered.

In essence, the structural balance of the Canadian system, in the medical and hospital service sectors, revolved around a central accommodation between the medical profession and the state. The nature of this accommodation varied province by province, but these provincial accommodations shared in common a version of the "implicit concordat" that Rudolf Klein has observed between the profession and the state in Britain (Klein 1995). Canadian physicians traded off their individual entrepreneurial discretion over the price of their services and accepted the role of the state in establishing overall budgetary parameters, in return for the preservation of a broad scope for clinical judgment in the allocation of resources within those parameters.

Private financial interests were essentially confined to health care sectors other than medical and hospital services: dental care, pharmaceuticals, prostheses, and nursing homes. Canada's "implicit concordat" differed from Britain's in one key respect: Whereas the British bargain was conceived in the context of a society whose expectations were still shaped by wartime austerity, Canada's was conceived in an era of plenty and high public expectations. An assumption of generous public funding underlay the provincial-level accommodations between the state and the medical profession. Governmental health expenditures stood at 5.4 percent of GDP in 1971, the first year in which Medicare was implemented in all provinces, and by 1990 this proportion stood at 6.8 percent.[6] But as in the British case, these accommodations gave governments the instruments of macro-level allocation to the health care system, while keeping microeconomic instruments largely out of the hands of state actors. Indeed, given the autonomous organization of providers, budgetary parameters were even more gross than was the case in the hierarchical pre-1990 NHS.

Provincial governments did not develop the capacity for nor incur the transaction costs of closely monitoring or managing the delivery system. Cost constraints, when they did come, were accordingly blunt and across the board. Governments did not, by and large, exercise their role as "purchasers" to specify contracts with providers.[7] Several provinces decentralized governmental authority in order to bring about horizontal integration in the hospital sector. These initiatives maintained the existing balance in the hierarchical, collegial, and market-oriented elements of the system, although they did represent a reorganization of the state hierarchy and a stronger assertion of the role of state actors in the structural balance in health care decision-making systems.

Providers, for their part, were concerned with maintaining their own discretion within budget limits. They did not enter into elaborate contracting arrangements with each other, nor did they develop horizontally or vertically integrated systems. The accommodations between the state and health care providers resulted in a system that was extraordinarily popular with Canadians, whether that popularity was viewed in comparison to Canadians' attitudes toward other public programs or in comparison to the attitudes of citizens of other nations toward their own health systems. Medicare became a defining feature of Canadian public mythology, and even more than was the case in other nations, tampering with the accommodations that underlay it carried great political risk.

There were thus a number of constraints on change in the institutional mix and the structural balance of the Canadian system: the provisions of the Canada Health Act (CHA), which limited the use of the price mechanism and the role of private finance; the accommodations between provincial governments and health care providers that created well-defined sets of roles based on interrelated tradeoffs; and public attitudes and expectations about the system that made tampering highly politically risky.[8]

In the mid-1990s, there was some reason to believe that one or more of these factors were changing in such a way that might lead to more fundamental change in the decision-making system in Canadian health care. One area in which some omens of change were developing was the framework of federal-provincial finance. The progressive withdrawal of the federal government from the financing of the system reduced its fiscal leverage to enforce the provisions of the CHA. The federal Liberal government's reiteration of its commitment to the principles of the act and its pledge to maintain federal financial participation at a minimum of $11 billion allowed it to maintain some enforcement leverage.[9]

However, the types of broad political change that would have been necessary to produce the major policy shift involved in changing the fundamental principles of the CHA—a shift in the partisan center of political gravity or a warming of the climate of federal-provincial relations—did not appear on the horizon in the mid-1990s. The hegemony of the federal Liberal Party, with its tight identification with the CHA, appeared secure in the face of a weak and divided political right. Federal-provincial relations, moreover, remained mired in acrimony in the wake of failed constitutional negotiations and provincial outrage over the unilateral actions of the federal government in dramatically reducing its transfers to the provinces for health, social assistance, and post-secondary education.[10] But even if such shifts in federal or federal-provincial politics were to occur, the degrees of freedom for policy change at the provincial level still appeared limited. Such change would have required the mustering of the political authority and will to make major policy changes in health care policy. And no province, not even Alberta, whose premier loudly chafed against the constraints that the CHA placed upon extra billing by private clinics, actually destabilized the status quo.

The existing accommodations and public attitudes that constrained change in the health care arena were nonetheless coming under stress, particularly as a result of the dramatic decline in public funding noted at the beginning of this chapter. Although health care spending was protected in most provinces relative to other areas of public spending, the health care arena nonetheless experienced what Klein described in the British case as "relative deprivation over time" (Klein 1995).[11] In Britain, this relative deprivation precipitated a breakdown of the "implicit concordat" between the medical profession and the state, which in turn triggered Prime Minister Thatcher's personal intervention and set in motion the process that led to the "internal market" reforms of the early 1990s. Such a breakdown is neither a necessary nor a sufficient condition for major policy changes directed at the institutional mix or structural balance of the system. Such changes, as noted, depend on the mobilization of political authority and will on the scale that Thatcher could accomplish in her third successive majority government.

In the mid-to-late 1990s, the strains in the profession-state accommodation in Canada were increasingly apparent. These developments varied across provinces, depending on the level of authority and will that provincial governments could muster. The Ontario government was at that time the most "Thatcherite" of Canadian provincial governments in severing its bargaining relationship with the Ontario Medical Association (OMA) and abolishing the government-OMA Joint Management Committee, in frustration with its stalemated processes. The British Columbia government, on the other hand, elaborated its accommodation with the British Columbia Medical Association (BCMA) to produce a fairly comprehensive joint-management process.

Meanwhile, the process of "relative deprivation over time" and the strains in the central accommodations within the health care system were having their effects upon the third factor constraining fundamental change, that is, public attitudes and expectations. The proportion of Canadian respondents to a cross-national poll who believed that "on the whole, the system works well and only minor changes are necessary to make it work better" fell from 56 percent to 29 percent between 1988 and 1994 (Blendon et al. 1995).

According to the same poll, Canadian levels of satisfaction converged with those of Germans. They remained higher than the satisfaction levels of Americans, but it is interesting to note that the proportion of Americans believing that only minor changes were necessary to their health care system actually increased from 1988 to 1994, after the failure of attempts to achieve comprehensive reform. The causal relationships between public opinion and public policy flow in both directions: The constraints of public opinion on public policy appear to be somewhat elastic in response to policy initiatives. To the extent that accommodations were unraveling and public satisfaction with the system declining, it appeared that Canada, after enduring the rhetoric of crisis in health care for years, might really be entering a critical phase.

IMPLICATIONS FOR MANAGING CHANGE, CONSUMER CHOICE,
AND RESOURCE ALLOCATION

The preceding sketch of the main features of Canada's health care system has consequences for the management of change, consumer choice, and the allocation of resources.

Managing Change

In the 1990s, change in the health care arena in Canada focused largely on restructuring the hospital sector, primarily through increasing horizontal integration, reducing the number of acute care beds, and to some extent building up capacity for community-based care. These policies had the effect of decreasing expenditures on hospitals from 40 percent of total health expenditures in 1990 to 37.3 percent in 1994 (OECD 1995). To put this 2.7 percentage point decline over four years in perspective, hospital expenditures as a proportion of total health expenditures had declined only 5 percentage points, from 45 to 40 percent, in the 20-year period from 1970 to 1990.

The mechanisms through which these changes were accomplished varied across provinces. In all provinces except Ontario, regional structures for the management of the hospital sector were established, although the organization and the mandate of regional boards varied widely. In Saskatchewan, a substantial amount of "downsizing"—the closing of fifty-two small hospitals—was accomplished by the provincial government before regional boards were established, so as to avoid encumbering the boards with such politically difficult tasks at their inception (Lewis 1996). Newfoundland and Manitoba followed similar strategies. In Alberta and New Brunswick, in contrast, an important part of the mandate of the newly created regional boards was to accomplish a significant reduction of the system. And in Quebec, the task of allocating budget cuts to institutions was implemented through a regional board structure that was established in the 1970s and revised and revitalized in the 1990s. In Ontario, regional bodies, the district health councils, remained purely advisory with no budgetary authority. But in 1996 the Ontario government established an arm's-length Health Services Restructuring Commission with executive authority to make decisions about hospital restructuring plans.

These restructuring processes have varied widely, according to the political cultures of various provinces and the partisan complexions of provincial governments. Saskatchewan's "populist" approach, including the direct election of regional boards and broadly consultative processes, contrasts with the "corporatist" approach characteristic of Quebec, where regional boards were elected by regional assemblies whose members are drawn from four "electoral colleges": (1) municipalities, (2) community health and social service organizations, (3) socioeconomic groups including business and labor organizations, and (4) health care institutions. Ontario's traditional managerialist approach to government appears to be taken to an extreme by the Conservative government elected in 1995, which seemed to view intermediate organizations as barriers to, rather than vehicles of, change.

All these processes had in common an increasing concern with the development of information on which to base policy decisions, although the capacity to do so was still in a nascent stage. The province furthest advanced in this respect was Saskatchewan, where the Health Services Utilization and Research Commission (HSURC) conducted studies of hospital utilization that informed restructuring decisions, and continues, among other things, to develop practice guidelines for various medical procedures based on health services research. In Ontario, the Institute for Clinical Evaluative Sciences (ICES) established in 1992 under the later-aborted "framework agreement" between the provincial government and the OMA, conducted health services and utilization research and, among other things, provided services to the provincial Health Services Restructuring Commission noted previously. Several provinces announced their intentions to allocate budgets to regional boards on a population needs-based formula. Again Saskatchewan moved furthest in this direction, with a per-capita formula adjusted for standardized mortality rates. The equity and incentive effects of such formulae, as well as their technical complexities, posed significant challenges that in turn paled in comparison to the political difficulties of reconciling "technocratically" generated evidence with democratically expressed preferences (Lewis 1996).

None of these restructuring efforts significantly touched physicians. In no case did the mandate of regional boards extend to physicians' services, although some maintained various types of medical liaison committees. Governmental control of medical services related almost entirely to issues of remuneration, although issues of supply began to rise on the agenda. The physician-to-population ratio rose 40 percent from 1972 to 1989, when it began to level off. Beginning in the early 1990s, medical school enrollments were deliberately reduced in the wake of an interprovincial agreement reached following a comprehensive and influential study of the medical workforce in 1991 (Barer and Stoddart 1991). The New Brunswick government negotiated an agreement with the NBMA on regional physician supply. The Ontario government passed legislation giving the Minister of Health extraordinary unilateral powers over physician supply by region, but these powers remained unexercised.

The organization of medical services remained much as it had been in the 1970s. Community clinics with salaried physicians were established in Saskatchewan and Quebec, and to a much lesser extent in other provinces in the 1960s and 1970s, but even in the two "lead" provinces these accounted for only a small proportion of practicing physicians and had not grown appreciably over time. Similarly, prepaid group practices serving defined rosters of patients existed only as perpetual pilot projects in Ontario. The Ontario government, taking up an initiative advanced by the OMA, began to consider a rostering model for primary care, ushering in an era of negotiation and experimentation within this sector that continued to the time of writing, as further discussed later in this chapter.[12]

Consumer Choice

As previously noted, Canadian consumers of medical and hospital services have free choice, not of plan, but of primary care provider at the point of service. In contrast to the British and American systems, which had already begun to generate a limited range of "performance indicators" to guide the choice of provider, no such information was systematically made available in Canada. Nonetheless, consumer satisfaction with health care services was relatively high—comparable to or higher than that of Americans or Germans. In a 1994 cross-national poll, 73 percent of Canadian respondents rated the quality of health care services available in their community as "excellent" or "good," compared with 72 percent in Germany and 65 percent in the United States. Waiting times had yet to emerge as an issue: Only 8 percent of Canadian respondents reported being unable to get needed medical care in the past year, and 16 percent reported having to wait more than one week to see a doctor.[13] Furthermore, Canadians' levels of expectation about what constitutes appropriate medical care appeared roughly similar to those of Americans and Germans (Blendon et al. 1995).

As individual consumers, then, Canadians in the mid-1990s were probably at least as satisfied with the hospital and medical services available to them as were consumers in other advanced industrial nations. This degree of satisfaction contrasts with attitudes toward the system as a whole, which declined precipitously between 1988 and 1994. Nonetheless, Canadians were still as content with their health care system as were Germans, and were considerably more so than Americans (Blendon et al. 1995).

One way of thinking about cross-national differences in this representation is to ask who exercises the consumer "proxy" in selecting the array of services available to individual consumers. In the United States this role is played largely by employers, in Germany by the sickness funds; in the Netherlands by a mix of sickness funds, employers, and individual consumers themselves; and in Britain by district purchasing authorities and General Practitioner (GP) fundholders.

Indeed, the increasing importance of relatively large, sophisticated, and aggressive "purchasers," exercising the consumer proxy in bargaining with providers, was a feature of most health care systems in advanced industrial nations in the 1980s and 1990s. In Canada, this process was very limited. Provincial governments held the consumer proxy, although this role began to be devolved to various degrees to regional boards. Under the terms of the profession-state accommodation previously outlined, provincial governments were fairly hard bargainers over the price of medical services, but bargaining over, for example, the volume and mix of services to be provided was restricted to a few hospital-based procedures.

For services other than medical and hospital care, such as dental care, out-of-hospital drugs and prostheses, most Canadian consumers participated in a private and largely employer-based system much like that in the United States. Managed-care firms intensified their marketing to employers with benefit plans covering these sectors, but their penetration remained limited.

Resource Allocation

Even before the fiscal constraint and regionalization measures of the 1990s, provincial governments had squeezed some capacity out of the hospital sector, largely through the blunt instrument of global budgeting. The number of inpatient beds per thousand population declined from 6.9 in 1979 to 6.6 in 1989, and the number of acute care beds per thousand population declined from 5.5 to 5.0 (OECD 1995). In the 1990s several provinces began to experiment with modification of global budgeting through funding formulae that reward efficiency, at least for some portion of the funding. But there was little explicit contracting for specific inpatient services.

In the medical services sector, negotiations between provincial governments and the medical profession continued to revolve largely around issues of remuneration. Over time, provincial governments came to negotiate not only across-the-board increases to medical fee schedules, but also global (and in some cases individual) caps on total physician remuneration (Lomas, Charles, and Greb 1992). The advent of this form of global budgeting for physicians had the effect of moderating increases in utilization (Tholl 1994). But despite the development of government-funded research bodies such as HSURC and ICES, provincial governments did not tie medical remuneration to the adoption of particular patterns of care or the following of clinical guidelines.

As previously noted, generous levels of public funding were a fundamental part of the accommodations at the center of Canadian Medicare. Even so, growth in private sector health care expenditures outstripped that in the public sector from the late 1970s onward. This growth is in part because of higher levels of price inflation for goods and services offered on private markets. In particular, pharmaceutical price inflation increased at a faster rate during the 1980s than did price inflation for medical and hospital services. Similarly, dental price inflation outpaced medical price inflation.[14] The relative growth of the private sector, however, also reflected a "passive privatization" of services—the effect of decreasing hospital capacity and utilization in a system in which some goods and services (notably pharmaceuticals and some forms of personal care) were covered by governmental health insurance on an inpatient basis but not on an outpatient basis.

The private sector share grew only a little over 5 percentage points as a proportion of total health expenditure from the mid-1970s to the mid-1990s. But this represented a 23 percent increase in the share of the private sector itself, and this expansion had its most concentrated effects on employment-based benefit plans. Accordingly, employers saw their benefit costs rise, and employer organizations increasingly expressed the fear that the competitive advantage they enjoyed by having the costs of health care spread across the tax base would be eroded (Alvi 1995; MacBride-King 1995).[15]

Business coalitions formed in response to these fears, generally expressing support for the maintenance of the five fundamental principles of Canadian Medicare while urging increased use of clinical guidelines, vertical and horizontally integrated delivery systems, and especially information systems to support such mechanisms (Employee Committee on Health Care [ECHC] 1995). These approaches were seen as efficiency enhancing, although the administrative costs of implementation received little or no attention. Clearly, however, one reason that the administrative costs of Canada's public system were as low as they were in international perspective lies in the limited roles that the monitoring of medical practice and the management of vertical and horizontal organizations played in the system.[16]

The design of decision-making systems in Canadian health care, in which provincial governments functioned as monopsonists for medical and hospital services while a range of other health care services were provided largely on private markets, proved remarkably stable over the 1970–1995 period. After the major episode of policy change in the 1960s that established the parameters of the existing system, the system was reinforced by provincial-level accommodations between health care providers, notably the medical profession, and the state. Under those accommodations, public funding was generous in international perspective, the state generally did not develop specific contracting and monitoring mechanisms for medical and hospital services, and providers continued to operate through collegial networks similar to those that predated Canadian Medicare.

In 1996, a major question was whether this stability would prove resilient and not brittle in the face of growing pressures. The accommodations that had grown up in the Medicare context resulted in a system with significant advantages, including broad clinical autonomy for providers, free choice of primary care provider for consumers, low administrative costs, and high levels of public satisfaction. But these accommodations rested on expectations of a continuing rate of increase in public funding—expectations that were deeply shaken in the 1990s. All participants in the system were adjusting to changing expectations in regard to funding.

The possibility of change in the basic parameters of the system appeared to be open to a greater degree than had been the case since the inception of Canadian Medicare. It was possible that different provincial systems could tip in the direction of a heavier weight for the state hierarchy (through state-enforced vertical or horizontal integration) or for market mechanisms (through contracting between the state and private providers or through the expansion of private markets for the purchase of services as a result of "passive privatization").

But British experience in the same period suggested that the health care decision-making system would show a considerable degree of resiliency. In Britain, a major and unilateral policy initiative in the form of the "internal market" reforms of 1990 significantly disrupted the established networks of health care decision making. In the face of the uncertainty and the high transaction costs generated by these changes, however, those networks began to reassert themselves (Le Grand 1994). Over time the reforms, largely through their effects on information flows, appeared likely to bring about changes in established relationships—as "new forms of mutual accommodation rather than a new balance of power" (Klein 1995). My prediction for Canada was similar: The logic of Canadian accommodation, like that of the UK, suggested a similar degree of resiliency in the face of the fiscal, technological, and social challenges. The remainder of this chapter will assess the degree to which that prediction was borne out.

The Experience Post-1996

The dramatic fiscal swing of the 1990s severely tested the stability of the system and the "resiliency" of the accommodations within it. It further exacerbated the growing acrimony between federal and provincial governments and reduced the possibility of achieving intergovernmental agreement on either the reinforcement or the modification of the system. It fueled conflict between provincial governments and health care providers over resources; placed provider organizations, especially medical and hospital associations, under extreme pressure to manage internal conflicts; and laid the ground for demands for "catch-up" increases as the first call on any new investment.[17] It reduced redundancy in the system, an essential condition for phasing in reforms in health care delivery. And although the limited evidence available suggests that restraint measures such as the restructuring of hospitals did not have a negative impact on health outcomes, they created an atmosphere of crisis that shook public confidence in the system and in the ability of governments to manage it.[18] Polls in the late 1990s and early 2000s consistently and dramatically demonstrated this erosion. The periodic cross-national survey previously cited showed that the proportion of Canadians reporting the health care system needed "only minor change," having plunged from 56 percent to 29 percent between 1988 and 1994, declined further to 20 percent between by 1998. Perhaps even more significant, public confidence did not rebound with increased public investment after 1997. By 2001, the proportion viewing "only minor change" as necessary still stood at 21 percent. By 2007, it had recovered only to 26 percent, despite the continuing upward trajectory of public funding (Blendon et al. 2002; Schoen et al. 2004, 2007). The proportion believing that the system needed to be "rebuilt completely," however, subsided somewhat from 23 percent in 1998 to 12 percent in 2007, but still remained well above the negligible level of 5 percent in the late 1980s (Figure 3.2).

Regarding their own interactions with the health care system, Canadians continued to present a somewhat more positive picture. They were more likely than respondents in Australia, New Zealand, the United Kingdom, or the United States to be somewhat or very confident that they could get quality and safe care when they needed it, and less likely than those in any of these nations except the United Kingdom to report problems in accessing health

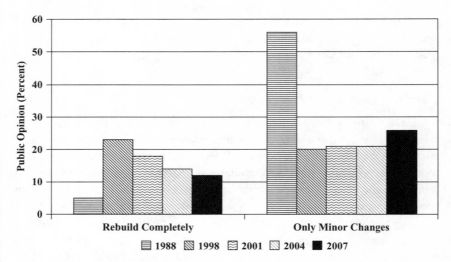

Figure 3.2 Public confidence: Canadian attitudes toward needed changes in the health care system, 1988–2007
Sources: Blendon et al. 2002; Schoen et al. 2004, 2007.

care for reasons of cost. The pressures on the system were apparent, however, in reports about the "safety valve" of emergency room (ER) care. Canadians had higher rates of ER utilization than respondents in any of the other four nations in the 2004 survey cited above, and they were most likely to have waited for two hours or more in an ER visit (Blendon et al. 2002; Schoen et al. (2004).

At the same time, however, changes in the broad political system, and at the intersection of the broader system with the health care sector, were coalescing to create the conditions for significant policy change. In the early 2000s, the apparent waning of the separatist threat in Quebec and associated constitutional wrangling, and the success of tax- and deficit-reduction strategies, diminished the salience of items that had dominated the policy agenda of the 1980s and 1990s. With the rise in public concern about health care in the wake of fiscal constraint and the growing alarm of provincial governments at the escalating share of their budgets consumed by health spending, health policy now came to define the climate of federal-provincial relations rather than being constrained by that climate as in the past. Meetings of "First Ministers" (the thirteen provincial and territorial premiers and the federal prime minister) were dominated by health care negotiations. For politicians at both levels of government, moreover, the changing public mood meant that the risks of inaction were seen as higher than the risks of action. As for relations between provincial governments and medical and hospital providers, fissures that deepened within both medical and hospital communities under the pressure of constraint created some footholds for support of reform, especially in primary care. And an era of reinvestment allowed at least in theory for flowing funding in such a way as to provide for some redundancy in transitional periods.

Accordingly, the first few years of the twenty-first century were a time of policy ferment in Canadian health policy. Governmental commissions in Alberta, Quebec, and Saskatchewan and two major inquiries at the federal level (one by a senate committee, the other by a federally appointed commissioner) explored a greater range of options than had been in play since the inception of Medicare in the 1960s. The system seemed poised for significant change. The key question was whether this change would occur within the parameters of the Canadian universal single-payer model or would entail remaking the model itself. In other words, was the "institutional mix" (of hierarchically structured, market-based, or collegially oriented instruments) or the "structural balance" (across state actors, private finance, and health care providers) to be changed, or could the necessary improvements occur without changing these fundamental parameters of the system? More specifically, increased roles for market instruments (by opening up the possibility of competition between private clinics and public hospitals for the provision of publicly funded services) and for private finance (by allowing for privately purchased alternatives to publicly funded services) were actively debated.

Nonetheless, although the rhetoric varied considerably, all of these reports made substantive recommendations that would maintain and enhance the essential mix and balance of the Canadian system. In Alberta, an option that would open the door to a greater degree of private finance as a matter of policy design—namely, the possibility of establishing medical savings accounts (MSAs)—was seriously considered. But even there MSAs were presented as an option that "warrant[s] further study" (Premier's Advisory Council 2002). Other reports, after canvassing a range of possibilities, rejected those that would enhance the role of private finance. The senate committee report (colloquially known by the name of the committee chair and driving force as the "Kirby report") saw the current model as sustainable only if key changes to improve performance (and in particular to shorten waiting times) were made. The senate committee and the Alberta report advocated greater competition within Canada's publicly financed "internal market" through more explicit contracting between public authorities and a range of not-for-profit and for-profit providers. Other reports, notably that of the federal commission (colloquially bearing the name of the commissioner, former Saskatchewan premier

Roy Romanow), argued against for-profit delivery. Both Kirby and Romanow advocated increased federal funding, primary care reform (bringing primary care providers together in groups to provide 24/7 care to defined populations, with population-based budgets) and building upon provincial drug plans and home care programs to provide more comprehensive and uniform coverage. Both also recommended the establishment of a national health council to monitor and report on the performance of the health care sector as a mechanism of accountability (Canadian Institute for Health Information [CIHI] 2003).[19]

In February 2003 and September 2004, the First Ministers reached agreements that committed the federal government to substantially increased cash transfers to the provinces for health care over a five-year period, beyond what had already been committed in 2000. Much of the increase was targeted at primary care reform, reducing waiting times for designated services, increased coverage for catastrophic drug costs and home care, and diagnostic equipment and information technology, although the expectation was that much of this funding would be rolled into the calculation of the base on which future federal transfers would be premised. A national health council, envisaged in the Kirby and Romanow reports as a body at arm's length from federal and provincial governments, emerged instead from the machinery of intergovernmental relations with its membership (half "government," half "nongovernment") determined by federal, provincial, and territorial ministers of health. It promises, nonetheless, to provide a vehicle for bringing a variety of perspectives within the health system to bear on the development and reporting of measures of performance.

In short, the Canadian model of health care finance passed a crucial test in the early 2000s. Some key conditions for major change had coalesced, yet decisions were made to reaffirm the essential institutional mix and structural balance of the system.

Then, in June 2005, the system was shaken by a major exogenous shock—a shock, that is, that had its source outside the federal-provincial and provider-state accommodations of the health policy arena. The Supreme Court of Canada, having unexpectedly agreed more than a year earlier to hear an appeal of a case challenging the Quebec legislation banning private insurance for publicly covered services, issued an even more unexpected ruling. In a four-to-three decision (there were at the time two vacancies on the nine-member court), the Supreme Court reversed the decisions of the lower courts in Quebec and struck down the legislation. Three of the four judges in the majority found that the provisions violated Section 7 of the Canadian Charter of Rights and Freedoms (guaranteeing a right to "security of the person"). The fourth ruled that it violated the Quebec Charter of Rights and Freedoms and did not rule with respect to the Canadian Charter. The question of whether similar cases in other provinces would succeed with a full nine-member Court and under the Canadian Charter alone remains open, but such challenges are almost inevitable (Flood 2006).

The *Chaoulli* decision did not prescribe a particular policy outcome—it allowed the Quebec government to come into compliance either by ensuring that patients did not experience undue waits in the public sector or by removing the ban on private insurance for publicly covered services. In other provinces, the policy implications are even more unclear, until the Supreme Court has decided a case under the Canadian Charter alone. By introducing a judicial imperative, the *Chaoulli* case and its successors may, however, reduce the political risk of making major changes in the institutional mix and structural balance of the Canadian health care system, and increase the likelihood that one or more provincial governments will form the will to do so.

Furthermore, provincial governments find themselves under increasing pressure to grapple with health costs. Various attempts to project the rates of increase in public health care spending shown in Figure 3.1 can engender reactions ranging from serious concern to panic on the part of those who keep the public finances. These projections, of course, depend upon the time frame chosen as the base for projection and various assumptions about other variables, notably the impact of an aging population.

One excellent attempt is by Jackson and McDermott (2004), who projected public health care spending as a share of GDP to 2040, taking into account the effects of an aging population on both health care expenditures and GDP. They found the following:

- Aging alone will raise public spending from 6.3 percent to 9.8 percent of GDP by 2040.
- Additional growth will depend on the "enrichment-to-productivity" ratio of health care spending (that is, the rate of growth in per-capita age-adjusted health care spending to the rate of growth in per-capita GDP).
- Projections based on the experience of the 1980s (a period of rapid increase in the enrichment-to-productivity ratio) would see public health spending rise to over 30 percent of GDP by 2040.
- Projections based on the 1975–2001 period (which includes periods of both expansion and constraint) take public health spending to about 16 percent of GDP.
- Keeping public spending to 10 percent GDP by 2040 would require replicating the enrichment-to-productivity ratios of the 1990s.

A 2005 forecast to 2025 by the Ontario Ministry of Finance (2005) makes the following assumptions:

- Public health spending in Ontario will grow at 6 percent per year—faster than GDP.
- Aging will account for just over 1 percent of this growth; most growth above GDP is the result of utilization (a highly uncertain variable).[20]

On these assumptions, public spending on health would rise from about 6 percent of GDP in 2009–10 to about seven percent in 2024–25. Accordingly, the health share of provincial program spending will grow from 45 percent to 55 percent.

An OECD working paper (2006) projected that public health spending in Canada would increase from 7.3 percent of GDP to 13.5 percent by 2050, taking into account demographic change and assuming that, over and above demographic effects, health costs increase at an annual rate 1 percent faster than income. If utilization rates were to be progressively constrained so that health costs grew only in line with income by 2050, public health spending would grow to 10.8 percent of GDP. The OECD study also makes it clear that Canada is not alone in facing these prospects, although it is above the OECD mean. On average, health care expenditures are projected to increase from 6.7 percent of GDP in 2005 to 12.8 percent (under the "cost pressure" scenario) or 10.1 percent (under the "cost containment" scenario) by 2050 across all OECD nations.

The pincerlike forces of public opinion on one side and a seemingly unsustainable trajectory of increasing costs on the other are driving health care to the center of provincial political agendas. In these circumstances, governments are increasingly likely to form the will to make major changes to the policy framework for health care. The forming of political will, however, is one of two conditions for major change in policy: The party in power must also be able to mobilize the necessary authority. Since June 2004, there have been three minority governments at the federal level—first Liberal, then Conservative. The Conservative government elected in January 2006 and again in October 2008 showed no more inclination to modify the CHA or to relax federal constraints (either symbolic or tangible) on provincial action than did the Liberals. The government's room to maneuver was limited by a minority Parliament populated by three other parties—the Liberals, with their historic commitment to the CHA model; the social-democratic New Democratic Party; and the Quebec separatist party, the Bloc Québecois. Should the Conservatives form a majority in the future, that development could represent the type of shift in the political landscape that is necessary for major change in the policy framework for health care.[21]

The relaxing of federal constraints makes such policy change easier at the provincial level but does not guarantee it. It should be kept in mind, moreover, that political factors at the provincial level are at least if not more important than those at the federal level: provincial governments are less constrained by the federal framework than they are by their own domestic situations, including popular support and accommodations with providers (Tuohy forthcoming). The provinces to watch in this regard, in both the short- and long-term, are Quebec and Alberta. The *Chaoulli* decision placed Quebec under the most immediate pressure to act, and historically Quebec has shown the capacity to pioneer changes, both on the delivery and the financing side. Furthermore, public opinion in Quebec in the run-up to the *Chaoulli* decision, and in the wake of the decision showed less opposition to paying for private alternatives in health care than was the case in most other regions of the country (although levels were similar in Alberta and British Columbia).[22] But the Quebec party system is highly and increasingly competitive: The 2007 Quebec election produced a minority government for the first time since 1878. That Liberal government faces a divided opposition, comprising the separatist and social-democratic Parti Québecois (the Bloc's provincial counterpart), which had loudly decried the *Chaoulli* decision, and the Action démocratique du Québec (ADQ), a right-wing populist party that made an unexpectedly strong showing in the 2007 election, having campaigned on a platform of greater reliance on the private sector in health care.

In the run-up to the tightly contested 2007 election, the Liberal government took incremental steps to allow for private insurance within a tightly regulated framework. It became the first among Canadian provinces to establish "wait-time guarantees" for specified procedures. If waits in the public system exceed established limits, the patient will be treated at public expense in a private or out-of-province facility. Furthermore, private insurance will be allowed to cover hip, knee, and cataract surgery—presumably appealing to those who wish to insure against the costs of accessing these treatments faster than they can be provided under the public wait-time guarantee. Especially critical in the Quebec framework is the continuation of the requirement that physicians function entirely within or entirely outside the publicly financed system. In the post-election 2007 budget, the Liberals announced the establishment of yet-another commission to review the health care system, this one, however, in the hands of a leading advocate of private sector mechanisms. The ADQ's moment of ascendancy appeared to pass quickly, however; and in the context of waning ADQ popularity the Liberal government quickly shelved the recommendations of the review, issued in February 2008. In the subsequent December 2008 election, the Liberals were returned with a majority and the ADQ was reduced to a rump.

In Alberta, the conditions for more major change could develop, although its fiscal cushion reduces the sense of urgency to act. Alberta, which has a Conservative government disposed toward market mechanisms and private finance, also has the least competitive party system among Canadian provinces. Oil and gas revenues also make Alberta Canada's richest province and swell the public coffers—and hence allow the province to sustain significant growth (at least up-front growth) in public health care expenditures as well. Under such circumstances, we could well see a move toward an integrated public-private financing structure for health care in which there are no losers—at least in the first instance. However, as long as the Conservatives are in a minority position in Ottawa, the Alberta government may be reluctant to jeopardize the electoral fortunes of its federal cousins by undertaking a dramatic reform of health care financing. Furthermore, a change in the leadership of the Alberta Conservative Party replaced a colorful and controversial premier who had advocated for a greater role for the private sector with a much more pragmatic premier who has clearly distanced himself from his predecessor.

The next several years are likely to see considerable experimentation at the provincial level in Canada. At its best, such experimentation could allow for an assessment and diffusion of new approaches to health care financing. But the take-up of different options will be very much conditioned by the political environment in each province and at the federal level.

Meanwhile, in all provinces, the accommodation between hospital and physician providers and governments continues to be elaborated. Regionalization of hospital facilities, including some degree of vertical integration with other community-based agencies and institutions, is proceeding—even in Ontario, where independent hospital boards continue to exist but are being incrementally drawn into "purchaser-provider" relationships with "local health integration networks." Primary care reform, focused on drawing family physicians into groups providing 24/7 access to care is also under way to various degrees across provinces. Information systems are being targeted for change. Together these developments amount to a pattern of cumulative incremental change in the institutional mix of hierarchical, market, and collegial mechanisms that could over time transform the system, albeit still within the structural balance of the single-payer model. The key question is whether and to what extent these developments will obviate or alternatively be overtaken by broader political developments that could lead to a major expansion of private finance. The testing of resiliency of the Canadian model, notwithstanding its affirmation under severe pressure in the 1990s and 2000s, is far from over.

Notes

1. Conference Board of Canada, *Performance and Potential 2001–2002* (Ottawa: Conference Board of Canada, 2001): 85–95.

2. Given the absence of reliable longitudinal data, it is impossible to know whether waiting times themselves actually increased in the mid-1990s and thereafter.

3. The original paper presented a framework that was subsequently more fully developed in my book *Accidental Logics* (Tuohy 1999).

4. The public share increased marginally after 1971 (the first year in which Medicare was implemented in all provinces) to a high of 77.1 percent in 1976 and then began a slow secular descent (OECD 1993, 252).

5. This observation underscores the importance of the timing of policy interventions and hence of the broader political context in understanding health care reform. Had comprehensive universal governmental health insurance been adopted when it was proposed by the federal government immediately after the Second World War, the resulting scheme would have borne a stronger resemblance to the British NHS than did the scheme that was ultimately adopted. The postwar federal proposals, however, fell victim to a climate of federal-provincial relations that was inhospitable to the development of cost-shared programs. It was not until that climate improved in the 1960s that a more propitious climate developed, by which time prevailing models of financing and policy ideas had changed markedly.

6. For comparative purposes, this proportion in 1971 was 4.0 percent in Britain, 2.8 percent in the United States, 4.5 percent in Germany, and 4.8 percent in the Netherlands. In 1990, the comparable figures were 5.2 percent in Britain, 5.2 percent in the United States, 5.9 percent in Germany, and 5.8 percent in the Netherlands (calculated from OECD 1993).

7. Government generally does not specify contracts with providers, but there are a few exceptions in the hospital sector. Although hospital global budgets are largely historically based, some provincial governments contract with hospitals to provide specified volumes of a few given procedures, such as coronary artery bypass surgery.

8. This portrait of stability should not obscure the other sources of conflict within Medicare's structure. Federal-provincial fiscal bargaining was (and is) highly charged, with blame shifting typical and wearing on the actors. Where long wait lists appear they provoke media interest and generate sharp disputes about the quality of what Medicare delivers (as opposed to promises). See (Maioni 2008); charges of excessive rationing follow quickly from wait list concerns and are part of the policy warfare within the Medicare world and across the Canadian-U.S. border (Marmor 2008).

9. One might wonder about the level of fiscal sanction necessary to maintain effective leverage. The political risk to provincial governments in incurring federal sanctions for contravening the CHA, however, has in the past magnified the effective influence of the act. All provinces, for example, eliminated "extra billing" in order to comply with the

act, even though the sanctions involved amounted to a small proportion (less than 1 percent) of provincial health budgets (Tuohy 1988).

10. The Canada Health and Social Transfer (CHST), which consolidated and reduced federal transfers to the provinces for health, post-secondary education, and social assistance, came into effect on April 1, 1996. The federal plan called for a negotiated agreement with the provinces on a set of principles to underpin the CHST and on an allocation formula across the provinces. But no negotiations were subsequently held on mutual principles, and the federal government established its own allocation formula in the absence of provincial agreement (McCracken 1996). Thomas J. Courchene, *Redistributing Money and Power: A Guide to the Canada Health and Social Transfer* (Toronto: C.D. Howe Institute, 1995): 92–93.

11. In the 1970s, public expenditures on health care in Canada increased in real terms (deflated by the price index for total domestic expenditure) by an average of 7 percent a year. In the 1980s the average annual real increase was 6 percent. Toward the end of the 1980s and the early 1990s, this rate slowed somewhat to about 4 percent, before plunging and then recovering as shown in Figure 3.1. This fiscal constraint is even more marked than that preceding the rupturing of the British profession-state accommodation in 1987. There, an average annual real rate of increase of 5 percent in the 1970s declined to about 1 percent in 1984 and 1985, before recovering to about 5 percent in 1987. In Britain, however, the annual change in the level of public spending had fluctuated much more widely than has been the case in Canada.

12. The OMA proposal was essentially a model for remuneration, not organization of delivery. Each general practice would be assigned a "benchmark threshold." The practice would bill the government plan on a fee-for-service basis until this threshold was reached. Thereafter only certain services such as obstetrics and anesthesia could be billed. This model was similar to the individual caps that had begun to be adopted in some provinces. The important difference is that the threshold would be assigned on the basis of the characteristics of patients on the practice's roster—a form of "needs-based" funding at the primary care level.

13. These figures compare with 12 percent and 15 percent of American respondents, respectively, and 6 percent of German respondents, respectively.

14. The average annual rates of hospital, medical, dental, and pharmaceutical inflation from 1980 to 1990 were 6.8 percent, 6.1 percent, 9.6 percent, and 6.6 percent, respectively (OECD 1995, 151).

15. The extent to which the existence of governmental health insurance provides firms with a competitive advantage is a matter of some dispute. Some economists maintain that health benefits simply form part of the compensation package for employees, and that as benefit costs decrease, wages will rise and vice versa (Fuchs 1993, 158–59). Others, however, point to the lower levels of health care price inflation and the lower administrative costs (for employers as well as public administrators) under governmental systems to demonstrate their cost advantages to business (Purchase 1996, 13). In the increasingly integrated North American economy, Canadian firms are more and more sensitive to such differentials.

16. It has been estimated that in the mid-1980s, the difference in the administrative costs of the two systems (including insurer- and provider-borne overheads but not over-

heads incurred by employers as purchasers or self-insurers) accounted for more than half the cost differential between Canada and the United States. Robert G. Evans et al., "Controlling Health Expenditures: The Canadian Reality," *New England Journal of Medicine* 320, no. 9 (1989): 571–77.

17. These demands relate not only to income but to numbers of personnel. As noted by the OECD, "the number of practising physicians and nurses per capita [at 2.1 and 7.5 per 1000 population, respectively, in 1999] is generally low in Canada by OECD standards, and this gap has widened during the cost-containment period of the mid-1990s. Between 1992 and 1997, the number of practicing physicians remained unchanged, while the number of nurses per capita actually declined. In most other OECD countries, these numbers continued to go up, albeit at a slower pace than in previous years." Organisation for Economic Co-operation and Development. 2001. *OECD Health at a Glance: How Canada Compares.* Paris: OECD.

18. See, for example, Marni D. Brownell, Noralou P. Roos, and Charles A. Burchill, *Monitoring the Winnipeg Hospital System: 1990–91 through 1996–97* (Winnipeg: Manitoba Centre for Health Policy and Evaluation, University of Manitoba, 1999).

19. These various reports are summarized in CIHI (2003, 5–7).

20. Because utilization is such an uncertain variable, the ministry also modeled the effects of higher and lower rates of utilization increase. The model is very sensitive to this assumption: Reducing the projected rate of increase in utilization from 1.5 percent to 1.0 percent per annum (in line with conference board projections) moves the government's fiscal position from a $7.2 billion deficit to a $4.5 billion surplus in 2024–2025, while raising the rate of increase to 2.0 percent (in line with background research for the Romanow Commission) nearly triples the deficit to almost $20 billion.

21. Arguably, there is a "catch-22" to this statement. In order to form a majority, the Conservatives might have to move so far toward the center that their election would no longer signify a major political shift. In this regard much depends upon the strength of competition they face—a question yet to be resolved as both the traditionally centrist Liberal Party and the social-democratic New Democratic Party struggle to reconcile internal tensions and factions.

22. See, for example, the annual Health Care in Canada survey reports for 2004 and 2005 conducted by the polling firm POLLARA (http://www.hcic-sssc.ca/index_e.asp). The reasons for this phenomenon have not been thoroughly explored. It may be that, having historically had the most interventionist public policies toward the organization of health care delivery, Quebec is now experiencing a backlash that places it in the company of regions of the country historically more supportive of market-based approaches.

References

Alvi, S. 1995. *Health costs and private sector competitiveness.* Ottawa: Conference Board of Canada.

Barer, M. L., and G. L. Stoddart. 1991. *Toward integrated medical resources policies for Canada.* Report prepared for the Federal-Provincial-Territorial Conference of Deputy Ministers of Health. Ottawa.

Blendon, R. J., John Benson, Karen Donelan, Robert Leitman, Humphrey Taylor, Christian Koeck and Daniel Gitterman. 1995. Who has the best health care system? A second look. *Health Affairs* 14 (4): 220–30.

Blendon, R. J., C. Schoen, C. M. DesRoches, R. Osborn, and K. L. Scoles. 2002. Trends: Inequities in health care; A five-country survey. *Health Affairs* 21 (3): 182–91.

Canadian Institute for Health Information. 2003. *Health care in Canada 2003.* Ottawa: Canadian Institute for Health Information.

CIHI. *See* Canadian Institute for Health Information.

Employer Committee on Health Care—Ontario. 1995. *A perspective on health care.* Toronto: Employer Committee on Health Care—Ontario.

Flood, C. 2006. Chaoulli's legacy for the future of Canadian health. *Osgoode Hall Law Journal* 44 (2): 273–310.

Fuchs, Victor R. 1993. *The Future of Health Policy,* Cambridge, MA: Harvard University Press.

Jackson, H., and A. McDermott. 2004. *Health spending: Retrospect and prospect.* Analytical Note. Economic and Fiscal Policy Branch, Fiscal Policy Division, Department of Finance, Government of Canada.

Kingdon, John W. 1995. *Agenda, Alternatives, and Public Policies.* Second edition. New York: HarperCollins College Publishers.

Klein, R. 1995. *The new politics of the NHS.* 3d ed. London: Longman.

Le Grand, J. 1994. Evaluating the NHS reforms. In *Evaluating the NHS reforms,* ed. R. Robinson and J. Le Grand. London: King's Fund Institute.

Lewis, S. 1996. Issues in the evolution of decision-making at regional levels. Paper presented at the symposium on Globalization, State Choices and Citizens' Participation in Canadian Health Care. York University, Toronto, April 1–2.

Lomas, J., C. Charles, and J. Greb. 1992. *The price of peace: The structure and process of physician fee negotiations in Canada.* Working Paper No. 92–17. Hamilton, Ontario: McMaster University Centre for Health Economic and Policy Analysis.

MacBride-King, J. L. 1995. *Managing corporate health care costs: Issues and options.* Ottawa: Conference Board of Canada.

Maioni, Antonia. 2008. Health care politics and policy in Canada. *One issue, two voices, issue nine: Health care in crisis: the drive for health reform in Canada and the United States.* Washington and Toronto: Woodrow Wilson International Centre for Scholars, Canada Institute on North American Issues, pp. 14–25.

Marmor, Theodore R. 2008. American health care policy and politics: Promises and perils of reform. *One issue, two voices, issue nine: Health care in crisis: the drive for health reform in Canada and the United States.* Washington and Toronto: Woodrow Wilson International Centre for Scholars, Canada Institute on North American Issues, pp. 2–13.

McCracken, Mike. 1996. *Federal transfer scenarios: What are the choices?* A paper delivered at the symposium on *Globalization, State Choices and Citizens' Participation in Canadian Health Care* sponsored by the Robarts Centre for Canadian Studies and the Centre for Health Studies, York University, Toronto April 1–2.

OECD. *See* Organisation for Economic Co-operation and Development.

Ontario Ministry of Finance. 2005. *Toward 2025: Assessing Ontario's long-term outlook.* Toronto: Government of Ontario.

Organisation for Economic Co-operation and Development. 1993. *OECD health systems: Facts and trends 1960–1991*. Vols. 1–2. Paris: OECD.

Organisation for Economic Co-operation and Development. 1995. *Internal markets in the making: Health systems in Canada, Iceland and the United Kingdom*. Paris: OECD.

Organisation for Economic Co-operation and Development. 2006. *Projecting OECD health and long-term care expenditures: What are the main drivers?* Economic Department Working Paper No. 477. Paris: OECD.

Premier's Advisory Council on Health. 2002. *A framework for reform*. Edmonton, Alberta: Premier's Advisory Council on Health.

Purchase, Bryne. 1996. *Health Care and Competitiveness*, paper presented at the National Health Care Policy Summit, Montebello, Quebec, March 15–19, 1996.

Schoen, C., R. Osborn, Michelle M. Doty, Meghan Bishop, Jordon Peugh, and Nadita Murukutla. 2007. Toward higher-performance health systems: Adults' health care experiences in seven countries. *Health Affairs*, Web exclusive (June 26): w717–w734.

Schoen, C., R. Osborn, P. T. Huyn, M. Doty, K. Davis, K. Zapert, and J. Peugh. 2004. Primary care and health system performance: Adult's experience in five countries. *Health Affairs*, Web Exclusive (October 28): W4–487–503. http://content.healthaffairs.org/cgi/content/abstract/hlthaff.w4.487.

Starr, P. 1982. *The social transformation of American medicine*. New York: Basic Books.

Tholl, W. 1994. Health care spending in Canada: Skating faster on thinner ice. In *Limits to care: Reforming Canada's health system in an age of restraint*, ed. A. Blomqvist and D. M. Brown. Toronto: C. D. Howe Institute.

Tuohy, C. H. 1988. Medicine and the state in Canada: The extra billing issue in perspective. *Canadian Journal of Political Science* 21 (2): 267–96.

Tuohy, C. H. 1999. *Accidental logics: The dynamics of change in the health care arena in the United States, Britain and Canada*. New York: Oxford University Press.

Tuohy, C. H. forthcoming. When is a single payer not a single system? Sub-national variation under a federal health policy framework. *Journal of Health Politics, Policy and Law*. in press.

White, W. D., J. W. Salmon, and J. Feinglass. 1994. The changing doctor-patient relationship and performance monitoring: An agency perspective. In *The corporate transformation of health care: Perspectives and implications*, ed. J. W. Salmon. Amityville, NY: Baywood.

Germany
Evidence, Policy, and Politics in Health Care Reform

MARTIN PFAFF

The complex and wide-ranging field of health policy making can be traversed along different routes and with different perspectives in mind. The route chosen depends, among other things, on an understanding of the very pattern of organization and operation, representing, as it were, the "lay of the land." Accordingly, this chapter starts with a brief description of the German health care system and its operation—its political dynamics and its recent evolution. Next, the chapter turns to the role of evidence and learning in general and in the German context in particular, citing examples of evidence versus interests and power as guiding principles in the policy-making process (the look within) and of cross-border learning for and from the German experience (the look across the fence).

Financing, Organization, and Operation of the German Health Care System in the Twentieth Century

The German health insurance system—often described as the Bismarck Model—is a mixed system. It combines contributions from employees and employers, co-insurance payments by the insured, private insurance premiums, and direct patient purchases and general taxes paid by citizens and foreign residents subject to taxation (Weinmann and Zifonum 2004, 454). In

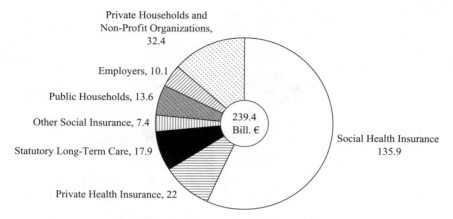

Figure 4.1 German health care expenditure by financing institution, 2005 (in billion euros)
Source: Figure based on data of *Statistisches Bundesamt* (Federal Bureau of Statistics), http://www.destatis.de/jetspeed/portal/cms/Sites/destatis/Internet/DE/Navigation/Statistiken/Gesundheit/Gesundheitsausgaben/Gesundheitsausgaben.psml, accessed July 7, 2007.

2005, total German health care spending (€=euro) amounted to €239.4 billion (or US$287.3 billion). Social health insurance accounted for the lion's share (€135.9 billion, US$163.1 billion, or about 57 percent of total health expenditure), followed by private households and nonprofit organizations (€32.4 billion, US$38.9 billion, or about 14 percent), private health insurance (€22 billion, US$ 26.4 billion, or 9 percent), and other sources of funds (see Figure 4.1).

These funds are channeled mainly through health insurance funds (or sick funds) to associations of providers. The latter distribute the money to individual providers in line with the health services they have provided. The government finances both the purely public health institutions (the public health service) and the fixed capital costs of public hospitals—mainly for investment in buildings and equipment—out of tax revenues (about 6 percent of funds in 2000). The sick funds and private insurers pay for the variable hospital costs and other medical care including prescription drugs. Patients mostly receive the health benefits (goods and services) as benefits in kind, in some cases also in cash (see Figure 4.2 for major categories of services and goods).

Some additional features of the system are noteworthy. Ambulatory care physicians must be members of their associations. They receive their remuneration through these associations, which submit the claims of individual doctors to the insurance funds for reimbursement. Since hospitals receive their funding in a "dual fashion"—investments mainly via the federal states,

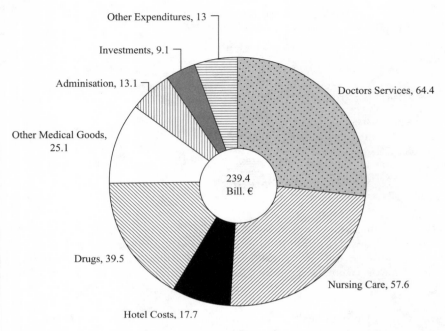

Other Expenditures, 13

Investments, 9.1

Adminisation, 13.1

Doctors Services, 64.4

Other Medical Goods, 25.1

239.4 Bill. €

Drugs, 39.5

Nursing Care, 57.6

Hotel Costs, 17.7

Figure 4.2 German health care expenditure by type of health care service, 2005 (in billion euros)
Source: Figure based on data of *Statistisches Bundesamt* (Federal Bureau of Statistics), http://www.destatis.de/jetspeed/portal/cms/Sites/destatis/Internet/DE/Content/Statistiken/ Gesundheit/Gesundheitsausgaben/Tabellen/Content50/Leistungsarten,templateId= renderPrint.psml, accessed July 7, 2007.

(Länder) current costs mainly from social insurance institutions—conflicts can and do arise. For example, with regard to the renovation of buildings and new equipment: Should this be the responsibility of the individual states or the sick funds? Moreover, hospital planning is the responsibility (and the right) of the regional state governments. Associations of sick funds have limited rights in this regard; they are only entitled to voice their interests in the planning process, without having to agree to the planning.

The state hospital associations and the (federal) German Hospital Association represent the interests of individual institutions. Unlike the physician associations, however, they hold only the status of private associations (Vereine) and cannot control the conduct of an individual hospital. Furthermore, while private nonprofit and private for-profit hospitals coexist, their interests and administration differ considerably (see also Chapter 8).

Since 1975 the government has attempted to control the costs of pharmaceuticals and even to regulate prices. The latter has always been an exercise in walking a tightrope. Irrespective of party preferences, the chief ministers of individual states generally have taken a protectionist stance whenever health policy interventions threatened to adversely affect "their" pharmaceutical companies. Fear of losing jobs plays a major role. Thus, national health policy measures are often subject to compromises in order to succeed in the second chamber of Parliament (that is, the chamber of the states, or Bundesrat). This experience is also illustrative of the particular tensions that arise in the policy making in federal systems.

Political Dynamics of Health Care Reform

Much as in other countries, forces and pressures from within the health care system itself as well as wider social change largely shape German health policy formulation. Not only observable facts but also stylized facts and traditionally held fictions play a role. The values and beliefs of the major actors and the framing by the media are powerful influences. The way the public at large sees all of those elements affects in turn the outcomes of the policy-making process.

Underlying this complex process are the economic interests of groups directly affected by health policy measures. The first are the insured: the members of various sick funds and private insured. The second are the providers of health services, generally in competition with each other for a share of health resources. The ability of each stakeholder group to pursue its interests is mainly limited by its power in the competitive struggle. At the same time, as in the Netherlands and other European countries, the German health policy arena has developed a remarkable culture of cooperation between the major actors and contenders that restrains the unbridled exercise of power of any one of them including government. Cooperation and competition are thus the twin poles of health policy making in Germany.

An emphasis on "evidence" has become part of this process. Governments and organized interest groups alike use central indicators of resource allocation, for example, to justify their claims or to ward off claims of others. Facts and fictions, values and beliefs enter the process of explicit and implicit bargaining.

It would be wrong to assume on the basis of these generalized remarks that all of this must necessarily lead to a chaotic, if charming, process of give-and-take. In fact, the German bargaining process is neither chaotic (taking place in a fairly organized and orderly fashion), nor is it charming (with actors quite serious in the pursuit of their—and their clientele's—economic interests). In other words, they are more interested in "taking" than in "giving."

International evidence became more prominent in the reform debate precisely for several of the reasons the editors of this volume allude to in their Introduction. Fiscal strain in periods of reduced economic and fiscal growth and the continuing and prolonged media critique of the welfare state rank among the foremost reasons. There appears to be a twenty- to twenty-five-year cycle in the critical debate of Germany's socially oriented state. Whenever economic growth turned down for one reason or the other—for example, in the wake of the first oil crisis—critics were quick to attack social welfare spending as the culprit, thus mixing up cause and effect in more than a cavalier fashion. This well-nigh orchestrated critique gained further momentum following the breakdown of the Soviet Union and the discrediting of the Socialist agenda. Thereafter, the welfare state elements present in Western industrialized countries seemed less needed to pacify the masses.

While the criticism of social welfare surely is only one among several motives, it provides part of the backdrop of the reform process in Germany. Most citizens associate the term "health care reform" not so much with a general increase in benefits but with a (continuing) process of retrenchment of the welfare state. A major reason is simply that neoliberal, even market-radical, reform proposals entail either an increase in co-insurance or an exclusion of benefits from the package hitherto financed on the basis of solidarity. In other words, individualization of benefits and financing, freedom of choice, or more competition invariably shift the financial burden from the stronger to the economically weaker segments of society. The redistributive effects of such proposals clearly violate the principle of contributions on the basis of ability to pay—one of the two founding principles of the Bismarck system (the other being utilization on the basis of need and not on the basis of ability to pay).

Behind the growing influence of neoliberal ideas, there were—and are—evidently vested interests—not only among well-organized groups but also private insurance companies trying to expand their share of the market. These trends appear to be fairly similar in most European countries but—as Rudolf Klein points out—the configuration varies from country to country.

Major Reform Acts, 1977–2007

Since the mid-1970s, cost containment has been the main (but not only) driving force of health care reform in Germany (Pfaff and Kern 2005, 203–6). The first Health Insurance Cost Containment Act took effect in 1977, followed—as can be seen from Table 4.1—by several other similar laws (such as the Hospital Cost Containment Act of 1981). Their common feature is the set of instruments aiming primarily at limiting prices and vol-

Table 4.1 Regulating social health insurance in Germany, 1977–2007

Regulation	Year
Health Insurance Cost Containment Act (KVKG)	1977
Retirement Pension Adjustment Act (RAG 1982)	1981
Cost Containment Amendment Act(KVEG)	1981
Hospital Cost Containment Act (KHKG)	1981
Regulation of Medical and Technical Aids (H&HMRI)	1982
Budget Support Act (HGB)	1983
Hospital Financing Act (KHNG)	1984
Hospital Reimbursement Regulation (BPflV)	1986
Improvement for Planning, Accreditation of Physicians Act (GVKBP)	1986
Health Care Reform Act (GRG)	1989
Health Care Structure Act (GSG)	1993
First and Second Health Insurance Restructuring Act (1.& 2.GKV-NOG)	1997
Improvement of Solidarity Act (GKV-SolG)	1998
Harmonization of Health Insurance Act (RanglG)	1999
Health Care Reform Act 2000 (GKV Reform 2000)	2000
Diagnosis Related Groups Financing in Hospitals Act (DRG-Einführungsgesetz)	2001
Risk-Structure Compensation Amendment Act (RSA-ReformG)	2002
Health System Modernization Act (GMG)	2004
Strengthening Competition in Social Health Insurance Act (GKV-WSG)	2007

Source: M. Schneider, "Evaluation of Cost-Containment Acts in Germany," in *Health: Quality and Choice* (Paris: OECD 1994), 63-81; and author's presentation.

umes, or else, for example in the 1977 law, to shift some of the costs of health insurance to the insured, specifically to patients in the form of the exclusion of certain benefits or increased cost sharing.

The earlier reform already contained efforts to bring about structural changes in the system. As exemplified in the 1989 Health Care Reform Act, reforms aimed to strengthen the participation of the major actors involved and to create wider consensus. The reform aimed to limit spending by setting revenue limits and prospective budgets. It also included measures to increase the transparency of the administration of benefits (information technology, standardization), co-insurance to influence the utilization of services, and uniform contract rules for health insurance funds and providers to improve efficiency.

On balance, many German experts considered these measures a limited success, at least when compared to the original policy aims of cost containment and structural reform. As a matter of interest, this perceived failure is also due to the lack of explicitly stated policy goals or specific indicators that could be applied to measure their effectiveness. More fundamentally, many of the measures were based on collective decision making of the national policy-making forum (the "Concerted Action in Health Care") that represented all major societal actors with interests in health care. Ultimately, most participants saw such "decisions" as only recommendations. No immediate sanctions could—or would—be applied towards interest groups that did not conform to the agreed-upon guidelines. The process leading to the formulation and enactment of the Health Care Reform Act of 1989 brought similar experiences. Opposition of affected groups, including the powerful states (as was the case with measures aimed to contain hospital costs), led to a "softening" of reform measures.

Health insurance funds and providers' associations shouldered the responsibility for implementing reforms to assure stability of contribution rates. The "self-management" by these actors was supposed to restrain both quantities and prices of health goods. The main instruments were an increase in the transparency of this process and new procedures for testing and controlling its efficiency. Evidently, the German policy makers vastly overestimated the capacity for resolving conflicts among and between "self-managing" representatives of health insurance funds and providers. Implementation of collectively agreed-upon guidelines proved impossible to achieve. At the same time, measures aimed at particular health care sectors proved inadequate to restrain the global level of health spending, and thereby contribution rates of social insurance.

Given the limited success of the measures aiming at the supply side, the attention shifted to the "utilization side." These included increased co-payments, the exclusion of benefits from social insurance coverage, "bonuses" to patients for nonutilization of services (when using preventive dental care) and no-claim-reimbursement of part of the contributions for non-use or lower use of services. Other efforts to change the organizational structure of the parties or to limit resource use more drastically showed even less success. Thus, the government often failed to put structural reforms into effect or meet the aim of cost containment largely because the instruments to influence providers' behavior proved to be too weak.

In the face of the successful efforts of vested interest groups to defend or expand their share of the economic pie, the use of macro indicators alone (in the form of economic or financial indicators of resource use) evidently have been insufficient—so it was felt—to curb expenditure growth since 1976. Similarly, the "self-management" of sick funds and providers' associations was not up to the task of resolving conflicts over distributional matters. In this regard, the Health Care Reform Act of 1989 proved to be just as ineffective as earlier cost-containment legislation. These outcomes, together with political pressure to stabilize the contribution rates in the face of an upcoming national election scheduled for 1994, shaped the perceptions of policy makers and media commentators. The stage was set, partly by the media and their influence on public opinion, for more drastic political intervention from the top down, often over the heads of the various central actors, to replace "self-management."

This picture may come as a surprise to some international observers. They would point to the fact that (private plus public) health spending measured as a percentage GDP has remained fairly constant in Germany since 1976. Germany was also relatively successful in curbing health spending within the statutory health insurance system since the mid-1970s. While that was the case at least since the early 1980s, the general public's and the policy maker's attention remained focused on the stability of the contribution rates. Because the share of wages as a proportion of GDP has declined (and the capital incomes increased), the financial basis of health care—the wage bill of dependent workers—has shrunk relative to GDP. This has caused a rise in contribution rates—highly unpopular not only with policy makers and employees but also with the employers, who pay approximately half of the contributions. In the employers' view, these increases in contribution rates added to labor costs, thereby weakening the competitive position of German exports in the world market. They exerted pressure for more drastic measures on the then-ruling coalition parties (Christian Democratic Union/Christian Social Union—CDU/CSU—and Free Democratic Party—FDP). The opposition Social Democratic Party (SPD) was tied in to all major social policy measures due to its powerful position in the Bundesrat, the upper chamber of Parliament in which the regional states are represented and whose consent is required for structural reforms (especially for reforms affecting hospitals). Indeed, the SPD made its support for cost-containment measures conditional on major structural reforms.

Given these economic, social and political pressures, the Health Care Structure Act of 1993 had two overall strategic policy aims. The first was to stabilize the precarious financial position of health insurance funds in the short run and to prevent a major increase in contribution rates. The second was to introduce structural changes as a base for more effective long-term cost containment. In spite of various budgetary measures, health insurance fund deficits amounted to around €7 billion in 1995. This experience reflected the "classical" pattern of the threefold effects of cost-containment legislation that has been observed time and again since 1976.

Phase One—The anticipation effect: Prior to the enactment of a new law, the parties affected (for example, patients or providers) anticipate the measure. Utilization (for example, for dentures) increases temporarily to avoid expected increases in co-payments later on, pushing up spending.

Phase Two—The implementation effect: After the implementation of a law (for example, the exclusion of benefits or increase in co-insurance), more discriminating utilization leads to a stagnation or even slight decrease in spending and stable (or even slightly decreasing) contribution rates.

Phase Three—The normalization effect: Since the basic forces giving rise to the dynamics of expenditure growth (excess capacity, nonrational systems of remuneration, duplication of facilities and services across different sectors, and so on) have not changed significantly, they tend to reassert themselves. The affected provider groups tend to increase their claims to compensate for the loss of earnings. Health spending rises again at an even higher growth rate than the initial stage.

All major cost-containment interventions of the period 1976–1998 took place in the year preceding a national election, and all of them helped stabilize contribution rates in the respective election year. As must be clear, it is the political cycle—based on public and political perceptions and fueled by media, as we noted before—that largely determines a subsidiary cycle of interventions in health policy.

The Evolution of the System since 1995

The First and Second Health Insurance Restructuring Acts of 1997 introduced "market-oriented" reforms, including increases in co-insurance and delisting of dentures for certain age groups. After the Social Democratic and Green Parties took office (the "Red-Green Coalition") in 1998, this coalition reversed these measures in part. The 2000 Health Care Reform Act continued the policy of structural reforms initiated by the 1993 Health Care Structure Act. It was very surprising to many observers that the 2004 Health System Modernization Act of the Red-Green Coalition, which was also supported by the CDU/CSU, contained several of the market-type elements that the same coalition had rejected in 1998—to the chagrin of many of their own party supporters. The party leadership proclaimed these measures as part of the "Agenda 2010." It considered this reform agenda necessary for Germany to regain its strength in the competitive global economy and to reduce the public deficit in order to adhere to the criteria of the European Union.

The main effect of the increase in cost sharing and partial exclusion of benefits was a further reduction in real disposable income for large segments of the German population, and thus a reduction of domestic demand. (At the international level, the German economy continued to prove highly competitive as evidenced by high trade surpluses.) The stagnation of domestic demand did not lead to a decline in unemployment (or stabilization of the funding base of sick funds). On the contrary, unemployment increased. Many sick funds incurred debts in order to avoid larger increases in contribution rates. Though the funds realized surpluses due to increased cost sharing and the exclusion of certain benefits, they were very hesitant to reduce the contribution rates (up to the latest health care reform of 2007, each sick fund used to set its own income-related contribution rate). The government called for a substantial reduction in contribution rates, but the funds argued that they first had to eliminate their debts before they could put into effect a substantial reduction in rates.

In the wake of federal elections in 2005, a Grand Coalition of CDU/CSU and SPD brought together parties that had thus far opposed each other, particularly in the field of health care policy, and that had divergent views of the reforms to be implemented. The coalition agreement of November 2005 contains as its major health policy goals: to secure an enduring and just financing of health care; to improve the continuing performance of the health care system via a stable financial structure; and to ensure high performance, solidarity, and demographic stability for the health care system in the long term.

It may come as little surprise that most observers conclude that the Strengthening Competition in Social Health Insurance Act of 2007 (GKV-Wettbewerbsstärkungsgesetz 2007) has failed miserably in attaining the lofty aims agreed upon at the start of the Grand Coalition. The coalition parties could not agree on a common concept for a meaningful reform of the financing system. Hence they diverted and reduced their avowed aims to a "strengthening of competition." But the measures enacted actually decreased the autonomy of the individual social health insurance organizations. They instituted measures that are likely to decrease the level of solidarity over time by introducing an individual "additional contribution" (Zusatzbeitrag) that is not subsidized by across-funds risk-adjustment transfers. Those who had hoped that the financing base would be strengthened by including other types of income beyond wages (that is, interest, rental income, and so on) and by including more well-to-do individuals in social health insurance via a system of "citizens insurance" (Bürgerversicherung) were disappointed. Similarly, others who had hoped for a greater individualization of financing through equal per-capita contributions and benefit provision were equally disappointed by the new act.

On the positive side, however, several meaningful measures were enacted as well. To name but a few: an obligation for the entire resident population to have health insurance coverage; the right of individuals to return to their previous health insurance fund, in which they had lost coverage (this right applies both to social health insurance funds and private health insurance organizations); extending the measures for integrated (cross-sectoral) health care provision; a liberalization of the rules governing contracts between social health insurance funds and providers; and a new system for remunerating ambulatory care physicians.

Most observers agree that instead of a reform of the financing system, the Grand Coalition in reality agreed on institutional reforms of social health insurance and partly also of private health insurance organizations. Among the former we find the following: the great ease with which social health insurance institutions may merge; the institution of a health fund (Gesundheitsfond) into which all contribution revenues from all social health insurance funds are to be paid and out of which funds are to be allocated on an equal per-capita basis to individual health insurance funds (the flow of funds, however, is to be modified by the risk-adjustment system); the creation of a top-level institution that binds together all social health insurance funds at the federal level (Spitzenverband Bund); the determination of a uniform contribution rate by the *state* rather than by individual social health insurance funds, as was the case in the past (this does not apply to the individual additional contribution determined by each fund, to make ends meet if the common allocation out of the overall health fund proves insufficient to cover expenditures).

The financial situation of social health insurance funds is improving markedly as a consequence of the upturn of the German economy, coinciding in time with the advent of the Grand Coalition. With rising wage incomes and decreasing unemployment, the income position of funds took a turn for the better. This economic revival—accompanied also by an upsurge of domestic consumer demand—will at least moderate the increase of contribution rates.

Some of the earlier reforms—for example, the institution of disease management programs or incentives to create integrated forms of health care provision (to mention but two measures)—take time to prove their beneficial effects. This factor reflects the classical political dilemma of democratic governments: They often pass short-run measures with an eye on the election cycle rather than necessary long-run measures whose benefits are invisible, if not illusive, in the short run and whose costs are seen as unwelcome burdens by the populace. There is therefore little doubt that political considerations rather than scientific evidence shape many health policy measures in Germany.

When looking at the overall health reform process, one is hard pressed to discern a consistent "evidence-based framework" for policy making. The dominant image that comes to mind is a process of trial and error and even of repeated shifts in policy direction under the varying influence of political parties.

It would thus be highly presumptuous to claim that evidence-based policy making represents the rule rather than the exception in German health policy making. Nonetheless, I maintain that the use of evidence to improve policy making is on the rise. I shall attempt to substantiate this claim below.

The Role of Evidence and Learning within and across National Boundaries
EVIDENCE—CLAIMS AND CRITICISMS

With the general rise in the level of education of legislators and—more often—of their legislative assistants, the very process of policy making becomes more sophisticated. Instead of continuing only with the time-honored process of trial and error, or of flying by the seat of your pants, policy makers increasingly try to base their decisions on evidence from both within the country or from abroad. After all one learns only from failure and criticism. Success and praise only confirm our existing images. Therefore, I wish to start by contrasting the ideal-typical role of evidence with some of the criticism raised in the small but growing literature on evidence-based policy making.

Niessen and others defined the ideal-typical role of evidence rather succinctly as "health policy and health care delivery driven by systematically collected proof on the effects of health-related interventions from the social and health services" (Niessen, Grijseels, and Ruttens 2000, 859). "Treatment guidelines supported by evidence on effectiveness and efficiency will be one essential element in this process" (866). To live up to this ideal, Biller-Adorno and others demand that health reform proposals should be evidence-based. They should demonstrate the social value of an intervention. And they require a context of randomized controlled clinical trials (besides systematic revision and meta-analyses) (Biller-Adorno, Lie, and TerMeulen 2003, 262; Norheim 2002, 310). In the face of these stringent formal requirements, many conclusions that standards of conventional wisdom would consider evidence fall by the wayside.

On the other side of the ledger, there is a more down to earth and also more critical view of the role of evidence, one that leads to several caveats. First, in real-world practice, "policy decisions are the outcome of complicated political processes among parties with different interests" (Niessen, Grijseels, and Ruttens 2000, 860). Second, "an important obstacle to evidence-based health policy is a clear understanding of policy objectives and the availability of relevant measurement instruments" (862). Third, evidence-based approaches meet resistance as they often serve as "a powerful instrument to bring about changes in power relations in health policy-making" (Biller-Adorno, Lie, and TerMeulen 2003, 263). Finally, they have "unintended discriminatory effects particularly in the care of older people," and "a bias of an evidence-oriented approach can be expected in favor of younger age groups, acute diseases, and drug therapy" (263–64).

Some observers are skeptical about the role of formal evaluation research as the basis for policy. "The history of evaluation research highlights the naïveté of the idea that evaluation findings from robust experimental studies would form the basis of a rational process of policy development" (Shadish, Cook, and Leviton 1991, 88). Others are particularly critical of the evidence-based approach to priority setting in health care. "The method is based on the assumption that life span can be multiplied by a weighting of quality of life and that one QALY always has the same weight, independent of applying it to young people or elderly, sick or healthy, one person or many. The basic design of the method is flawed, and the flaw is that it portrays a wrong model of political decision making" (Biller-Adorno, Lie, and TerMeulen 2003, 263). Norheim points in a similar direction: "Evidence should not replace values. Evidence and values must be combined in decisions limiting access to health care. People affected by such decisions have conflicting values and interests" (Norheim 2002, 315). Rudolf Klein concludes that "in the case of policy, evidence tends to be something of a Delphic oracle—difficult to decipher and apt to be misinterpreted. The platitude is that policy should be *informed* by evidence . . . The nonsense is that policy should be *based* on scientific evidence" (Klein 2003, 429).

To my mind, there are therefore at least two levels at which a definition of *evidence* can be attempted in the context of health care policy. At the *subjective level* of the individual decision maker, evidence refers to any information (whether derived from descriptive material, statistical work, or analytical or fully integrated comparative studies) that the decision maker relies on in the context of his or her reference model of the process to be controlled. At the *objective level,* however, evidence may be defined more narrowly as information that was systematically collected using statistical procedures or various forms of systematic comparative studies. One test of the latter approach may be found in the question whether different investigators using the same method would arrive at the same conclusion.

Similar considerations seem to underlie the scale judging the "hardness" of evidence as formulated by the Agency for Health Care Policy and Research (AHCPR). Accordingly, evidence ranges from meta-analyses of randomized control studies, those without randomization, quasi-experimental studies and nonexperimental descriptive studies (including comparative studies, correlation analyses and case-control studies), to the report of expert commissions or opinions or clinical experience of recognized authorities (Lauterbach 1998, 101).

My own view on the role and value of evidence is shaped by my experience in German policy making. Firstly, data in themselves are not information. Data acquire value only in the context of the reference model of the policy maker. Secondly, the "implementation problem" means that recommendations of the researcher or policy adviser do not always result in action by policy makers. For these recommendations are based—explicitly or implicitly—on the reference model of the researcher or policy adviser, not that of the policy makers. Thirdly, national policy makers—whether at the legislative or executive branch—will favor evidence that serves their perceived interests. They favor policies that enhance the political careers or the personal power of particular policy makers. Fourthly, evidence-based policies seldom make explicit or even implicit reference to a particular model of the *goals* of the proposals, the *instruments* employed in the pursuit of these goals, the nature and timing of the *control process* (including control limits and critical levels of the controlled process), or the types of policy responses required if the process gets out of control. And lastly, very rarely indeed do such general policy concepts specify which type of alternative control is to be employed if the process remains out of control. It is to these requirements that I turn next.

THE USES OF EVIDENCE IN THE CONTROL
OF HEALTH-RELATED PROCESSES

A rational approach to health policy making does not, in principle, differ from any other field of endeavor. It presupposes a willingness to explicate the goals to be pursued, the instruments employed in the pursuit of these goals and the control process. In other words, it generally requires a reference model of the controlled process that identifies causal relationships and acceptable levels of deviation of the outcome from the preset reference levels.

It also requires a clear identification of parameters to be changed when the process gets out of control.

If one applies such a generalized information-and-control model to health policy, three types of evidence (or "control levels") are required for improved policy making. The first control level consists of the monitoring of an ongoing process. The controlled or outcome variable has to stay well within upper and lower limits of acceptable variance. For such purposes, evidence-based policy making requires real-time reporting on indicator values and outcomes, for example, objective and subjective indicators of health status or patient satisfaction. Generally, a slight deviation in itself does not call for immediate interference, merely increased vigilance. The second control level is called for when the variables reach the upper or lower control levels without showing a trend toward reversal. Here parameter change is clearly called for. If this results in a reversal of the trend so that outcomes remain within pre-established limits, the process can be said to be "under control." An example of the second control level is effectiveness studies of particular interventions as the basis for adjustment. The third control level is called for if the above steps do not suffice to bring the process back "under control." Here a change of the entire control model is needed—with a renewed specification of goals, instrumental or control variables, measures of outcomes, the timing of the control process, upper and lower control limits, and so on. International comparisons of health care systems that focus on financing, production, and organization are examples of this control level.

As might be expected, evidence required for higher levels of control are more crucial, more complex, and harder to acquire than that required for lower levels. The change of the very control model itself entails the most "political" of exercises. It relates to contending actors' worldview (Weltanschauung) to the very foundations of their political reference model.

In Germany, as in other OECD nations, there are always competing groups within political parties, parliamentary fractions, and interest groups. As a consequence, the democratic process requires coalitions within and across party lines. The product of such a policy-making process seldom reflects the unadulterated worldview of one particular group. Rather, it generally results from a compromise between conflicting interests. In such situations, evidence-based policy making becomes complex and sometimes seemingly impossible when level-three control measures are called for. In such situations, the classical conflict resolution mechanisms prevail and powerful interests usually override the less powerful ones. I shall return to these real world lessons later.

Far from these "idealized" functions of evidence in controlling health-related processes, most types of comparative health policy analyses fall essentially into the categories sketched out by the editors of this volume in their Introduction. In Germany, the greatest share of comparative studies appears (at first sight) to consist of "mostly descriptive material, organized by country," followed by "statistical work." Other types of comparative studies, such as "analytical comparative studies" or even "fully integrated comparative studies," are quite rare. This claims requires, however, more systematic substantiation.

Such a distribution of study types can perhaps be explained by the purposes that they are expected to serve. In reference to the purposes mentioned by the editors in their Introduction, "learning about health policy abroad" probably ranks first, followed perhaps by the hope "to draw lessons for policy." Less likely "causal explanations" are sought in a rigorous manner. The latter would require a far greater knowledge of the total system and the interdependencies of its various parts—a requirement for anyone who truly wants to "understand" how these systems function.

THE LOOK FROM WITHIN
Evidence-Based Policy Making in Germany

Germany has not yet created a true culture of evidence-based policy making, but there are some hopeful beginnings. Thus, we find an increasing transfer of research-derived knowledge into the conception, execution, and public justification of government policy. Furthermore, we note a strengthening of the infrastructure of research aimed at providing guidance to policy makers.

Some examples can be cited right away (others will be cited later in this chapter). First, the annual reports of the Advisory Council for Concerted Action in Health Care, established in 1985, have had manifold impacts on the legislative process and the implementation of policy. Second, the system of health reports formulated at various levels of the federal system has also influenced policies. Third, the Ministry of Research and Technology has sponsored medical networks for information and cooperation designed to link research to practice. These networks have dealt with specific diseases or fields of treatment, such as cancer, chronic diseases, neurology, and psychiatry.

Research-based evidence is gaining weight in policy making. Lawmakers increasingly recognize the complexities of the proposals they have to consider. They increasingly recruit academic assistants from universities and scientific research institutes. The public debate on legislative proposals in the first decade of the twenty-first century frequently refers to scientific evidence. Some disillusioned observers of the German scene may receive the latter conclusion with some skepticism. Therefore, I find it more appropriate to state my case by giving specific examples rather than generalized claims about the scope and the limitations of using scientific evidence in health policy making.

Examples of Evidence-Based Policy Making in the Legislative Process of Germany

In the following section, I shall summarize the German experience of evidence-based policy making with some examples of policy making that were preceded and accompanied by lively public debates. In so doing, I shall employ what Pawson would call a "narrative review" (Pawson 2002) rather than the alternative strategy of a "meta-analysis." However, one should be aware of Pawson's argument that "they share common limitations in their understanding of how to provide a template for impending policy decisions" and that "the lessons currently learned from the past are somewhat limited" (157–58).

Presumably the very effort entailing a "narrative review" raises a host of methodological questions about the process of inference, about fallacies potentially arising in comparative work, and about methodological issues. Since these questions, fallacies, and issues are not specific to the examples (case studies) cited but more general, I shall summarize them in the Appendixes to this chapter.

Let me present three examples of policy issues where evidence played a crucial role: first, the role of risk adjustment as a prerequisite for competition amongst social health insurance funds; second, the introduction of disease management programs to improve the treatment of chronic diseases; and third, the allocation of resource flows within health care, given the requirement laid down by law for the Ministry of Health to submit to the German Parliament the recommendations to be made by Germany's Advisory Council for Concerted Action in Health Care.

Risk Adjustment as Prerequisite for Competition among Social Health Insurance Funds

The balance between revenue and expenditures determines the financial position of a social health insurance fund. The revenue is based on contributions paid by its members (and thus by the wage level). Expenditures mostly depend on the level and pattern of morbidity of its insured (members plus dependents). Given different risk structures, there is little surprise in the finding that competition among unequal contenders is likely to lead to unsatisfactory outcomes. In a regime where, by law, benefits are well-nigh equal for all insured, a fund's competitive success is determined not so much by the efficiency of its operation but largely by the composition of its members (by income, age, and morbidity).

The Health Care Structure Act of 1993 was passed in response to a recommendation of Germany's Advisory Council for Concerted Action in Health Care. It provided for risk adjustment among the insurance funds as a basis for extending freedom of choice to the insured. The risk-adjustment formula provided the basis for transfers between funds characterized by "better risks" (members with higher income, fewer dependents, fewer females, younger age, fewer disabled) and funds with more "bad risks" (members with lower income, more dependents, more females, more elderly, and more disabled).

During the first years, those risk-adjusted transfers led to a narrowing of the gap in the contribution rates of funds. However, risk selection ("cream skimming") was not eliminated completely. By focusing on "good risks," newly founded health insurance funds could change low contribution rates, distorting the rules of competition.

Scientific evidence from studies commissioned by the Ministry of Health led to changes in the risk-adjustment scheme. For example, it will include direct measurement of morbidity. Further, it will provide financial incentives for the introduction of disease management programs (DMPs, see below) and provide for risk pooling of certain high expenditures. It can be concluded that scientific evidence, together with goal-oriented political action, led to changes in health policy both for the first reform of 1993 and the "reform of the reform" put into practice. While it is generally true that a government often collects "evidence" to support its already decided-upon policies and also that it often tends to overlook "inconvenient" evidence, these types of errors in evidence-based policy making did not, in my judgment, occur in the cases cited.

If the success of evidence-based measures is judged by changes in policy, then one can argue that the recommendations of scientists led to a successful outcome. If, however, the ultimate success of the changes of transfer formula depends on changes in competitive outcomes—or even of health outcomes (which is yet to be accomplished)—judgment will have to be postponed by a few years. As observed by Okma and de Roo in Chapter 5, policy measures take time to "mature," or to bear fruit.

Disease Management Programs to Improve the Treatment of Chronic Diseases

As a part of the Risk-Structure Compensation Act (RSA-ReformG) 2002, the German Parliament decided to provide financial support for the development of DMPs for selected types of illnesses. This measure goes back to the recommendations of the Advisory Council for Concerted Action in Health Care to remedy deficiencies in the quality of treatment of chronically ill patients, in particular those with diabetes mellitus, breast cancer, coronary heart disease, or bronchial asthma. The council had argued that the treatment of those patients had not sufficiently taken into account the scientific evidence.

Financial incentives are provided for accredited DMPs with proven quality standards, which are to be evaluated from time to time. The incentives focus on chronically ill patients who have (voluntarily) subscribed to a DMP. The standardized expenses associated with this group are the basis for additional risk-adjustment payments. Health insurance funds are thus provided with financial incentives to compete not only for "good risks" but also for chronically ill persons subscribing to DMPs.

As a rule, DMPs have to follow evidence-based guidelines based on scientific studies of their effectiveness, safety, and benefits for particular forms of treatment. They have to frame specific treatment plans for each individual patient and to cooperate with different types of providers of health services (for example, general practitioners, specialists, hospitalists). Such collaboration is expected to benefit the patient. These providers have to participate in quality-tested training programs.

Treatment guidelines in Germany consist mainly of scientific studies that, according to the scale of the AHCPR, would be classified as "level four" studies—"evidence on the basis of expert-commissions or expert opinions, and clinical experience of recognized authorities" (Lauterbach 1998). Some have argued that these guidelines should also consider the benefit-cost ratio of therapies if they are to gain greater acceptance by practitioners and health politicians (106).

For the second example of evidence-based policy making we may also conclude therefore, in a similar vein as in the case of the first example, that scientific evidence has decidedly influenced policy making, but we have yet to wait for the consequent improvement of health outcomes.

The Allocation of Resource Flows to the Health Care Sector: Scientific Evidence to Be Reported Regularly to the German Bundestag

The most generalized call for the use of scientific evidence is found in the Health Care Reform Act 2000, which deals with the "Concerted Action in the Health Field." This body, which consisted of a cross-section of government levels, associations of health insurance funds, providers associations, and representatives of employees and employers associations, was to give regular recommendations (on the basis of medical and economic reference data) about particular health sectors, including excess supply or deficiencies. It was also to make recommendations on fees for providers.

Biannual reports of the Advisory Council for Concerted Action in Health Care in 2004 were to serve as the basis for such recommendations, with the first recommendation due by April 15, 2001. The Federal Ministry of Health submits this evidence to the legislative bodies at the federal level. The Ministry must also comment on the scientists' reports. The report of the Ministry of Health to the legislative bodies must be submitted every three years, making reference to the development of contribution rates of the social health insurance funds and also to the implementation of the recommendations of the Concerted Action in Health Care concerning the level of performance, effectiveness and efficiency in health care. This surely implies a general enhancement of the power of scientific evidence in policy making. The very government coalition that passed these laws, however, abolished the Concerted Action in Health Care, while keeping the Advisory Council with its previous obligations.

A LOOK ACROSS THE FENCE: EXAMPLES OF CROSS-BORDER LEARNING
FOR AND FROM GERMAN EXPERIENCE

This section employs a comparative perspective, focusing in particular on the process of cross-border learning in German health politics. This variant of comparative analysis essentially starts by posing the following questions: What has Germany learned from other countries' experience, particularly from the U.S. experience with market-type reforms? What have other countries— particularly the post-Soviet states in Central and Eastern Europe—learned from the German experience with the functioning of its Bismarck Model of social insurance?

Foreign Role Models in German Health Policy Debates

The claim that the German health policy debate is influenced by the experience of health care systems of other countries fortunately need not rest on subjective impressions or observations alone. Zentner and Busse analyzed the references to foreign health care systems during the debate on the Health System Modernization Act of 2004 (previously mentioned; Zentner and Busse 2004, 24–34). Their analysis is based on a model of the policy process, starting with ideas, followed (at times) by a pilot project carried out at the local or institutional level, leading to a process of legislation (involving again several steps), and culminating in the implementation and practical application of the law and possibly in a—more or less formal—form of evaluation.

In the empirical analysis, they concentrated on the legislative phase (June 2003 through November 2003), analyzing official documents, protocols of five parliamentary hearings, and 195 written statements. The aim was to find out which (industrial) countries were mentioned to support or reject a particular reform element of the Health System Modernization Act of 2004. The study measures the frequency with which particular countries' experience was cited and also the frequency with which specific reform proposals were mentioned by specific actors.

Foreign experience was mentioned 332 times. The major reference countries were the United States and Switzerland (each was mentioned in 22 percent of country-specific references), the United Kingdom (11 percent), and France (9 percent). The other countries account for less than 4 percent of the references.

Among the specific reform proposals, the British National Institute of Health and Clinical Excellence (NICE), which basically provided the model for the Institute for Quality and Efficiency (Institut für Qualität und Wirtschaftlichkeit im Gesundheitswesen, IQWiG), was the most referenced with ninety-three referrals, followed by mail-order pharmaceuticals with seventy-two referrals. The other reform proposals were mentioned distinctly less often. What may surprise some is that 28 percent of written and oral statements submitted for the hearings made reference to health care systems of other countries.

Zentner and Busse conclude: "The reference to international experience has become a standard instrument of German politics and actors; [. . . however,] models derived from other countries are thus, firstly, adapted to the German context which is characterized by federalist and corporatist structures and cultural values . . . Experiences of other countries serve, secondly, also as a powerful instrument to assert health policy interests" (2004, 33).

The case example cited is by no means unique. Reference to other countries' experience has a long tradition in German health policy debates. But it is my impression that since 1990 this trend has become more pronounced, as noted in this volume's Introduction. Some specific legislative measures that are in effect, or still under discussion, and that clearly are based on foreign influences include diagnosis-related groups (DRGs), for which Germany adopted the Australian variant (AR-DRGs); disease management programs (U.S. influence); primary care along the Dutch model (with gatekeeping general practitioners); capitated contributions (along with tax subsidies for lower-income individuals) in line with Swiss practice (under discussion in the middle of this decade); and case management methods as practiced in the United States. Reference to cross-national learning would be incomplete without mentioning the increasing influence of the European Union on individual nations' health policy (Riesberg, Weinbrenner, and Busse 2003, 36).

The German Model (Bismarck Model) as a Blueprint for Reforms in Central and Eastern Europe

Multiple causes account for the fact that all ten countries that gained membership in the European Union in 2005 have discarded their former centralized health care systems. Most, if not all, replaced that model with a pluralistic model based generally on social health insurance principles (Bismarck Model).

Among these causes we find, first, historical ties and traditions in particular for some countries formerly part of the Austro-Hungarian Empire; second, distrust of centralized government structures based on experiences during Communist rule; and third, the expectations of the powerful group of physicians to increase their incomes (as is the case in countries with social health insurance systems) via the application of a fee-for-service system of remuneration (Busse 2002, 41–50).

There is considerable variance in the specific form of financing, production, and organization of health care in the ten countries. Only Latvia has relied on pure tax financing for its health insurance funds. All others employ a mix of contributions (which cover about 65 percent of total health care expenditures), co-payments, and other forms of individualized (often sub-rosa, or under the table) payments to individual providers (Busse 2002, 50).

The return to the social health insurance principle thus appears to be based not only on the current influence of Germany in Central and Eastern European (CEE) countries but perhaps no less importantly on the historic evolution of ties with Germany and Austria. Since the start of the twenty-first century the influence of other countries' experience has become more evident. "[In this context] there is not only special interest [among CEE countries] in the health reforms in Germany, but also developments in the Netherlands, in Switzerland, in Scandinavia, in the USA and in Canada play a major role" (Knieps 2002, 38).

Recent experience of the CEE countries with their variants of SHI systems have reflected problems of financing resulting from major economic transition and economic stagnation as well as with organization and control. Most of these problems—and perhaps some others—would also have arisen if they had moved from their centralized systems more in the direction of a national health service model (Beveridge Model).

For the focus of this chapter, the point can be made that there has been an extensive process of transfer of health policy ideas from Germany (and other countries) to CEE and other post-Soviet states since the nineteen-nineties. This trend is likely to continue.

Some Conclusions
EVIDENCE VERSUS INTERESTS AND POWER IN THE POLICY-MAKING PROCESS

More than a quarter century's experience with cost-containment policies and, more generally, with the legislative process of change in health care ought to give rise to some lessons about the role of evidence, consumer choice, and the process of resource allocation in the area of health care.

In an open society, the policy process in the area of health care is essentially—and must necessarily be—a "public" process. The media— "published opinion"—play a major role in determining the way in which the success or failure of policies is judged and thereby in influencing public acceptance (or rejection) of cost-saving and other measures. By the same token, the reform process is an eminently political process.

In the German context, the legitimacy and acceptability of drastic measures of cost containment or of structural change is vastly greater if it is a bipartisan or even "multipartisan" effort. For most of the 1980s and 1990s, health reforms reflected a compromise between the liberal-conservative governing coalition (CDU/CSU and FDP) and the SPD. The situation changed somewhat when the Red-Green Coalition (SPD-Green) was voted into office in late 1998. Some subsequent reform proposals faced the opposition of the parties out of power (CDU/CSU and FDP). On the other hand, the new coalition rescinded some of the earlier measures with the stated aim of restoring and reinvigorating the social insurance principles upon which the German social health insurance system has been based. Its version of structural reform (the Health Care Reform Act of 2000) sought to stabilize and improve the system without recourse—as was the case with earlier laws—to benefit exclusions or increases in co-payments. Only three years later, however, the Health System Modernization Act of 2004 returned to the consensus process. And in the ruling Grand Coalition, former antagonists have been obliged to arrive at a consensus, whether they like it or not.

Interest groups play a major role in German health policy making. They represent a broad spectrum of opinion from outright opposition (including public campaigns against anticipated legislation or even against the implementation of specific elements of existing laws) to implicit or explicit support. The policy process involves elements of a dialogue or even of implicit bargaining between major actors and the political parties. Generally, the earlier these actors are involved in the process leading up to a new reform act, the more likely is their acceptance of the measures ultimately arrived at (though even then there may be exceptions).

The same lesson applies to the process of gathering evidence in the context of systematic research. When conflicting interests of different policy makers and groups are involved, the research is well advised to include them in the conception and conduct of the study. While this inclusion in the early steps surely makes a researcher's life more difficult in the short run, it improves the odds of acceptance of the evidence generated at a later stage.

There has been a trend towards an increase in consumer choice, leading also to an increase in competition for consumers' favor. This process was given its real momentum by the 1993 act. However, there is serious concern lest the broader goals of the social health insurance system (utilization solely on the basis of need and financing on the basis of the ability to pay, resulting in major distributional effects in favor of the old, the sick, women, families with children, and lower-income groups) will be watered down or even dissolved if consumer choice is extended further. Accordingly, a careful balancing of the advantages and risks of consumer choice will have to be part and parcel of future deliberations about the social health care system. Meanwhile, the role of intermediaries and of consumer advocacy can and must undoubtedly be expanded.

The debate about competition-based versus command-and-control-based models for resource allocation somehow does not take into account the central experience of Germany since the mid-1970s. Simply, both elements coexist in a mixed form in Germany's health care system. Indeed, it is arguable that both elements must be present if we are to pursue multiple objectives at the same time (more distributional equity in the provision of health care as well as greater efficiency in the production of health goods). For example, the Health Care Structure Act of 1993 combined extensive use of budgeting with an increase in consumer choice for insurance fund members. Furthermore, it is fairly well established that even the more extensively competition-based systems require a regulatory framework that defines the forms and limits of competition. As I shall point out in my concluding comments, the evidence available from cross-national comparisons cannot be cited as proof of the superiority of market reform as vehicles of cost containment. And I would add that the same observation also applies to the specific case of competition as an instrument to improve efficiency.

Evidence certainly plays a major role in the process of policy formulation and in the process of "societal bargaining" that precedes the enactment of legislation or follows its implementation. However, every interest group uses information—not surprisingly—in a fashion conducive to self-interest, however defined. There are, therefore, radically different qualities of information present in the public debate or in what I have described as "published opinion."

Information gathering—and its dissemination even more so—is a major part of the competitive process. Information itself becomes a commodity to be bought and sold, and there is therefore a premium on "objective" information. By definition, such information should be gathered by agencies not immediately party to the resource-allocation process. It is scientific and scholarly sources (universities, research institutes, and the like) that come closest to this requirement. As was pointed out and is worth noting, in Germany since 1985 the Advisory Council for Concerted Action in Health Care has been charged with providing economic and medical guidelines in support of a more rational process of resource allocation. While initial experience with the implementation of its recommendations was mixed, it can be shown that all major elements of the 1993 act appeared earlier in one of the council's annual reports.

As described in this chapter, the "why" of health reforms has mostly to do with presumed financial, economic, or political necessities as perceived by the government in power. The "how" of health policy formulation, however, is often guided by evidence, information, and policy advice. But even this process is "political" in the sense that the interests of the actors involved strongly influence the conception and implementation of particular measures.

In my experience, health policy formulation in the practice of a parliamentary democracy generally entails a quarrel within Parliament between political parties, but also outside Parliament between lobbies, associations, and interest groups, and between scientific and policy advisors favoring competing and sometimes conflicting reference models. These processes within and outside Parliament are interlinked. For the extra-parliamentary actors, at the surface, the quarrel is about competing goals, competing instruments, and competing organizational arrangements. But behind this visible quarrel about goals, instruments, and organizations, there are different interests and, linked thereto, different worldviews (Weltanschauungen) about cause-effect relationships or—in the language of science—between different reference models and the diagnoses and therapies related thereto.

Not surprisingly, many observers complain about the seemingly chaotic nature of the process. The dynamics of health policy formulation seemingly follow no consistent concept but are driven mainly by what is perceived as short-run political necessity. In Germany, this picture may be explained by three main "drivers." First, health policy formulation fails to appear as a consistent and complete exercise following an overall concept since in practice it is the result of political coalition: The interests and perceptions of different interest groups and parties combine in intra- or extra-parliamentary coalitions. This results in what appears to be a pragmatic compromise of seemingly opposite elements rather than a totally consistent whole. The reason for such an outcome is evident: If every party to a compromise were to derive its demands from an overall, consistent ideology, compromises would become well-nigh impossible. But compromises are often made, as long as they do not compromise the core goals of the actors. A policy of "muddling through" must thus be seen as the logical outcome of the pre-existing, fragmentized pattern of power and interest.

Second, there is a fundamental reason for outcomes judged as suboptimal by any particular goal. In health policy, several goals are being pursued simultaneously that are often only partly consistent. Almost all major German health reform laws of the last two decades address not one but several different issues. Third, a good part of policy making can be seen as a response to short-term political necessity. Laws designed to stabilize contribution rates in election years (preceded by exclusion of some benefits, by increased co-payments, and so on) are typical examples of such measures.

Quite apart from these eminently "political" reasons for the limitations of a clear-cut, comprehensive, and consistent transfer of scientific evidence into policy making, there always remain the restrictions within the scientific evaluation itself. Whitehead and others put these rather succinctly emphasizing "the complexity of evaluating policy change because so many other factors are changing at the same time. Furthermore, it is often difficult to separate the impact of the policy from underlying trends" (Whitehead, Gustafsson, and Diderichsen 1997, 938). But it is for these reasons that more stringent methods, particularly experimental or quasi-experimental designs, are called for as a basis for the evaluation of studies.

For men and women of practical affairs who wish to go beyond purely "political" arguments, at the bottom line there always remains the question: What else, if not scientific evidence (for all of its limitations), is one to use when formulating health policy? Evidently this field of human endeavor, too, requires a learning process, consisting of a step-by-step journey, albeit (with hope) in the right direction. In this limited sense, I agree with Murray and Frank's conclusion about the general desirability of building an evidence base over time. "The evidence base is a long-term investment that will require a steady process of refinement and application of measurement methods. Assessment and performance of health systems with the best available evidence will fuel this development" (Murray and Frank 2001, 1700). Unfortunately, this caveat was not given sufficient attention when the authors attempted to rank countries (as will be commented on later in this chapter).

SOME LESSONS LEARNED FROM TAKING A COMPARATIVE PERSPECTIVE

The dictum often applies to international comparisons: What you (think you) see is not what you get (after a more painstaking inquiry). In other words, what strikes you at first sight as a significant aspect of another country's health care system—or a major point of difference when compared to your own—becomes more abstruse on closer inspection.

There are therefore not many easy lessons to be learned. And the lure of simple generalizations can lead one astray. The reason may be found in the presence of one or more fallacies or else in the application of an inadequate methodology. (See Appendixes 4A and 4B.)

Appendix 4A: Fallacies in International Comparisons

On reflection about the discussions characterizing many international meetings (including the Four Country Conferences), I come up with an—admittedly subjective—listing of at least six actual or apparent fallacies.

1. The fallacy of definitions: Some words unambiguously translated with the help of a dictionary simply do not mean the same thing in the context of different countries (for example, "primary care" or even "medical specialists").

2. The fallacy of comparing parts at the neglect of the whole: The division of labor within countries' health care systems differs. As a consequence, comparing particular subsystems across countries may lead to erroneous conclusions if the role of that subsystem in the overall network is ignored. For example, looking at infant mortality rates in hospitals may lead to false conclusions when one neglects the fact that, say, in one country almost all child births occur in hospitals while in another country it is customary that most children are born at home.

3. The fallacy of the implicit ceteris-paribus assumption: When a particular dimension or aspect is used for comparisons, quite often it is assumed that the ceteris-paribus assumption holds. The impact of not explicitly considered variables on the target variable is thereby simply ignored. Ideally, statistical analyses should eliminate all such exogenous differences for purposes of comparison. Only the impact of the "experimental variable" on the target variable should be examined. As is evident, at best this ideal can only be approximated in empirical work relying on secondary data.

4. The fallacy of either inadequate or excessive methodological rigor: Associating differences in an output or outcome variable of health processes with differences in a particular input variable—while neglecting other determinants—may lead to spurious correlations and a wrong attribution of causality. At the other extreme, relying solely on randomized controlled trials, for example, will limit the scope for international comparisons severely. Rarely if ever will decision makers in two countries consent to subject their process of health policy formulation to the rigorous requirements of a health policy researcher trying to apply criteria derived from the scientific method. Occasionally, however, such com-

parisons of policy across two countries or regions are possible. Fortunately, there are several forms of systematic inquiry available to comparative health policy researchers that do not conform to either of the extremes cited.

5. The fallacy of excessive simplification in formulating typologies: By necessity, the formulation of ideal types of health care systems entails the suppression of complexity and a concentration on central features. But what constitutes an essential aspect is often subject to a researcher's or an observer's judgment. And the latter is colored by what one wants to see. Motivation often distorts perception; excessive motivation distorts excessively. For example, the classical typology of health care systems differentiates between tax-financed systems (the Beveridge Model), contribution-financed systems (the Bismarck Model), and privately funded systems. For the third type, the United States is generally—and often rightly so—cited as a deterrent to health policy makers elsewhere. Thereby, however, the fact is neglected that the share of public health spending in the United States has reached a level that is not compatible with such a simple typology.

6. The fallacy of misplaced ideology: Individual policy makers, or even individual scholars, only too readily transfer generalized views about what works—or does not work—in society or economy in general to particular aspects of the health care system. Given the complexity of overall societies or economies, what works in one part does not necessarily work in another. Such inconsistencies are a fact of life. For example, most Western observers are convinced of the superiority of market-type competition as compared to centralized planning or collective provision. However, in most areas of health care provision, "willingness and ability to pay" cannot be accepted on social policy grounds as the sole criterion for the allocation and distribution of health services. In juxtaposition, the rejection out of hand of competitive elements in social health insurance systems would be a similar mistake, as long as the overriding health and social policy goals (in particular the goal of distributive justice) are not violated thereby. In some areas of the production of health goods (for example, pharmaceuticals and medical-technical aids), even market-type competition among providers is considered by most to be superior to monopolistic or oligopolistic market structures. Clearly, even this discussion entails the type of value judgments that are generally inspired by ideological positions. However, the researcher performing comparative analyses, to my mind, is well advised, firstly, to explicate the values or

criteria that are being applied to the task and, secondly, when in doubt to compare a country's performance with its own values laid down in its constitution and its laws.

Appendix 4B: Issues in the Application of an Inadequate Methodology

As was pointed out previously, to limit comparative research solely to the formal requirements for designing experiments (for example, randomized controlled studies) would impose severe limitations on what must be considered to be a growing field of inquiry. To repeat, reality rarely presents us with opportunities for conducting such rigorous experiments with health policy or health reforms of entire countries or regions ("deterministic causality").

However, the real world situation contains considerable variance within and across countries that can be used by the researcher for hypothesis testing. It can be treated as a quasi-experiment that allows some linking up of what (probably) is cause and effect ("probabilistic causality").

Similarly, the measurement of instrument and target variables cannot always rely on interval- or even ordinal-scaled data, even though such "objective indicators" would generally be more useful to researchers and policy makers alike. However, "subjective indicators" (employing ordinal or even nominal scales for measurement) often provide for additional and highly relevant evidence (for example, patient satisfaction with hospitals or long-term care institutions).

One of the most common methodological shortcomings of comparative analyses is the lack of sophistication in dealing with subjective indicators of health (sub)systems' performance. Typically, the attributes of a particular type of health service are investigated through survey data derived from the application of ordinal-scale measurements (for example, satisfaction with hospital services, measured on a five-point scale from very satisfied to very dissatisfied). Thereafter, a cardinal value (say, from five to one) is associated with each point of the ordinal scale; the values of individual items are summed up, divided, and compared across countries. The results lead to some considerable surprises, as was the case with a effort by the World Health Organization to rank countries.

To arrive at meaningful results, comparative studies employing subjective indicators have to successfully answer several questions:

1. The representation problem: Which attributes of a health service or good are considered to be important, and by which socioeconomic group of

the population? The attributes used to represent an object must themselves be chosen in a representative fashion. Evidently, there is no universal consensus about relevant dimensions for comparing health systems.

2. The scaling problem: What type of scale is necessary or available for measuring particular attributes?

3. The weighting problem: Which weight is to be associated with scale values (for example, nonmetric scaling procedures, such as Guttmann-Lingoes procedures)?

4. The aggregation problem: How are individual indicators to be combined to arrive at overall indicators of health system quality or performance?

As several comparative researchers have treated such questions either in a cavalier fashion or ignored them altogether, comparative health policy research has been associated with an image that it should not deserve.

By relying solely on objective indicators of health system performance, and by using the variance present in the values of those indicators in different countries, some statistical analyses can be performed that yield—at the very least—some provocative insights for health policy. An example serves to illustrate this possibility. The focus is on the relationship between exogenous factors (for example, a country's wealth and the share of the aged) as well as endogenous factors subject to policy decisions (for example, the transfer rate versus the co-insurance rate or quasi-price in financing, or the coverage rate) and health spending.

Some of the results are as follows:

1. "The analysis confirms the conventional wisdom that the major explanatory of cross-country differences in health expenditures is simply found in differences in per-capita wealth, as measured by GDP per capita . . ."

2. "In addition, differences in the share of the aged population play a minor role in helping to explain the differences found . . ."

3. "Turning to the transfer rate [=share of health expenditure paid out of public funds, that is, the converse of the (quasi-)price or co-insurance paid by the individual at point of utilization of health services]: The results . . . clearly contradict the theoretical propositions derived from microeconomic demand theory about the rationing function of prices and cost sharing. Countries with higher transfer rates are not generally characterized by higher expenditures, and countries with a preponderance of private funding generally do not have lower expenditures than countries which rely more on public sources of funds. Furthermore, countries

characterized by more universal coverage generally show lower expenses than those with less universal coverage."

4. "[T]he record thus far cannot be cited . . . as proof of the superiority of market reforms as vehicles of cost containment . . ."

5. "Evidently, a greater degree of public penetration offers a better chance for control of health spending, particularly in periods of austerity" (Pfaff 1990, 20–22).

The most severe restriction on this type of systematic inquiry is found in the paucity of comparable and reliable time series for a multitude of countries. This paucity results from the fact that different institutions employing different statistical conventions are collecting the data; they treat some aspects of health care provision differently. However, substantial inroads are being made to redress this deficiency.

Till then, the truism continues to hold that the best baker is helpless if he lacks the ingredients to bake the pie.

References

Biller-Adorno, N., R. K. Lie, and R. TerMeulen. 2003. Evidence-based medicine as an instrument for rational health policy. *Health Care Analysis* 10 (3): 261–75.

Busse, R. 2002. Health care systems in EU pre-accession countries and European integration. *Arbeit und Sozialpolitik*, 5–6: 41–50.

Klein, R. 2003. Evidence and policy: Interpreting the Delphic oracle. *Journal of the Royal Society of Medicine* 96 (9): 429–31.

Knieps, F. 2002. Osteuropa: Zwischen Altlast und Aufbruch. *Gesundheit und Gesellschaft* 5 (2): 31–39.

Lauterbach, K. 1998. Chancen und Grenzen von Leitlinien in der Medizin. *Zahnärztliche Fortbildung—Qualitätssicherung (ZaeFQ)*, 92: 99–105.

Murray, C., and J. Frank. 2001. World health report 2000: A step towards evidence-based health policy. *Lancet* 357 (9269): 1698–1700.

Niessen, L. W., W. M. Grijseels, and F. F. H. Ruttens. 2000. The evidence-based approach in health policy and health care delivery. *Social Science and Medicine* 51 (6): 859–69.

Norheim, O. F. 2002. The role of evidence in health policymaking: A normative perspective. *Health Care Analysis* 10 (3): 309–17.

Pawson, R. 2002. Evidence-based policy: In search of a method. *Evaluation* 8 (2): 157–81.

Pfaff, M. 1990. Differences in health care spending across countries: Statistical evidence. *Journal of Health Policy, Politics and Law* 15 (1): 1–68.

Pfaff, M., and A. O. Kern. 2005. Public-private mix for health care in Germany. In *The public-private mix for health,* ed. A. Maynard, 191–218. Oxford, UK: Nuffield Trust and Radcliffe Publishing.

Riesberg, A., S. Weinbrenner, and R. Busse. 2003. Gesundheitspolitik im europäischen Vergleich: Was kann Deutschland lernen? *Aus Politik und Zeitgeschichte,* 33–34: 29–38.

Shadish, Jr., W. R., T. D. Cook, and L. C. Leviton. 1991. *Foundations of program evaluation: Theories of practice.* London: Sage Publications.

Weinmann, J., and N. Zifonum. 2004. Gesundheitsausgaben und Gesundheitspersonal 2002. In *Wirtschaft und Statistik,* 4: 449–62.

Whitehead, N., R. A. Gustafsson, and F. Diderichsen. 1997. Why Sweden is rethinking its NHS-style reforms. *BMJ,* 315: 935–39.

Zentner, A., and R. Busse. 2004. Das Ausland in aller Munde: Eine systematische Analyse zum Einfluss anderer Gesundheitssysteme auf die deutsche Reformdebatte. *Gesundheits- und Sozialpolitik,* 9–10: 24–34.

The Netherlands
From Polder Model to Modern Management

KIEKE G. H. OKMA AND AAD A. DE ROO

This chapter focuses on how managers in Dutch health insurance and health care have addressed the challenges of a rapidly changing business environment. It starts with a brief description of health care in the Netherlands at the beginning of the twenty-first century. That system shares some features with other European countries, but it also has particular characteristics. For example, the long tradition of health care funded and provided by nongovernment actors has shaped the administrative arrangements still visible today.[1] The typical Dutch neocorporatist policy-making style, with extensive consultations with organized interest groups, often bears the label of the Dutch Polder Model. It has traditionally limited the ability of government to introduce major change without support of the main stakeholders. However, institutional change in the policy arena—in particular the elimination of direct stakeholder representation in advisory bodies in the 1990s— has eased the way for the government to pass through major policy change with less resistance than in earlier times.

The chapter next discusses the (only partially implemented) reform proposals of the 1980s and 1990s. As in other industrialized countries, the oil crises and economic stagnation in the 1970s triggered extensive debate on the future of the welfare state. With some delay, the debate also turned to a reassessment of health care funding, contracting, and governance. The reform proposals of the 1980s reveal a major shift in ideological thinking.[2] After decades, if not centuries, of consensual policy making combined with widely accepted government control, the focus shifted to models of individualized and decentralized decision making. While those health reforms did not succeed directly, they helped change the political climate and opened the way for new forms of private care that did not have much public support before. Managers in health insurance and in health care adjusted their attitudes and behavior in reaction to—and in anticipation of—announced government policies even while some of that policy was never implemented. And once such changed behavior became visible and generally accepted, it also encouraged the government to change its course and to take up reform proposals that failed in the 1990s. In 2005, with surprisingly little political debate or public opposition, Dutch Parliament passed a law that introduced a new form of population-wide health insurance. In essence, the law was similar to earlier proposals that had failed to gain lasting public and political support. But it meant a further push towards privatization of health insurance. The chapter characterizes the positions of patients and consumers: they, too, face new options, and have reacted in quite different ways.

The Dutch experience illustrates that health policy making takes place within the constraints of national traditions, national culture, and national institutions. Formally stated policies can differ substantially from actual developments. Sometimes, even after passing formal law, the government changed its actual implementation for a variety of reasons. This experience confirms the importance of clearly distinguishing policy proposals as announced plans from implemented ones. Terms such as "policy" or "health care reform" are usually poorly defined.[3] Moreover, policy proposals unacceptable at one time gain support later as some of the main stakeholders change positions and show anticipatory behavior.

The chapter describes how government policy interacts with the behavior of groups affected by that policy. Announced reforms (even partially implemented) and anticipatory behavior by health providers and insurers alike have reshaped the Dutch health care landscape and opened the way for new directions in government policy.[4] Still, new developments are tested against strong popular support for universal access without undue barriers, as well by a strong sense of social equality in Dutch society. Both public and private actors feel the restraint of such cultural factors and are quick to assure the Dutch population that innovation will not lead to erosion of solidarity. When facing public outcry over developments that are generally seen as unfair, the government is quick to act and impose restrictions or to reverse its policies.

One important finding regards the time dimension of policy change. Policy ideas take time, sometimes much time, to "mature" and to transform into programs, legislative steps, and policy measures. Policy proposals that were unacceptable in Dutch society at one time became more acceptable in a later period.

As a matter of interest, the partially implemented health reforms of the 1980s and 1990s and the new 2006 health insurance did not replace existing governance models or policy directions. Since the early 1980s, successive governments have emphasized the need for more competition in Dutch health care and health insurance. At the same time, the government has kept, if not strengthened, its position in the health care arena to safeguard universal access to health insurance without undue financial barriers, to monitor health insurers and the quality of health services, to stimulate innovation and to support the development of patient information. The Ministry of Health (MoH) continued to seek close collaboration with organized stakeholders, in particular the national association of health insurers, the medical association, other provider groups, and in some cases, the federation of patients' associations to realize its policy goals. It is noteworthy that the elimination of direct interest group representation in the "neocorporatist" policy arena has not led to more adversarial relations between the government and those groups. The main organized stakeholders have shown great willingness to sit down with the government and share the responsibility over a wide range of policy issues. Thus decentralized decision making, strengthened state control, and continued "consensual policymaking" (Lijphart 1968) in Dutch health politics go hand in hand (Okma 1997a).

There are different ways of framing general conclusions about that experience. For example, some authors use the term "shifting discourse" to indicate major shifts in ideological thinking or shifting paradigms in social policy (Grit and Dolfsma 2002). Others emphasize the importance of "policy learning" of stakeholders that can lead to a greater willingness and capacity to accept and actually implement policy change (Helderman et al. 2005). Still another notion is that of "institutional complementarity" (Helderman 2007). The common element in those approaches is that they provide a vocabulary to help understand the current landscape of health care and health insurance in the Netherlands. It is an interesting and complicated mix of state control and deregulation, of patient autonomy and paternalistic government, of market competition and market concentration, of individual choice and collective action, and of universal health insurance and rapidly growing collective, employment-based health insurance arrangements. But the current landscape not only reveals a succession of policy directions, it feels like an erratic layering of broken and partially overlapping continental shelves that continue to move and that are not stable. Managers have to find their way through this volcanic and uneven landscape of diverging policy directions.

Common Principles and Diverging Administrative Arrangements in European Health Care

Most Western European countries share the same basic underlying principles of their health care systems: universal (or near-universal) access to health services and health insurance, equity (or fairness) in payments by patients and insured, and good quality of services (OECD 1992, 1994,).[5] As the major share of health funding is public, cost control has become one of the overriding concerns of governments as well. Beyond that, most industrialized nations regard patient satisfaction and patient choice, as well as professional autonomy of physicians, as important goals.[6]

Nonetheless, there is a wide variety in administrative arrangements for the funding, contracting, and governance of health care. In all countries of Western Europe (and North America), social health insurances and general taxation (including tax expenditures and tax subsidies) provide the largest share of health care funding. In the United Kingdom, Italy, Spain, and the Scandinavian countries, the main funding source is general (earmarked) taxation; in Austria, Belgium, Germany, France, Luxembourg, and the Netherlands, the main funding source is social health insurance. Germany and the Netherlands (until 2006) restrained access to social health insurance to groups with incomes below a certain ceiling. Higher income groups had to seek coverage in the private market. Germany (since 1994) and the Netherlands (since 1968) have separate population-wide social insurance schemes for long-term care. The two countries share several institutional features of health care funding, contracting, and governance. Both systems are, in fact, hybrids between the employment-based Bismarck Model and the universal Beveridge Model; they combine employment-related schemes with population-wide health insurance. In both countries—similar to other European ones—the population strongly supports universal access to health care, and expects government to safeguard that access, regardless how. The European countries combine, in varying degrees, public health care and other services run and owned by government with self-employed health professionals and other independent providers, both non-profit and for-profit. There is also wide variety in the dominant modes of governance.

Specific Characteristics of Dutch Health Care

Aside from the elements Dutch health care shares with other European countries, there are three important characteristics that traditionally set it apart: (1) the relatively high share of private funding, (2) the long tradition of private provision of care, and (3) the typical Dutch consensual style of social policy (the Polder Model).

The first important characteristic is the predominance of private funding. Until January 2006, the mandatory sickness fund insurance Ziekenfondswet (ZFW) covered about two-thirds of the Dutch population. The ZFW entitlements included acute medical care in hospitals and by general physicians, prescription drugs, and some other entitlements. One-third could opt to take out voluntary private health insurance. In all other OECD member states, with the exception of the United States, the share of privately insured persons was (and is) much smaller. Though private insurance was voluntary, the rate of noninsurance was only about 1 percent of population (MoH 1996).

Box 5.1 The 2006 Dutch health care changes

In 2006, Dutch health care changed dramatically with the introduction of a new health insurance law, Zorgverzekeringswet (Zvw), that replaced the former public and private health insurance schemes.* As of January 2006, all residents have to take out basic health coverage with any of the forty or so insurers of their choice. Insurers have to accept any applicant for that basic coverage. The "invisible" part of contribution is the insurance charge levied by employers as earmarked taxation and channeled via the Tax Department. This amount covers about 50 percent of their revenue. For the remaining 50 percent of their income, insurers charge a flat-rate premium directly to their insured. Premiums may differ between insurance companies, but not between individuals who have selected the same plan. To compensate for risk differences in their portfolio (for example, when they have a relatively high share of elderly or chronically ill patients), insurers receive extra funding so that, in theory, they will focus less on selecting the most profitable clients. The assumption is that premium levels solely reflect variations in efficiency or quality. Patients pay modest user fees. Out of the total amount of €50 billion (€=euros) of health expenditure in 2007 (or about €3,000 per person per year), €46.4 billion came out of tax and insurance contributions, and patients paid €3.9 billion in user fees (less than 10 percent of total health expenditure). On average, the insured paid about €1,000 per year for the Zvw directly to their insurer, about €1,000 for the income-related contribution for the

Zvw, and €980 for the long-term care insurance, Algemene Wet Bijzondere Ziektekosten (AWBZ; Ministry of Health 2006). Low-income groups can apply for fiscal subsidy and about six million (out of sixteen million) Dutch citizens are eligible to do so.**

The new scheme aims to strengthen market competition in Dutch health care and to create a "level playing field" for sick funds and private insurance. In a striking departure from earlier reform proposals (discussed later in the chapter), it removed the not-for-profit requirement of health insurance. A second major change is that the scheme cannot legally be labeled as "social insurance"; all residents are required to take out insurance but are not automatically registered as beneficiaries.

---

* There is no agreement on the question of whether the new health insurance is, in fact, public or private. The only authority to determine its nature is the European Court of Justice, which will only give a ruling if someone brings a case to court. Such a case has not (yet) happened. At first, the Dutch government presented the new insurance model as private, but when it realized that such privatization might be in conflict with several international treaties that prescribe that governments must safeguard coverage of a minimum share of populations by social insurance, it reversed its position and labeled the scheme public. There are no universally agreed-upon definitions of "public" and "private" insurance, but "social insurance" usually means mandatory participation for certain population groups, income-related contributions, non-means-tested use of health care. and government control of entitlements, contribution rates. and other conditions (e.g., not-for-profit status of sick funds).

** For the purpose of the basic health insurance, 40 percent of Dutch families or six million out of a population of sixteen million qualify as "low-income" and are eligible for tax subsidy. For the administration of this subsidy, the Tax Department had hired over 600 staff to check the incomes of the recipients every month. In 2007, the Ministry of Health announced it would simplify the procedures to reduce the administrative burden.

The second important characteristic of Dutch health care is the dominance of private provision of services.[7] Like other Western European countries, the Netherlands has a long tradition of voluntary, nongovernmental organizations providing collective goods. Their origins trace back to medieval guilds offering financial protection to their members in case of illness or death and to local communities, churches, and monasteries setting up hospitals for the homeless, the elderly, the sick, and the mentally ill (De Swaan 1988). That tradition of public services by nongovernment actors is still visible in the early 2000s. Most Dutch hospitals and other health care institutions are owned and run by charities, nonprofit foundations, and religious orders, even while waves of hospital mergers in the 1980s and 1990s have blurred their denominational backgrounds.

State intervention in Dutch health care was modest until the Second World War, largely limited to public health measures, consumer protection, and the regulation of health professionals. In the first three postwar decades of reconstruction and the development of the modern welfare state, successive governments stepped in by mandating sickness fund membership for low-income wage earners. This expanded the scope and coverage of social health insurance. The state also expanded its role in the allocation of resources and planning of health facilities. As a logical consequence, this led as well to efforts to strengthen government control over health expenditures. However, the management of health facilities remained largely nongovernmental. Most general practitioners, dentists, and physiotherapists continued to practice as self-employed health professionals. Policy shift of the 1980s and 1990s—inspired by a general ideological preference for more market competition and less government intervention—also encouraged the expansion of for-profit health care and for-profit health insurance. That shift does not sit easily with the tradition of not-for-profit organizations sharing the responsibility over the shaping of social policy with the government. Dutch hospitals and other providers suddenly have to act like market players, a role in which they do not always feel comfortable (Rosenberg 2006, 2007).

The third important characteristic of Dutch health care has been its tradition of neocorporatist policy making (Lijphart 1968; Hill 1993; Schut 1997; Okma 1997a). In the 1950s and 1960s, the health care system expanded through the creation of a wide array of advisory bodies, with formal representation of many interest groups. In those bodies, health insurance agencies and providers of care held a dominant position. Ironically, this form of engagement of all the major stakeholders in the shaping and implementation of social policy—sometimes labeled the Dutch Polder Model in reference to the centuries-long tradition of collective action to keep the Low Lands below sea level dry by building dykes and windmills and systems of decentralized water management—was vilified as one of the main contributing factors of the tenacity of the "Dutch disease" (the booming state expenditure based on the windfall of natural gas and oil revenues) in the 1980s as a main cause of stagnating economic growth and high unemployment. Then again, it was heralded as the "Dutch miracle" when in the 1990s, economic growth turned higher (and unemployment lower) than in neighboring countries in Europe (Visser and Hemereyk 1997). The system provided veto power to organized interests that enabled them to block proposals they felt detrimental to their status or incomes (De Roo 1995). In several instances, that veto power derailed or slowed down planned or announced health reforms. At the same time, the involvement of a wide array of private organizations also contributed to the remarkable stability of Dutch politics.

In the 1980s, inspired by debates about a broader reassessment of the Dutch welfare state, there was mounting criticism of the Polder Model. The critics emphasized its ample opportunity for organized interests to slow down, thwart, or veto government policy altogether (Visser and Hemereyk 1997). In the early 1990s, Dutch Parliament commissioned a study on the role of advisory bodies and found there were several hundred expert committees in the domain of health policy alone. The Parliament decided to reduce drastically the number and size of those external bodies (as well as its own standing committees) and to eliminate stakeholder representation altogether (Okma 1997a). The change in this advisory structure also meant that the scope for organized interests to influence health policy sharply declined. The relatively easy passing of the 2006 Health Insurance Law illustrates that the dismantling of the neocorporatist structures has made life easier on the government. Substantially, the law is very similar to the earlier Dekker reform proposals of the late 1980s that failed largely because of stakeholder opposition. It pushed the market orientation even further by allowing for-profit health insurers to offer the basic insurance. In 2005, when the new law passed Parliament, there was remarkably little public debate or opposition to the proposals. The Senate, or First Chamber of Parliament, even passed the bill in one day (the day before summer recess), a stunningly short time for passing such far-reaching change in social health insurance.

However, the Polder Model mentality has not completely disappeared. Associations of health providers and other organized interests still show a remarkable willingness to sit down with the government and to discuss social policy (even while their members do not always adhere to informal agreements). The 2007 budget document (MoH 2006) for health care mentions several efforts where the Ministry of Health has joined forces with stakeholders to realize policy goals of increased quality, efficiency, and cost control. The ministry has taken the lead in the development of a countrywide electronic patient record but works together with other parties in health care. It encourages collaboration between acute hospital care and ambulatory care (while also creating conditions for greater competition) and provides subsidy for education, experiments to improve efficiency of care, and innovation of general practice (while emphasizing the importance of the private sector). The "covenant" illustrates the close ties between government and private associations in Dutch social policy-making. Covenants play a major role in Dutch social policy (Klee and Okma 2001). Less than formal law and more than an

> Box 5.2 *Characteristics of Dutch health care*
>
> With a population of 16 million, the Netherlands has over 100 general hospitals, 9 teaching hospitals, and 34 specialized hospitals (data for 2002). The 7,000 or so general practitioners work in 3,500 GP offices and act in principle, if not always in practice, as gatekeepers to secondary and tertiary care by prescribing drugs and referring patients to hospitals and specialist care. The long-term care insurance, Algemene Wet Bijzondere Ziektekosten (AWBZ), created in 1968, fueled a surge of investment in nursing homes, psychiatric hospitals, and other long-term care facilities. In the early 2000s, the system of long-term care included 76 psychiatric hospitals, with a capacity of 25,000 beds, and 148 regional institutions for ambulatory psychiatric care. There are over 1,000 retirement homes, with 115,000 residents, and 326 nursing homes and psycho-geriatric institutions totaling over 55,000 residential places. The 130 or so facilities for patients with severe mental disabilities cater to almost 34,000 residents. Finally, over 140 home-care organizations (both nonprofit and for-profit) provide extensive home nursing and home help. They serve over 600,000 clients per year.

informal agreement, the government regards covenants as a convenient way to engage and involve major stakeholders in realizing its goals. For example, when the actual expenditure for hospitals surpassed the budget estimates in 2004, the Ministry of Health signed a covenant with the hospital association and national association of health insurers (*Rijksbegroting 2007*). There are similar covenants with pharmacists and the pharmaceutical industry (MOH 2005).

Box 5.2 and Table 5.1 provide a brief overview of the core characteristics and financial data on Dutch health care. The budget for total health care expenditures in 2007 surpasses €50 billion, or over 9 percent of gross domestic income (MoH 2006).

Dutch Health Reform Efforts of the 1980s and 1990s

In 1987, an expert committee headed by the CEO of Philip's Electronics, Wisse Dekker, proposed a major overhaul of the Dutch health care system (Commissie Dekker 1987). The committee signaled several problems including the fragmented funding, lack of financial incentives to consumers, providers, health insurers to contain the growth of health expenditures and offer good quality care, and rigid regulation inhibiting a flexible organization of services. The committee proposed to integrate existing funding

Table 5.1 Funding sources and spending categories of Dutch health care, 2000–2007

A. Funding health care in the Netherlands, 2000–2007 (in billion euros and percentages)

Funding sources	2000	Funding sources	2006	2007
Long-term care insurance (AWBZ)	12.9 (38.0)	Long-term care insurance (AWBZ)	21.0 (44)	20.9 (41.8)
Sickness fund insurance (ZFW)	12.5 (36.9)	Basic health insurance	25.7 (48)	23.6 (47.2)
Private health insurance	4.8 (14.1)			
Government subsidy and government provision*	1.5 (4.4)	Government tax subsidy	1.9 (4.1)	1.9 (3.8)
Direct payments	2.3 (6.7)	Direct patient payments	3.9 (8.0)	3.9 (7.8)
Total	34.0 (100)	Total	46 (100)	50.1 (100)

*The total amount of tax subsidy is higher as Dutch government also provides funding for both acute care and long-term care insurance, for example, to compensate for the fact that young insured under eighteen do not pay premiums. It also covers for some overhead, the fiscal subsidy for insured since 2006, and other expenses.

B. Allocation of financial resources over subsectors of Dutch health care, 2000–2007 (in billion euros and percentages)

	2000	2006	2007
Prevention	0.7 (2.1)	0.5 (0.5)	0.05 (0)
Hospitals, general practitioners, and other medical care	13.4 (39.3)	18.7 (42.5)	18.0 (35.3)
Nursing homes, retirement homes, and home care	7.8 (23.2)	11.5 (26.1)	11.4 (22.4)
Pharmaceuticals and medical aids	3.7 (11.0)	4.9 (11.1)	6.2 (12.2)
Care for handicapped	3.0 (9.0)	5.7 (13.0)	4.9 (9.6)
Mental health care	2.8 (8.2)	3.6 (8.0)	3.6 (7.1)
Insurance, administration	2.5 (7.4)	1.2 (2.7)	1.2 (2.4)
Total	34.0 (100)	44.1 (100)	50.1 (100)

Source: MoH 1999; MoH 2006 (in 2006, one euro equaled about US$1.2; there is a small ex ante difference between total funding and total spending).

streams into one mandatory health insurance for the entire population, covering the risks of both acute medical care and long-term care.

In itself, this problem analysis was not new. Earlier reports had pointed to those weaknesses and proposed an amalgamation between private and public insurance schemes (Okma 1997a). What was new, however, was the shift in emphasis from state control to decision making by competing insurance agencies and competing providers over the allocation of (public) funding. The report reflected changing ideological views about the roles of the state and private sector (Williams 2005). It advocated strengthening the role of sick funds as third-party payers in health care and increasing consumer choice and exit. (Consumer voice, however, did get short shrift as the dismantling of advisory bodies in the early 1990s also led to the elimination of the direct representation of patient and consumer groups.) The proposals further included free choice of health insurer, reduction of the mandatory coverage of social health insurance, partial replacement of income-related contributions by community-rated nominal premiums, and options for deductibles or co-insurance in exchange for lower premiums.

The Dekker Committee wanted to reduce the role of government by deregulating the existing planning and tariff legislation. Basically, it recommended the introduction of an "internal market" within the framework of social health insurance (Schut 1997; Schut and Van de Ven 2005). This recommendation did not eliminate the role of the state in health care altogether, however, as the government would still determine the coverage of the mandatory health insurance, set the budgets of the health insurers, and monitor insurance and the quality of health services. The responsibility for negotiations over the quality and prices of health services was to shift to (competing) health care providers and (competing, but not-for-profit) health insurers.[8]

At first, the proposals caused considerable uproar in the world of Dutch health care. After lengthy debate, the Parliament accepted the proposals, and the Ministry of Health framed an ambitious four-year implementation plan for 1989 to 1992 (MoH 1988). In the end, however, it only realized a few (but important) steps. For example, ambulatory mental care, prescription drugs, and some other entitlements shifted from the public and private health insurance schemes to the long-term care insurance, AWBZ, which was to become the new universal social health insurance. The government further relaxed the rules for planning and setting fees. Other steps included the abolishment of regional boundaries of the working areas of the sick funds (so they could expand their activities countrywide and offer the Dutch insured a choice of sick fund) and selective contracting of self-employed health professionals by the funds (with the announcement that mandatory contracting of health facilities would end later). Local authorities lost control of the opening of new practices of family doctors, and tariff ceilings replaced fixed tariffs for health services. These measures increased the room for insurers to negotiate with providers over volume, price, quality of services, and to selectively contract with providers.

Erosion of Support and the Demise and Revival of Dutch Health Reforms

After the first steps of implementation of the reforms in the early 1990s, opposition of organized stakeholders resurfaced, public support eroded, and the political backing became more and more hesitant (Okma 1997a). After accepting (albeit in adjusted form) the legislation for the second reform phase in 1991, Dutch Parliament shelved the discussion over the next steps. Ultimately, this delay led to the total demise of the reforms. After general elections in 1994, a new governing coalition—consisting of the surprising combination of Conservatives (VVD), Labor Party (PvdA), and Liberal Democrats (D66)—stepped into office. For the first time in over half a century, the Christian Democrats were out of office. The governing manifesto of the new "Purple Coalition" stated that it would no longer continue the reforms but would shift to incremental adjustment of the existing system instead (*Regeerakkoord 1994*). Four years later, the same coalition continued its reign and maintained the same policy course (*Regeerakkoord 1998*). However, this time it also announced a study of the need for structural reform of the health insurance system and framed its intentions to introduce a universal basic health insurance in the policy paper "Vraag aan Bod" ("Demand at the Center," MoH 2001).

In December 2001, the Purple Coalition stepped down from office over the political fallout of the tragic events in Srebrenica, where a small and insufficiently armed battalion of Dutch soldiers were not able to defend the village's population. As they fled, the Serbian attackers murdered all 5,000 or so male Muslim inhabitants. General elections of May 2002 brought a sweeping gain for the new party Lijst Pim Fortuyn (LPF) only a few weeks after the murder of its populist leader Fortuyn. This surprising election brought the Christian Democrats (CDA) back into power, together with the Conservatives VVD and LPF. The new coalition presented its governing manifesto in June 2002 (*Strategisch Akkoord 2002*). But escalating internal conflicts led to its rapid demise. After the January 2003 elections, in spite of a large electoral gain of the PvdA, CDA and VVD switched partners and replaced the LPF with the Liberal Democrats D66. This combination, in effect, re-created the dominant coalition of the early 1980s. The new coalition presented its plans in the governing manifesto in May 2003 "Meedoen, Meer Werk, Minder Regels" ("Participation, More Work, Less Rules"; *Hoofdlijnenakkoord 2003*). In health policy, the program included a striking mix of "old" and "new" instruments: delisting of entitlements, new or increased co-payments and deductibles, strict budgetary ceilings, increased efficiency and, again, the intention to introduce a universal health insurance based on the principle of "regulated market competition" (without defining or explaining that term in detail).

The change in political coalitions and the shift from structural reform to incremental policies, however, did not kill the core elements of the Dekker reforms. In that regard, Dutch health policy has shown a remarkable degree of continuity. For example, the 1989 Cabinet continued the implementation of the new capitated budget model for sick funds (which still is in place in 2009 as the base for determining budgets for health insurers) and abandoned the territorial borderlines of the regional sick funds. In the 1990s, almost all of the thirty funds had expanded their activities countrywide. Since 1991, sick fund insured can choose to change funds. To encourage this mobility, the Dutch government has sponsored websites that enable consumers to compare health insurance policies. Initially, very few actually switched funds and until the early 2000s, mobility of insured remained very modest (Laske-Aldershof et al. 2004). The number of insured who did go to another fund changed dramatically with the introduction of the Health Insurance Law of 2006.

In contrast to earlier Dekker reform proposals, the new insurance scheme excludes the long-term care insurance AWBZ. For this segment of health care, the government initially proposed to shift budgets and decision-making power to local authorities. But in 2007, it announced a moratorium on those changes, and in early 2009 it is not yet clear what categories of services will remain under central government control.

Table 5.2 provides a brief summary of important policy steps in Dutch health care reform from the 1980s to the late 2000s. One of the interesting features is the fact that changes in political coalition do not appear to have much direct impact on health policy. For example, after the presentation of the Dekker reform plans by the Christian Democrat-Conservative coalition in 1987, the next CDA-PvdA-D66 coalition actually started to implement the plans under Deputy Minister Hans Simons. The 1994 surprise coalition that excluded the Christian Democrats formally abandoned further implementation but with a few exceptions, did not undo steps already taken; actually, it continued most of its predecessor's policies but relabeled structural reform as incremental adjustment. The comeback of the Labor Party in 2007 neither stopped nor reversed the introduction of the universal health insurance.

Table 5.2 Dutch health care reforms from 1987–2007

Year	Governing coalition	Health reform steps
1987–1989	CDA-VVD (Deputy Minister Dees)	1987 Dekker proposals: population-wide social health insurance including long-term care
1989–1994	CDA and PvdA (June 1989; Deputy Minister Hans Simons)	1991 first steps of implementation (e.g., end of regional borders of sick fund, end of local planning of general practitioners' offices)
1994–1998	First Purple Coalition: VVD, PvdA, and D66 (Minister Borst-Eilers)	Formal abandonment of Dekker reforms, but continuation of some steps; shift to incremental policy
1998–2001	Second Purple Coalition: VVD, PvdA, and D66 (Minister Borst-Eilers)	Continuation of incremental policy, announcement of feasibility study on universal health insurance
2001	Fall of Purple Coalition	
2002	CDA, VVD, and LPF (Minister Bomhoff)	Proposals for universal health insurance (excluding AWBZ) allowing for profit insurers
2003	CDA, VVD, and D66 (Minister Hoogervorst)	Continued preparation of universal (private) insurance
2004	CDA, VVD, and D66 (Minister Hoogervorst)	Second Chamber of Parliament passes (public) Basic Health Insurance Law, administered by former sick funds and private health insurers
2005	CDA, VVD, and D66 (Minister Hoogervorst)	First Chamber of Parliament passes Basic Health Insurance Law

(continued)

Table 5.2 (continued)

Year	Governing coalition	Health reform steps
2006	CDA, VVD, and D66 (Minister Hoogervorst)	January 1, 2006: Basic Health Insurance Law into effect
2007	CDA and PvdA (Minister Klink)	Continued implementation of basic health insurance, but moratorium on changes in AWBZ

The New Policy Environment Facing Managers of Dutch Health Care and Health Insurance

At the Cabinet level, there are different, competing, and conflicting policy goals dealing with employment creation, education, public infrastructure, social security, or health care. Since the 1991 Maastricht Treaty, E.U. countries have to meet budget deficit criteria for joining the European monetary system. That sets a ceiling to public spending. At this level, macroeconomic policy considerations—rather than the policy goal of improving health—are the driving forces of health policies and reform. Here, the main issue is not so much the "health of the population" but the "health of the nation's budget." One of the main policy goals has been to restrain labor costs by containing taxes and social insurance premiums (including health insurance contributions) in order to reduce unemployment. In spite of changing governing coalitions with different ideological orientations, reining in the growth of public spending has remained one of the dominant concerns since the 1980s.

Successive Dutch governments have explored a variety of cost-containment instruments—including competition in social insurance, budgetary mechanisms at different levels, delisting entitlements from social insurance, and measures aimed at restraining consumption. Budget reforms included annual spending ceilings for health expenditures (both public and private) and the allocation of financial resources over different sectors and regions, as well as setting budgets for individual hospitals, institutions, and sick funds (Scheerder 2005; MoH 1994; Van het Loo et al. 1999). One crucial change in policy direction was the shift from the underlying assumption that health care is mostly a public good with strong government responsibilities to viewing health care as a market good. The new idea is that of health services as largely private, with patients as customers and health care providers as business administrators. This difference marks, in other words, a shift from a "public administration paradigm" toward a "business paradigm" (De Roo 1993, 2002). In the 1960s and 1970s, managers of sick funds and providers acted mostly as administrators of licensed organizations, with guaranteed incomes based on public funding and legally protected domain monopolies. Strategic decisions of the licensing agency (*in casu* government) determined their playing field. Public support for the dominant position of government provided ample opportunity for rolling off financial and access problems to higher levels of hierarchy.

The (partial) creation of internal markets brought growing uncertainty over incomes and continuity of clientele. The reform legislation introduced entrepreneurial risks to players who before had enjoyed high levels of certainty and income protection. Since 1991, health insurers are receiving fixed budgets based on numbers of insured and particular risk factors instead of the open-ended reimbursement that had characterized the sick fund model of the mid-twentieth century. In a way, the new budget model heralded the restoration of independent risk-bearing insurance agencies by breaking up the wider pool of social insurance and shifting the insurance risk (back) to individual health insurers (Okma and Van der Burg 2004). In addition to the income-related contributions (levied by employers and channeled to individual funds via the Central Fund administered by the Treasury), sick funds have had to charge a (modest) flat-rate premium directly to their members since 1991. In 1997, the insured paid on average about €100 per person per year and in 2000, 170 euros (MoH 1999). Still, most of the sick fund budgets came from the common public pool.

As of January 2006, all health insurers (both the former sick funds and the private health insurers) receive a budget that covers about 50 percent of expenditure. The budget allocation criteria include numbers of insured, age, gender, and health status. This share is paid by employers as an income-related earmarked tax and by government for welfare recipients and certain categories of insured without income. For the other half of their revenue, insurers charge their customers flat-rate premiums.

The rules of the game in social policies changed, but the new rules did not replace the old ones. In the early 2000s, a certain degree of internal inconsistency in Dutch health policy emerged (perhaps reflecting a somewhat weak belief in the cost-controlling capacities of market competition in health care). The government turned its attention, once again, to a reassessment of the benefit package of social health insurances and a shift from public to private funding by delisting services and introducing or increasing deductibles, co-payments, and coinsurance (Scheerder 2005).[9] The government encouraged providers and insurers to compete but at the same time kept control over health expenditure and the allocation of public funds. In fact, the policy changes created a complicated and sometimes inconsistent overlay of governance models based on quite divergent notions of the role of the state and citizens. This also created managerial dilemmas for Dutch health care providers and insurers. They have to invest in improving services and expanding market shares but face growing uncertainty over future clients and income streams. They have to act as entrepreneurs but also have to sit down with government to discuss policy results. They compete and face increased financial risks, but the government also wants them to collaborate with their colleagues in the region. They have to attract and keep their patients and their insured, but they also have to please governments at different levels.

Managerial Response in Dutch Health Insurance

Health insurance managers in the Netherlands have tried different approaches to address those dilemmas. They sought to defend and expand their market shares and to gain strategic market positions by marketing and advertising, merging with others, and improving and expanding (sometimes contracting) their coverage.

But they did not engage in such activities evenly. In 2005 and 2006, most health insurers focused their activities on expanding or maintaining market shares rather than on negotiations with providers over quantity, quality, and prices of health services. They spent massive amounts on marketing, advertising, improved administration, and other measures to satisfy their insured, but not necessarily much more on improving the quality of services. In the years before and after the introduction of the new insurance in 2006, many insurers set their premiums below cost. On average, premiums rose about 10 percent in 2006, and experts expected a further hike in 2008 of at least 15 percent as several insurers were in the red (Smit and Mokveld 2007). The competition between insurers has clearly not yet resulted in lower prices.

While the 2006 health insurance is "mandatory," there are few effective sanctions if one does not take out insurance.[10] Moreover, private health insurers can bar someone who has not paid his or her monthly premium for over three months. In early 2007, the national association of health insurers announced that as of July, their members would start to delist delinquents. According to the rules, uninsured who would need hospital care would face the hospital bill themselves but also would have to take insurance and pay premiums retroactively. Later that year, the MoH persuaded insurers to keep the delinquents on their rolls while the parties sought a solution for the problem. After a study by the national bureau of statistics (Centraal Bureau voor de Statistiek, CBS) revealed that (predictably) young immigrants, single parents, and welfare recipients were overrepresented in this group, the government turned to another solution (CBS 2006). It announced that in the future, local welfare offices would withhold the flat-rate payments for the welfare recipients, a solution already proposed by the cities of Amsterdam and Rotterdam in 2005. Another proposal was to set up a separate risk pool for this group of uninsured, but this separation clearly would defeat the notion of a "universal" scheme (MoH 2006).

In principle, the ending of regional monopolies of sick funds encouraged competition by allowing new entrants into the social health insurance field. In practice, however, it fueled a rapid process of mergers and acquisitions that, if it did not eliminate, sharply reduced competition. In fact, this process heralded the demise of the sick fund. After providing coverage and income protection to their members for over a hundred years, independent Dutch sick funds have all but disappeared. The number of independent funds went down from over sixty in the early 1980s to thirty in 1999 (www.ZN.nl; Okma 2001). Membership ranged from a few thousand to over one million insured. In that year, there were about forty private insurers. In 2005, after a rapid process of mergers and informal collaboration between public and private insurance, there were forty-three health insurers in the Netherlands; that number dropped to thirty-one in 2007. Many of those operated as part of broader conglomerates. For example, five main health insurance groups (Achmea, VGZ-IZA, CA, Menzis, and Agis) covered eleven million insured, or over 60 percent of the Dutch population (Rengers and Van Uffelen 2005). The process of mergers and acquisitions has not yet stopped. After further consolidation and market concentration, the two largest conglomerates, VGZ-IZA and Agis-Menza, covered over 50 percent of the population. The next stage of this development has been the rise of international insurance conglomerates in the European Union offering both public and private health insurance, a development that has already made its first (but thus far not very successful) appearance. Within a few years of entering the Dutch market in the late 1990s, both the German DKV and the French AXA left again.

Some health insurers successfully focused on the market for collective insurance contracts. Almost 60 percent of those who changed their health insurance in 2006 did so as members of collective employment-based plans (Smit and Mokveld 2007). In 2007, this share had risen to over 80 percent (even though in that year less than 5 percent of the Dutch insured were switching). Clearly, there has been a trend towards collective employment-based health insurance, in a way strengthening rather than weakening the employment base of Dutch health insurance. In some cases, the collective contracting included collectivities of patients or other special groups, a new phenomenon in Dutch health care. Insurers do not have to accept every group seeking coverage, and some patient groups have been turned down. Some insurers even offered a "collective contract" for insured without access to another collectivity (Smit and Mokveld 2007). The growth of collective contracting and the strengthening of links between health insurance and other employee benefits pushed up the premiums for individual coverage (to prevent a widening of this gap, health insurers cannot offer more than a 10-percent discount. In general, people who belong to collective groups represent better risks and are more attractive to insurance companies. But thus far, there are no signs of large-scale risk selection or self-selection by insured.[11] Similar to the former private insurance market, Dutch health insurers feel bound by social norms that condemn such behavior, and they never applied risk rating that fully reflected the risk of certain groups (Okma 1997a).

Some insurers became active in efforts to reduce wait lists and waiting times by contracting for-profit clinics, pressuring hospitals to work more efficiently, and streamlining their administrations. Others offered new services, such as twenty-four-hour call centers and preferred-provider arrangements (that never became very popular with Dutch patients). In the latter option, the insured face higher charges when they prefer to go to a provider outside the contracted network of their health insurance. Some health insurers have been creative in widening their supplemental coverage by including preventive services such as sports clinics or regular checkups.

As a latest step in this development in the 1990s, insurance agencies explored forms of integration of health services. This step, in effect, led to the creation of some sort of "health maintenance organization" (HMO), the model that started in the United States in the 1970s. In a broader historical perspective, the HMO model is very similar to the traditional nineteenth-century sick funds that combined income protection arrangement for their members with the ownership of health facilities and employment of physicians. But the development of such forms of such "integrated plans" in the Netherlands has been slow.

Managerial Responses in Dutch Health Care

Providers of health care in the Netherlands are facing challenges similar to those of the health insurers. After the abolishment of mandatory contracting, insurers no longer have to contract every self-employed health professional (since 1991) or hospital (since 2005). While Dutch insurers have shown themselves reluctant to break off long-standing contract relations (to avoid angry reactions of their insured), this measure decreased the power of providers of health care. In some areas—in contrast to health insurance, where there have been few newcomers in the market—new providers entered the market offering substitutes for traditional health services. For example, the number of home care organizations went up from 170 to 264 between 1998 and 2005 (CBS 2006). After the government stopped providing loan guarantees for investments of hospitals and health facilities, they had to look for alternative funding sources in the capital markets. Under the long-term care insurance (AWBZ), patients have the option of a cash benefit instead of receiving services in kind (discussed later in this chapter). This cash benefit (the so-called *persoonsgebonden budget,* or personal budget) has shifted purchasing power to patients as they can chose to contract nontraditional services. The development of independent, expert-only assessment committees in the mid-1990s implied a further encroachment upon the professional autonomy of Dutch health care providers. At first, those assessment committees functioned under the control of local authorities, but ending this form of decentralization in the early 2000s, central government resumed control by establishing a countrywide and uniform system to assess patients' needs. All those factors have contributed to the growing income insecurity of Dutch health care providers.

Health care managers—like the health insurers—have reacted in different ways to these challenges (De Roo 2002). They tried to secure future income by attracting patients and discouraging clients from switching to rivals by improving their services. Next, they built up financial buffers to overcome lean periods. They created financial reserves by improving their efficiency, realizing economies of scale or finding substitutes for labor-intensive services. Some providers sought to differentiate and broaden their range of services, for example, by expanding office hours, opening sports clinics, and collaborating with insurers in setting up phone services. Others focused on the most promising market segments and, like insurers, reduced their financial risks by "cream skimming" of patients (selecting the wealthiest, healthiest, and cheapest groups), for example, in setting up health clinics for employees to provide rapid access. Public polls and debates in Parliament reveal strong opposition in Dutch society to such queue jumping or services limited to certain groups only. In the late 1990s, the Health Minister announced measures to limit the activities of private clinics and to prohibit those forms of preferential treatment altogether. A few years later, however, that opposition seemed to have faded. In fact, Dutch government saw the rise of private clinics or "independent treatment centers" (*zelfstandige behandelcentra,* ZBCs) as a solution to the problem of long wait lists as they added to total capacity. Not all of those centers fared well, and after a few years, some closed their doors again (see also Chapter 8 by Okma and Decter in this volume). And finally, health care providers strengthened their market position by processes of horizontal and vertical integration of their services. This strategy has become popular. Many Dutch hospitals expanded their activities by formal mergers and informal networks of similar institutions as well as collaboration with nursing homes, retirement facilities, and extramural care. In particular, providers of care for the elderly and mental health have shown themselves to be eager entrepreneurs.

Such regional collaboration has sharply reduced the number of independent providers, reducing consumer choice at the local level. In some instances, this rapid and ongoing process of market concentration has led to virtual regional monopolies, defeating pro-competitive government policies. This market concentration has also created tension between the contracting role of health insurers (based on the assumption that they negotiate with competing providers over contracts) and efforts of the Ministry of Health to encourage regional collaboration between health care services (Boot 1998).

The 1990s and early 2000s witnessed a spread of all these management approaches in Dutch health care. Health facilities reined in labor costs by differentiation of functions and by replacing qualified staff by less expensive labor (faced by budgets squeeze after the local authorities had taken on the contracting for home care services, the home care organizations dismissed thousands of workers in 2007 and 2008). They created subsidiaries to offer commercial services, shifted from standardized to customized care, and added luxury care and extended services to the standard package of benefits. Some providers ventured into new areas of health-care-related for-profit services, including extensive home care, meals on wheels, gardening, and extended home help. They reacted to critical media coverage over unduly long waiting times by working more efficiently and improving their administration.

On the financial side, hospitals and other facilities contracted out maintenance and hotel functions, and they engaged in collective purchase of medical goods. Pressured by budget restraints and new payment methods, hospitals shifted from inpatient to outpatient care, from long-term care to short interventions, from high-skilled personnel to lower-skilled (and lower-paid) labor. Finally, providers and health insurers alike engaged in risk selection and risk shifting, even while Dutch society frowns upon such activities, which sometimes provokes direct government intervention.

To illustrate these developments, Box 5.3 presents a selection of collaborative activities in Dutch health care in the early 2000s. The leading journal on health care information and finance in the Netherlands, *Zorg en Financ-*

*Box 5.3 Announced mergers, actual mergers, and divorces
in Dutch health care, 2002–03*

The regional hospital Coevorden-Hardenberg announced its intended
merger, at some time in 2004, with the Hardenberg-Gramsbergen foundation. They will become part of the larger group including the Harden-
berg hospital, day care hospital Aleida Kramer and nursing homes
Aleida Kramer, Clara Feyoena Heem, Oostloorn and 't Welgelegen. The
merger creates a strong regional position, but the hospitals and nursing
homes will "keep their own identity and culture." The Woonzorg foundation West-ZeeuwsVlaanderen consisting of woonzorgcentra Rozeno-
ord and Ter Schelde, and nursing home De Stelle will merge with care
center De Burght, the latter part of Ouderenzorg in West Zeeuws Vlaan-
deren foundation. The psychiatric hospital Duin and Bosch has signed
an agreement to merge with the regional groups for mental care RIAGG
Midden-Kennemerland and Zaanstreek/Waterland. They intend to fully
merge early 2004. In the Gooi region east of Amsterdam, existing ambulance services Broeder de Vries, the GGD and the Central Post Ambu-
lancevervoer will integrate in 2004, creating a regional ambulance
monopoly. The vegetarian nursing home Felixoord will merge with the
housing and care group Rijnoeverhoven that also includes the retirement
homes Molenberg, Overdal, Beekdal, Mooi-land, De Sonnenberg and
Heidestein. In Nijmegen, the Sint Maartenskliniek and Sport Centrum
Papendal announced their future collaboration in the area of sports-
related medical care. The health minister insisted that the merger of the
IJsselmeerziekenhuizen in Lelystad and Almere has to continue. No
other hospital has agreed to merge with either of the institutions.

. . . ARE HAPPY TO ANNOUNCE THE MARRIAGE OF . . .

CZ health insurance signed an agreement with the regional German
sickness fund AOK Rheinland. The agreement is also signed by a group
of regional hospitals. In Meppel, five housing corporations signed up
with two larger care institutions Icare and Sensire to offer a range of
housing and care services. Medisch Centrum Alkmaar, hetWestfires
Gasthuis Hoorn and Gemini hospitals created the hospital network De
Noordwester to create a common policy without a formal merger. In
contrast, all nursing homes in the Westland region have merged as of
November 2002. The Oosterschelde hospitals, Oosterschelde Home
Care and Home Care Netherlands have signed an agreement for jointly
providing transmural care. In Haarlem, mental care and addiction clinics will work together with Jeugdzorg Foundation, Salvation Army,

Box 5.3 continued

Jeugdriagg-NHz and other institutions in a regional group. In 2000, the regional sickness fund RGZ and health insurer Geové merged into the health insurance group Geové RGZ. The group has since become part of the Menzis group that also includes Amicon and Prové Reïntegration. Health insurer DSW acquired the pharmacy Ketel, opened its own pharmacy in Schiedam and announced the opening of another one.

... SADLY HAVE TO INFORM ...

The Rabobank subsidiary Interpolis broke off the joint venture (and also, the abortion of the announced full merger) with VGZ health insurance. The intended merger between Ooosterschelde Home Care and Arcus care Centra is delayed. The merger between the group practices of obstetricians of the Catharina hospital and the Máxima Medical Centre, both in Eindhoven, was cancelled. Both groups now intend to set up their own clinic (*zelfstandig behandelcentrum*). Similarly, freelance physicians and nurses created a new venture 'Skills for Care' offering health professionals serviced by the hour.

The large-scale merger of local health authorities GGD offices Rijnmond met with political hesitance to continue the collaboration. And in Brabant, the merger process of regional assessment offices (RIOs) has slowed down. In Rotterdam, mental hospital Delta and the TBS clinic De Kijvelanden cancelled merger plans as the Justice Minister refused to agree with the plans. In the east, the Neijenborch foundation had also to stop plans to integrate with other elderly care institutions because of failure to reach agreement over formal decision powers of regional group's board.

Source: *Zorg en Financiering*, various issues, 2002 to 2006.

ing, presents a regular overview of announced, failed, and implemented mergers in health care and insurance. This special rubric reads like a crossbreed between the *New York Times* wedding announcements pages and glossy magazines' pages about failing marriages and divorces.

New Roles for Patients and Consumers in Dutch Health Care

Consumers have taken a new role too. In the early 1990s, the main consumer association in the Netherlands, Consumentenbond, started to publish systematic assessments of costs and quality of health care and health insurance.

The weekly *Elsevier* published lists of the "best and worst" hospitals in Holland. The national daily *Algemeen Dagblad* gained fame by publishing detailed lists of waiting times for certain medical procedures, encouraging patients to actively shop around when faced with unacceptable wait lists. Government-sponsored websites offer comparative information about health care and health insurance. The rapid growth in comparative information, however, seems to have had very limited effect on patient behavior. There is no evidence that star ratings or similar rankings of hospitals have led to a shift in patient streams, and Dutch citizens seem rather weary of the bombardment of new information (Okma and Ooijens 2005).

Interestingly, the area where consumer action has affected services most is not acute medical care, but rather long-term care (Okma 1997b). In this domain, organized patient groups (for example, the "lunatics movement" of psychiatric patients in the 1960s and parents and relatives of mentally handicapped patients) have successfully demanded better quality of services. Since the mid-1990s, the long-term care insurance AWBZ has offered the option for certain categories of patients to take vouchers that allow them to contract providers outside the traditional institutions. Within a few years of their introduction, those vouchers became very popular. By the end of 2003, over 50,000 patients had actually chosen this option, receiving an average amount of about €20,000; in 2006, the total budget for those vouchers was almost €1 billion, or about half as much as the entire budget for home care that served over 600,000 persons (MoH 2006).

There is some backlash against the rise of "consumerism" in Dutch health care. Not everyone is able or willing to spend time to compare the quality of health services or the insurance coverage and financial conditions (Okma and Ooijens 2005). With the growth of complexity of choices in supplemental insurance coverage (the basic coverage is the same for all), levels of deductibles and co-insurance combined with premium rebates, it has become much harder to compare insurance policies. Public polls show that most Dutch citizens prefer a wider choice in the provision of care rather than a broader choice of insurance plan. The first year after the introduction of the new universal health insurance, almost 20 percent of the Dutch population switched insurers. But that share went down to 5 percent in 2007, and experts do not expect a rise of that share in the future (Smit and Mokveld 2007). Most of that switch was based on employment-based collective insurance contracts, not really expressive of individual preference.

In general, Dutch patients and citizens show substantial loyalty to hospitals (particularly to hospitals with a religious background) and to the former regional sick funds (Laske-Aldershof et al. 2004). This loyalty seems to confirm

Herbert Simon's assumptions of "satisficing behavior"; most people limit their choice to the first few alternatives they can clearly comprehend (Simon 1957, xxv). They do not want to spend too much (travel) time and effort to look at all possible options and simply refuse to go much beyond the first option that seems reasonable. The bombardment of information provided by government-sponsored or commercial websites, newspapers, specialized journals, or other media has not done much to change that satisficing behavior. In general, Dutch hospitals have a strong regional (and sometimes still denominational) base for attracting their patients as well as staff.

Thus, "voice" and "exit" did become two effective strategies in long-term care. In acute medical care, Dutch citizens express far less interest in exiting the range of care with which they are familiar. Exit in health insurance seems to have been a one-shot event in 2006, mostly as part of collective employment-based arrangements. Interestingly, Dutch government policy is mostly focused on increasing competition in acute care. The government seems least convinced of the market power of consumers in long-term care. In 2007, it announced a moratorium on processes of change in the AWBZ and will keep the long-term care insurance under strict central government control.

Concluding Remarks: Change, No Progress?

At the beginning of the twenty-first century, Dutch health insurance agencies and providers of care demonstrated a mix of anticipatory and defensive behavior. They anticipated shifts from centralized, consensual policy making under government control to decentralized decision making and the creation of internal markets. At the same time, they sought ways to limit competition by merging and creating new strategic alliances on the regional level, in several cases effectively limiting or eliminating competition altogether. The verdict is still out on whether and to what extent these activities contributed to the improvement of the quality and diversity of Dutch health care services.

The health policy "discourse" has shifted as well, but the new orientation on market competition has clearly not replaced former notions of social solidarity in Dutch society. Thus managers face a complicated overlay of several competing and often conflicting notions of public and private governance roles in health care. They have to compete and to negotiate over contracts, but the government also expects them to collaborate with others on the regional level. They face increasing uncertainty over their future income stream but also political demands and patient pressures to act like "social entrepreneurs" and engage in collective efforts to improve the quality and efficiency of

Dutch health care. These uncertainties and contradictions are not likely to disappear soon.

The creation of the "internal market" in Dutch health care has not led to a reduced presence of government. On the contrary, competitive markets require extensive regulation and supervision, and in spite of an announced shift from "supply regulation" to "demand regulation," it now seems that both categories of government regulation are firmly in place. It has become clear that Dutch citizens expect a strong governmental role in safeguarding access to good quality care and stepping in if needed. Rising numbers of uninsured (even while modest compared to, say, the United States) rapidly prompt the government to take action. Similarly, complaints about the delisting of health services from the coverage of the basic insurance caused the government put some of those entitlements back on the list again (Maarse and Okma 2004; Ministeraad 2007). The government has extended its presence in monitoring health care quality and health insurance and encourages innovation and the development of information technology (by providing ample subsidy).

Some critics have voiced concern about the potential effects of the market-driven change (Okma and Ooijens 2005; Kreis 2005). The main actors seem to be focused on gaining strategic market positions and cutting costs or shifting costs, rather than on increasing consumer choice or improving the quality and efficiency of health care. In particular, two strategies have attracted much critical public (and political) attention: the rise of commercial-investor-owned for-profit services and agreements between hospitals and employers for preferential treatment of employees.

The strategic behavior of health insurance and health care providers—itself shaped by government policy—has reshaped the Dutch health policy landscape. This new landscape has created new problems. For example, the announced amalgamation of the funding for acute care and long-term care insurance schemes encouraged managers to seek vertical integration of hospital and nursing services. In 2006, the government reversed this plan. It left the long-term care out of the entitlements of the basic insurance and announced that local authorities instead of health insurers will have greater say over long-term care (and actually shifted some entitlements to the local level). Thus, the integrated services face another split in their revenues and have to deal with different negotiating partners. For example, after merging with other providers, the Parnassia organization decided to "de-merge" and split itself (again) into two legal entities for acute and long-term care.

It is interesting to note the extent to which modern management ideas and strategic market considerations have become stronger forces of change in

Dutch health care than government policy, technological change, or demographic transitions. Those managerial changes, however, have affected government action, for example, in opening the way to a greater role of for-profit health care and for-profit health insurance.

Even after major change in neocorporatist institutions, the main stakeholders in Dutch health care exhibited great willingness to continue their participation in government efforts to increase efficiency and quality and to contain health expenditure, both public and private.[12] The association of the Dutch health insurers, Zorgverzekeraars Nederland (ZN), has kept a prominent presence in a wide range of collaborate efforts in the health care system. Likewise, the hospital association and the medical association are keen to keep their presence. In a political sense, they clearly have not "exited" from the small country's health policy arena where the leaders of all the main stakeholders (as well as leaders of large businesses) continue to meet regularly.

As to the next decade in Dutch health care, we see some general trends. Efforts to engage in risk selection by insurers and providers on a large scale will likely face strong resistance by society as well as government action. It is not yet clear whether this resistance will change if (or perhaps rather, when) international insurance conglomerates decide to enter the market (again), in particular when those businesses do not share the traditional business norms of Holland. Thus far, efforts to develop commercial services have only been successful on a modest scale. There is "consumerism" in the margin, but there is no sign of widespread acceptance of rising inequality in access to health care, and there is no evidence that Dutch citizens will embrace "consumer-driven health care." They have strong feelings about universal and fair access to health care. Patients and relatives of elderly and handicapped patients are willing to take an active position to increase their choice of provider (as seen by the rapid growth of the cash benefit scheme). The trend towards greater market concentration in health insurance and health care will continue to reduce effective competition (and thus drive up costs unless government steps in again). Such market concentration may also reduce the effectiveness of consensual policy making as larger insurers or providers with strong market positions will feel less bound by covenants or other informal agreements with government.

Notes

The authors express their gratitude to Joseph Rojas, Avi Feller, and Nick Gerry-Bullard, students at Yale, for their editing support.

1. Anyone who has visited the Rijksmuseum in Amsterdam or the Frans Hals Museum in Haarlem will remember the large seventeenth- and eighteenth-century paint-

ings of the boards of directors of orphanages, hospitals, and other institutions providing care and shelter to orphans, homeless, elderly, and disabled persons. The city elites of those centuries considered board membership as part of their civic duty as well as a status symbol, not unlike the modern-day membership of the New York Metropolitan Opera or Lincoln Center boards.

2. Alan Williams frames such a shift, in its polarized form, as a shift toward libertarian ideology that advocates freedom of choice as a good in itself, as well as rewards for achievement. It also prefers private charity over collective mechanisms and, if they conflict, absolute freedom over equality (Williams 2005).

3. The term "policy" can mean a set of standard activities and behavior of certain agencies ("it is our policy not to smoke in this office"), a broad set of policy goals ("we want to improve the health of the nation"), specific intentions to change ("the government policy aims to eradicate smoking in this country"), or programs and policies actually in place ("smoking in public buildings is prohibited") (Palmer and Short 1989).

4. Rudolf Klein observed that "incremental change" means two quite different things: first, a step-by-step adjustment that, in the end, can result in substantial change or reform; and second, random step-by-step change into different directions (Klein 1997).

5. In the context of health insurance, the term "equity" has different meanings. It refers to the sharing of the financial burden of health insurance. In a narrow (most common and least-questioned) sense, "equity" means everybody faces the same burden and has the same access to medical services when he or she needs them. The measure for "the same burden" usually is taken as the same share of family income; thus, proportional tax is fully equal, while community-rated flat premiums are regressive as higher income groups pay a lower share of their incomes than people with lower incomes. Another meaning of "equity," however, is the commonsense notion of the absence of an insurmountable financial burden for everybody. For example, the early European sick funds charged the same contributions to all their members and offered equal medical services to all. Likewise, the late-twentieth-century German social insurance meant that all members of one particular sick fund paid the same contribution rates (but until the mid 2000s, the rates varied little between the funds). The community rating served as an equalization mechanism between the members, not between the funds. In contrast, until 2006, members of sick funds in the Netherlands all paid the same income-dependent contribution. The British NHS gets most of its funding from general taxation. The notion of equity thus depends on the redistributive working of the tax system. Those are three examples of funding mechanisms that, in general, were perceived as fair or equitable by the general populations.

6. The notion of "consumer choice" in health care has taken on two quite distinct meanings. For most patients, in most countries, "choice" refers to their ability to see a physician or other provider of their own choice. In modern-day health policy making, the term often refers to the possibility to sign up with (or to switch to) the health insurance or health plan of one's own choice. Paradoxically, the increase of the latter has sometimes reduced the former: as insured can choose their health insurance plan, they may find that that particular plan has not contracted their preferred provider, say, their long-standing family physician or dentist.

7. "Private provision," generally speaking, includes both for-profit health care facilities and not-for-profit providers. In North America, the term usually refers to investor-owned clinics and facilities, whereas in Western Europe (and in particular the Netherlands), it assumes nongovernmental actors, both for-profit and not-for-profit.

8. Interestingly, the Dekker report itself does not refer to comparative studies of international experience. The staff of the expert committee wrote the report largely based on internal discussions. Afterwards, some claimed that Alain Enthoven's "consumer choice plan" served as a model for the report (Enthoven 1978, 2008; Enthoven and Van de Ven 2007; Schut and Van de Ven 2005). But there is no evidence of such parentage. There is in fact another more likely explanation for similarities between reform proposals in different countries, namely, the limited number of options available for any country seeking to combine universal access with efficient management. On the funding side, earmarked general taxation and mandated contributions for social health insurance fulfill the requirement of income-related payments that can safeguard universal coverage. On the contracting side, there are three modes: (1) the integrated model of the British NHS, (2) the reimbursement model of private insurance, and (3) the long-term contractual relations between third-payers and providers (OECD 1992). Therefore, the search for models that combine universal access to health care with a fair distribution of the financial burden and increased efficiency of health care will only come up with a limited number of models. The dominant experience in the 1980s and 1990s was the shift towards the "public contracting model," with public funding and independent health care providers.

9. As in other countries, user fees met with fierce resistance and to soften the impact, the government regularly exempted certain groups such as the elderly or chronically ill or reversed the measure altogether. In fact, the story of efforts to reduce the coverage of social insurance reads like a "catalogue of failure" (Maarse and Okma 2004).

10. The story of the sanctions against nonpayment is exemplary of Dutch health policy. At first, the government decided that, when hospitalized, persons who had not taken out health insurance would have to pay for hospital care themselves; they also would have to take insurance on the spot and face both retroactive premiums and a fine. But faced with an increased number of noninsured, this course of action did not appear such a good idea and the government shifted to micromanagement instead. The controversial announcement that health insurers would drop their nonpayers mid-2007 prompted the Ministry of Health to reframe its position quickly and to propose a common risk pool for this group by imposing a system of prepayment. It also promised subsidies to insurers if they agreed not to drop the nonpayers.

11. One of the hotly debated questions in the reform process since the 1980s was whether allowing persons free choice of health plan would lead to risk selection by insurers and self-selection by insured (see Van de Ven and Ellis 2000; Lamers, Van Vliet, and Van de Ven 2003). Even while Dutch private insurers started to offer cheaper policies to (young and healthy) students, triggering a spiral of risk selection, they never set the premiums at rates that fully reflected risks; and there have been few if any examples of excluding pre-existing conditions of care on a large scale. Public opinion in Holland seems a major barrier to such behavior (Okma 1997a).

12. One of the interesting features of Dutch social policy is that even while Parliament has no say over private insurance, the annual budget document *Rijksbegroting* (2007) presents figures of both public and private health insurance. In fact, the government treats the total health expenditure as a quasi-budget.

References

Boot, J. M. 1998. Schaalvergroting en concentratie in het Nederlandse ziekenhuiswezen [Concentration and increase in operational scale of Dutch hospitals]. *Bestuurskunde* 7 (1): 28–37.

CBS. *See* Centraal Bureau voor de Statistiek.

Centraal Bureau voor de Statistiek. 2006. Health and welfare. http://www.cbs.nl.

Commissie Dekker. 1987. *Bereidheid tot Verandering* [Willingness to change: Report of the Committee on Health Care Reform]. The Hague: Distributiecentrum Overheidspublicaties.

De Roo, A. A. 1993. De Zorgsector als bedrijfstak in wording [Health care as emerging market branch]. Lecture at Catholic University, Brabant.

De Roo, A. A. 1995. Contracting and solidarity: Market-oriented changes in Dutch health insurance schemes. In *Implementing planned markets in health care,* ed. R. B. Saltman and C. Von Otter. Buckingham, UK: Open University Press.

De Roo, A. A. 2002. Naar een nieuw zorgstelsel? [Towards a new health care system?] Lecture presented at Tilburg University.

De Swaan, A. 1988. *In care of the state: Health care, education and welfare in Europe and the USA in the modern era.* Oxford: Polity Press.

Enthoven, A. C. 1978. Consumer-choice health plan, a national health insurance proposed based on regulated competition in the private sector. *New England Journal of Medicine* 298: 709–720.

Enthoven, A. C. 2008. A living model of managed care competition: A conversation with Dutch health minister Ab Klink. *Health Affairs*, web exclusive 27 (3–4).

Enthoven, A. C., and W. P. M. M. Van de Ven. 2007. Going Dutch: Managed competition health insurance in the Netherlands. *New England Journal of Medicine* 357 (24): 2421–2423.

Grit, C., and W. Dolfsma. 2002. The dynamics of the Dutch health care system: A discourse analysis. *Review of Social Economy* 60 (3): 377–401.

Helderman, J. K. 2007. *Institutional complemetarity in Dutch health care reforms: Going beyond the pre-occupation with choice.* Paper presented at the meeting of the European Health Policy Group, Berlin, April.

Helderman, J. K., F. T. Schut, T. E. D. Van der Grinten, and W. P. M. M. Van de Ven. 2005. Market-oriented health care reforms and policy learning in the Netherlands. *Journal of Health Politics, Policy and Law* 30 (1–2): 189–209.

Hill, M. 1993. *New agendas in the study of the policy process.* New York: Harvester Wheatsheaf.

Hoofdlijnenakkoord 2003 [Governing manifesto]. Kamerstukken II, 2002–2003, 28637 nr. 19. The Hague: SDU.

Klee, M., and K. G. H. Okma. 2001. Convenanten: nieuw instrument van beleid? [Covenants: New Policy Instrument?]Z & V, no. 1: 8–20.

Klein, R. 1997. Learning from others: Shall the last be the first? *Journal of Health Politics, Policy and Law* 22(5): 1267–1278.

Kreis, R. 2005. Marktwerking maakt zorg niet beter of goedkoper [Market competition does not make care better or cheaper]. *De Volkskrant,* February 22.

Lamers, L. M., R. C. J. A. Van Vliet, and W. P. M. M. Van de Ven. 2003. Risk adjusted premium subsidies and risk sharing: Key elements of the competitive sickness fund market in the Netherlands. *Health Policy,* no. 65: 49–62.

Laske-Aldershof, T., E. Schut, K. Beck, A. Shmueli, and C. Van de Voorde. 2004. Consumer mobility in social health insurance markets: A five-country comparison. *Applied Health Economics and Health Policy* 3 (4): 229–41.

Lijphart, A. 1968. *Verzuiling, pacificatie en kentering in de Nederlandse politiek* [Pillarization, pacification, and changes in Dutch policies]. Amsterdam: J. H. De Bussy.

Maarse, H., and K. G. H. Okma. 2004. The privatization paradox in Dutch health care. In *Privatisation in European health care: A comparative analysis in eight countries,* ed. H. Maarse. Maarssen: Elsevier gezondheidszorg: 97–116.

Ministerraad. 2007. Tandarts terug in het basispakket. [Dental care returns to basic coverage]. Press release of Council of Ministers. May 26. http://www.regering.nl/actueel/nieuwsarchief/2007/05May/25/0-42-1_42-97663.jsp.

Ministry of Health. 1988. *Verandering Verzekerd* [Change assured]. Kamerstukken II, 1987–1988, 19945. The Hague: SDU.

Ministry of Health. 1994. *Kostenbeheersing in de zorgsector* [Controlling health care expenditures]. Kamerstukken II, 1994–1995, 24124. The Hague: SDU

Ministry of Health. 1996. *Financieel Overzicht Zorg 1997* [Financial survey health care 1997]. Kamerstukken II, 1996–1997, 25004. The Hague: SDU.

Ministry of Health. 1997. *Financieel Overzicht Zorg 1998* [Financial survey health care 1998]. Kamerstukken II, 1997–1998, 25604. The Hague: SDU.

Ministry of Health. 1999. *Zorgnota 2000* [Health budget paper 2000]. The Hague: SDU.

Ministry of Health. 2001. *Vraag aan Bod* [Demand at the center]. The Hague: Ministerie van Volksgezondheid, Welzijn, en Sport.

Ministry of Health. 2005. Geneesmiddelenconvenant 2006 and 2007 levert 1,8 miljard op. [Pharmaceutical Agreement for 2006 and 2007 will save €1.8 billion] Press release. December 11.

Ministry of Health. 2006. *Rijksbegroting Volksgezondheid, Welzijn en Sport 2007* [Health budget 2007]. The Hague: Ministerie van Volksgezondheid, Welzijn, en Sport.

MoH. *See* Ministry of Health.

OECD. *See* Organisation for Economic Co-operation and Development.

Okma, K. G. H. 1997a. *Studies in Dutch health politics, policies and law.* PhD diss., University of Utrecht, the Netherlands.

Okma, K. G. H. 1997b. Concurrentie, markten en marktwerking in de gezondheidszorg. [Competition and markets in health care]. *Tijdschrift voor Politieke Ekonomie* 2: 164–78.

Okma, K. G. H. 2001. *Health care, health policies and health care reform in the Netherlands.* The Hague: Ministry of Health.

Okma, K. G. H., and H. Van der Burg. 2004. Das Budgetmodell der niederländischen Krankenkassen [Budgeting Dutch sickness funds]. *Die BBK: Zeitschrift der Betrieblichen Krankenversicherung,* no. 92: 36–39.

Okma, K. G. H., and M. Ooijens. 2005. De patient centraal: Zijn de Verenigde Staten ons voorland? [Patient centered care: the United States as our example?] *Tijdschrift voor de Sociale Sector* (June): 26–29.

Organisation for Economic Co-operation and Development. 1992. *The reform of health care: A comparative analysis of seven OECD countries.* Health Reform Studies no. 2. Paris: OECD.

Organisation for Economic Co-operation and Development. 1994. *The reform of health care: A review of seventeen OECD countries.* Health Reform Studies no. 5. Paris: OECD.

Palmer, G. R. , and S. D. Short. 1989. *Health care and public policy: An Australian analysis.* South Yarra, Australia: MacMillan Co. of Australia.

Regeerakkoord 1994 [Governing manifesto 1994]. Kamerstukken II, 1994–1995, 23715. The Hague: SDU.

Regeerakkoord 1998 [Governing manifesto 1998]. Kamerstukken II, 1997–1998, 26204 nr. 9. The Hague: SDU.

Rengers, M., and X. van Uffelen. 2005. Het zorgstelsel is een sigaar uit eigen doos [The new health system as a "Dutch treat"]. *Volkskrant,* October 22.

Rosenberg, E. 2006. Ziekenhuizen moeten hard zijn [Hospitals must be hard]. *NRC Handelsblad,* January 18.

Rosenberg, E. 2007. Concurrentie in de zorg blijft uit [Competition in health care does not materialize]. *NRC Handelsblad,* May 15.

Scheerder, R. 2005. Kostenbeleid 2005. [Cost Control Policy 2005]. *Zorg & Financiering* 193 (2): 8–28.

Schut, F. 1997. *Competition in Dutch health care.* PhD diss., Erasmus University, Rotterdam.

Schut, F. T., and W. P. M. M. Van de Ven. 2005. Rationing and competition in the Dutch health-care system. *Health Economics* 14: S59–74.

Simon, H. A. 1957. *Administrative Behavior,* 2nd ed. New York: The Free Press.

Smit, M., and P. Mokveld. 2007. *Verzekerdenmobiliteit en keuzegedrag* [Mobility and choice in Dutch health insurance]. Zeist: Vektis.

Strategisch Akkoord 2002 [Governing manifesto 2002]. Kamerstukken II, 2001–2002, 28375, nr. 5. The Hague: SDU.

Van de Ven, W. P. M. M., and R. P. Ellis. 2000. Risk adjustment in competitive health plan markets. In *Handbook of health economics,* ed. A. J. Culyer and J. P. Newhouse. Amsterdam: Elsevier Science, 755–845.

Van het Loo, M., J. P. Kahan, and K. G. H. Okma. 1999. Recent developments in health care costs containment in the Netherlands. In *Health care and cost containment in the European Union,* ed. E. Mossialos and J. Le Grand. London: Ashgate, 573–603.

Visser, J., and A. Hemereyk. 1997. *A Dutch miracle: Job growth, welfare reform and corporatism in the Netherlands*. Amsterdam: Amsterdam University Press.

Williams, A. 2005. The pervasive role of ideology in the optimisation of the public-private mix in public healthcare systems. In *The public-private mix for health*, ed. A. Maynard. London: Nuffield Trust.

6

The United Kingdom
Health Policy Learning in the National
Health Service

MARK EXWORTHY AND RICHARD FREEMAN

Health systems can be seen as the way a country assumes and then exerts collective responsibility for protection against the risks of injury and illness. Those risks include the maintenance of health as well as the medical and financial consequences of falling ill. Everywhere such arrangements rest on political settlements of different kinds: between the state and economic actors, principally employers and employees, about how to finance the system and whom it should serve; and between the state and doctors about the conditions under which to provide and pay for health care. In combination, these effectively define the extent of public and private activity in the health sector. Underpinning them all, of course, are assumptions about the appropriate scope and structure of the state.

The United Kingdom reached a distinctive set of such settlements in 1946 with legislation that established the National Health Service (NHS). The NHS was to be "universal and comprehensive," providing a full range of health care to all residents of the United Kingdom. It was to be funded by general taxation, making it "free at point of use" for patients. It was to be guided by the Minister of Health and organized for administrative purposes into geographical units (or Health Authorities). These authorities owned and ran hospitals and other facilities. Specialist physicians, though retaining some freedom to practice privately, held salaried contracts with the NHS for work in NHS hospitals. General practitioners contracted independently with Health Authorities according to the number of patients they covered. A strict referral system governed the relationship between specialists and generalists; patients had to consult a general practitioner to obtain a referral to hospital (that is, specialist) care. A distinctive ethos of equality has dominated the NHS, which for most of its lifetime and for most actors within it has meant uniformity.

In comparative perspective, these settlements have meant that the NHS has been remarkably centralized, and public, with an unusual configuration of the relationship between the professions and the state. Since the 1940s, the political settlements have been, of course, variously renegotiated and remade. The characterization remains largely valid; what it means has changed over time.

The purpose of this chapter is to describe the NHS and its politics and to make sense of it in comparative terms. We have already implied that the NHS's history is crucial, and we begin by reviewing that history. We describe a pattern whereby reform meant to realize the original vision gives way to attempts to modernize it. It also created a continued process of frantic change, much to the frustration of providers in the NHS. Our principal concern is with the politics of modernization. We focus on relations along three axes: between center and locality, public and private, and government and professions in turn. In keeping with the theme of this volume, we address the following question: To what extent have such "modernizing" developments been informed by learning? Our answer comes from describing its sources and styles, prospects and limits.

In passing, however, we should note the "beacon effect" that the NHS appears to hold in international policy debate. This international prominence is rarely simple or straightforward, though it is significant. Whether praised for efficiency or decried for severe rationing, its influence abroad is considerable (Koeck 1998). In comparative perspective, then, what is interesting is the extent to which the NHS learns but also offers "lessons." Its size and history give it iconic status as the "first" National Health Service. The key features of the NHS's organization at inception, such as tax financing, public ownership of facilities, and central government direction, mean that it serves as an ideal-typical counterpoint to not only the United States but also to continental social insurance models. The relatively sophisticated management practice the NHS has fostered may explain some of its influence, if only in contrast to developments in the United States. As a managerial and policy "leader," the NHS, like the United States, also supports a health service research community that constitutes a minor industry in itself, and the production and dissemination of that work in English. What all of this means is that policy makers in the United Kingdom and the United States, to the extent that they are concerned with what goes on elsewhere, are primarily interested in each other. This comparison might be labeled as a "most different system comparison." The scope and effect of that Anglo-American interest is the topic this chapter addresses in closing. What is important now is the suggestion that the NHS might be an object of learning precisely because it is a subject of learning. The interest in learning from the NHS may arise in part from the perception that the NHS is itself engaged in learning.

The National Health Service, 1950–2000

The NHS emerged from the post-1945 consensus on the role of the welfare state that lasted until the late 1970s. The Emergency Medical Service that operated during the Second World War had demonstrated that a national public scheme could be effective, though the form it should take was clearly shaped by professional influence and interests (Peckham and Exworthy 2003; Klein 2006). Its principal inpatient organizational unit was the Hospital Board, while Executive Committees (later called Family Practice Committees) governed general practitioner (GP) services. Hospital consultants were salaried whereas GPs received a basic salary, plus capitation payments and fees-for-service. This difference reflected the GPs' status as independent contractors. Incorporating both voluntary and municipal hospitals, the NHS effectively removed the latter from local government control, though the municipalities remained responsible for public health and for some community health services. The result was not an integrated system but a tripartite structure (of hospitals, general practice, and local government). It represented what was feasible rather than ideal (Ham 2004; Klein 2006). It also illustrates that there are limits to what central government could do.

This description immediately challenges the view of the NHS as a monolithic organization with a top-down, relatively rigid command-and-control planning model, with decision making vested in elected officials at the national level (Exworthy, Powell, and Mohan 1999; Saltman and von Otter 1992). The irony is that the political cost of bringing the NHS into being was that government control of it would be limited. The NHS, certainly in its early incarnation, was essentially a collegial system run by professional interest groups. Hospital consultants were powerful actors in determining the quantity and quality of local services. GPs' independence left them largely semidetached from NHS planning initiatives (and in this respect independent doctors in local practice were more like other European systems than is commonly assumed).

The command-and-control model of the NHS in this period was a facade (Holliday 1995). Policy was made largely by exhortation, though backed by financial clout (Exworthy, Powell, and Mohan 1999).

The NHS became more hierarchical following the 1974 reorganization, when planning and strategy increased in prominence. The newly introduced Health Authorities provided the government with a missing link to local action. This so-called unified structure, however, applied only to hospital and community health services, not general practice. By removing the last vestiges of medical provision (such as community nursing) from local government, the 1974 reforms further separated the NHS from other welfare services and from the local state.

For its first thirty-five years, Hospital Management Committees, dominated by doctors, ran the local NHS. In 1974, although multidisciplinary consensus teams took over local management responsibilities, administrators played no more than a "diplomatic" role because doctors still held the power of veto (Harrison 1988, 1999). However, a Royal Commission on the NHS that reported in 1979 made recommendations to develop its managerial capacity at the same time as a new Conservative government came to power. In 1983, Prime Minister Margaret Thatcher asked Roy Griffiths, head of the Sainsbury grocery company, to lead a small team (also drawn from the private sector) to inquire into NHS "manpower." Its twenty-four-page report argued that the NHS had been "under-managed," suggesting, "if Florence Nightingale were alive today, she would be wandering the hospital corridors trying to find out who was in charge" (National Health Service Management Inquiry 1983, 22). Griffiths recommended that executive decision making replace consensus management, and general managers were appointed at all levels of the NHS in 1985.

A second key impulse to organizational change was the introduction of the so-called internal market in 1991. Until then, geographically based Health Authorities were in charge of the management of hospital and community health services. By separating planning and strategy from operational management, the Health Authority became a "purchaser" of services from organizationally independent hospitals known as Trusts. At the same time, GPs (in group practices) could elect to hold their own budgets for some hospital services by becoming "fundholders" (Le Grand and Robinson 1994). Contracts between purchasers and providers were supposed to enhance (technical and allocative) efficiency and improve the quality of care. Although purchasers could in theory commission services from any provider, the majority contracted with their local providers (Exworthy 1998). And while some gains were evident, the incentives set by the internal market were insufficiently strong to generate the improvements hoped for (Le Grand, Mays, and Mulligan 1998).

The new Labour government elected in 1997 initially sought to remedy the fragmentation the internal market had wrought. While emphasizing a "one-nation NHS," more collaborative than competitive, Labour in fact maintained many of the market-style structures and processes. It did adjust the language. Hospital providers now made "agreements" (not contracts) with "commissioners" (not purchasers). Meanwhile, organizational amalgamation began to shift the way these internal markets worked. General practice fundholding was abolished and all GPs were included within newly formed Primary Care Groups (PCGs, later Primary Care Trusts, or PCTs). The effect of this policy was to integrate general practice into the NHS for the first time in its history. All these changes in turn reinforced a need for and commitment to service management.

"Modernization" was the key metaphoric term of the NHS white paper (Department of Health [DoH] 1997). When the NHS Plan for England in 2000 restated the commitment to management, modernization became its mantra (Rivett 2005). What this focus on modernization seemed to mean was that health services should work as efficiently as business systems. They should employ comparable administrative and managerial tools, and be as capable as other services of satisfying customer (or user) preferences. Drawing in part on ideas and techniques proposed by the U.S. Institute for Healthcare Improvement, the project was to be advanced through a new Modernization Agency. At its height (in 2004, and before a government decision to reduce the number of such Agencies), the Modernization Agency employed 760 people on a budget of £230 million. Demonstration sites, case studies, and pilot projects all promulgated the tenets of modernization throughout the NHS.

Meanwhile, political devolution in the United Kingdom from Westminster to Scotland, Wales, and Northern Ireland gave territorial governments responsibility for health and health care policy. In each case, health has been a notable political priority (Jervis and Plowden 2003), in part because the performance of the NHS was a matter of concern. But the more limited policy range of the devolved administrations also made health a greater part of government and parliamentary business.

Center and Locality

The structure of the NHS presents the government with a distinctive political problem. A chain of command runs (at least in theory) from the Secretary of State for Health via intermediate administrative tiers to the managers of local services, traditionally based around a local district general hospital. The classic hierarchical model vests the key ministers at its apex with unusual authority. As a result, it also makes them unusually accountable (and this holds whether ministerial instructions are commands or merely exhortations). The nature of the public service and its centralized decision making turns what might be local, technical decisions into national, political ones. Even where ministers delegate decision making, they risk remaining (or are seen to remain) accountable for what goes on at the periphery.

At first, this arrangement seemed to present few problems. As Aneurin Bevan (secretary of state in the 1945 Labour government that founded the NHS) famously stressed, "When a bedpan is dropped on a hospital floor, its noise should resound in the Palace of Westminster" (Powell 1998, 58–59). From its inception in 1948 until 1974, the organizational structure of the NHS in England remained largely unchanged. However, since then, organizational restructuring has taken place every few years, irrespective of the government in power. The role and size of local Health Authorities have changed frequently on both vertical and horizontal axes. Along the vertical axis, connecting the locality to the center, District Health Authorities were first grouped into Areas and Regions in 1974. The NHS then abolished the Areas and reduced the fourteen Regions to eight in 1994. And in 2002, Health Authorities merged into a smaller number of Strategic Health Authorities.

Other changes crosscut this process as Health Authorities integrated primary, secondary, community, and public health services. Operational and strategic functions led to further reordering. Reform in 1974, for example, was meant to integrate secondary and community health services, with public health becoming an NHS function following the Acheson review in 1988. In 1991, with the separation of purchasing and provision, Trusts received a degree of organizational and managerial autonomy. In turn, some hospitals have gained greater operational devolution as Foundation Trusts as they showed good clinical and organizational performance. This arrangement gives managers increased freedom in financial management as well as in service design, recruitment, and setting rates of pay. Foundation Trusts are accountable not to the Secretary of State but to Monitor, an independent regulator set up specifically for them.

Health Authorities merged primary care with Family Health Service Authorities (FHSAs, then responsible for GP services) in 1996. Since then, Primary Care Groups responsible for service delivery have evolved into Trusts, some of which have merged. Many local agencies have pre-empted central directives by forming proto-agencies or introducing ad hoc arrangements. While PCTs are responsible for about 80 percent of the NHS budget, their scope for independent action is limited by national guidelines, targets, and financial constraints. Service pricing, for example, is determined by Healthcare Resource Groups (HRGs), the equivalent of Diagnosis-related Groups (DRGs). HRG tariffs are effectively a national tariff designed to make sure that various providers compete on quality and efficiency rather than on price. This arrangement belies the extent to which, in the continual search for efficiency and legitimacy, local change reflects change at the center.

Since the 1980s, the Department of Health (DoH) created a series of executive agencies to separate operational and ministerial accountability (Pollitt et al. 2004). Operational matters were devolved to a new NHS Executive in Leeds, a geographic shift that symbolized a formal and a physical separation from the DoH in London. The appointment of a Chief Executive (in addition to the Chief Civil Servant at the DoH) emphasized this division, although these separate posts have since been recombined. The DoH also established other agencies at "arm's length" from government. Nevertheless, the centrality of the NHS in British politics has always made a sharp distinction between policy making and administrative implementation difficult if not impossible (Day and Klein 1997).

Two agencies in particular reflect the tension between local variations and national standards. They also mark a shift toward more explicit "evidence-based" national standards and regulation. The National Institute for Clinical Excellence (NICE) is the independent organization responsible for providing national guidance on clinical standards, including the promotion of good health and the prevention and treatment of ill health. The Healthcare Commission (formerly the Commission for Health Improvement [CHI]) monitors the performance of NHS organizations. It uses "National Service Frameworks" and guidelines developed by NICE for selected clinical services (such as those for coronary heart disease and mental health) to assess performance.[1]

The agenda drawn up by the still-new Labour government in 1998 clearly indicated that it wanted to direct attention to learning how to improve the quality of NHS care (Secretary of State for Health 1998; Davies and Nutley 2000). It proceeded in two ways. The Healthcare Commission first set targets and awarded performance ratings for NHS agencies and organizations in a way that was top-down and directive and perhaps closer to teaching than learning. This strategy was most crudely visible in the "star ratings" given to Trusts in England (star ratings were abolished in 2006 and replaced by an "annual health check"). NICE developed guidelines for different clinical procedures. In accordance with its proclaimed spirit of modernization, the NHS at the same time commissioned a review of work on organizational change (Iles and Sutherland 2001) and developed new initiatives. The Policy

Collaborative was one example, described as a bottom-up, "let's try something different" part of the DoH Corporate Change Programme, and of which the stated purpose "to learn."[2] Meanwhile, the NHS Confederation, the independent association of agencies comprising the NHS, became increasingly explicit about its role in promoting learning and organizational development as well as lobbying.

The difficulty in all of these efforts is that the conditions required for learning are generally different from those inculcated by oversight (Davies and Nutley 2000).[3] For the DoH, as for NHS management, there is a tension between the need to encourage learning and the need to exert control. Learning from research, studies show, is best promoted by dialogue and communication between those who produce it and those who use it (Elliott and Popay 2000; Innvaer et al. 2002). An organizational culture of targets, guidelines, and ratings, by contrast, is monologic rather than dialogic, top-down not bottom-up. Meanwhile, devolution presented quite different opportunities for learning, both in scale and kind.

DEVOLUTION

The promotion of autonomy and accountability were two fundamental arguments for devolution in the United Kingdom. The Scottish government, for example, was newly free to develop "Scottish solutions to Scottish problems." The assumption was that it could respond more appropriately to circumstances north of the border than had been possible under direction from London. Local control meant more responsiveness, the argument went, to the demands and values of Scottish voters and other organized interests. Similar processes in Wales and Northern Ireland would produce a degree of policy diversity across the United Kingdom (Greer 2004), constituting a domain of innovation and experimentation from which different actors in different contexts might learn.

But the policy diversification on which this learning depended is neither new nor unlimited. For example, the territorial administration of health and social care in the United Kingdom has always been slightly different in different countries. As a consequence, initiatives such as primary care commissioning normally worked somewhat differently in local environments (Exworthy 2001). What difference devolution makes is itself subject to experiment. For some time after 1999, health policy communities, one can say, engaged in a process of meta-learning about the properties of devolution itself. Policy makers have tried to work out not just what they and their voters want, but what is politically, administratively, and not least, financially possible in devolved public policy making. Distinct territorial policy networks have formed around the new assemblies. The relationship between them and key professional networks in medicine—which remain U.K.-wide in their scope—however, is not wholly clear. And perhaps most important, policy differentiation has been barely tested by political difference between territories. From devolution in 1999 until 2007, Labour held sway in government across England, Scotland, and Wales (the party system in Northern Ireland has always been different from that in the rest of the United Kingdom). However, the May 2007 elections to the Scottish Parliament heralded a Scottish Nationalist (SNP) First Minister, and the changed government in Scotland seems likely to present new challenges for Westminster.

Meanwhile, there has been a devolution dividend in policy experimentation. Wales abolished prescription charges, and Scotland declared personal care for older people an NHS entitlement. In Scotland, too, the Millan commission heralded a progressive redesign of mental health legislation (Freeman 2007). The freedom to experiment in the new "policy laboratory" is of course partly constrained by the increased accountability that came with it. The U.K.-wide debate prompted by the proposal to extend entitlement to personal care exposed an obvious tension between territorial autonomy and diversity on the one hand, and a commitment to the equity and universalism that are the NHS's cultural markers on the other. This tension makes for a constrained learning or learning within parameters. In time, those parameters may be set in Europe as much as among the countries of the United Kingdom (Freeman and Woods 2002; Greer 2004; Woods 2004).

For the rest, a more critical learning, just as in the relationship between research and policy, depends on the quality of information available to participants and then on the quality of their communication. Policy design is hampered, first, by a lack of comparable data across the countries of the United Kingdom even on key indicators such as spending and waiting times (Alvarez-Rosete et al. 2005). Beyond that, the institutional mechanisms of communication between different jurisdictions remain rudimentary at best. For example, a Joint Ministerial Committee on Health (JMC[H]) took shape in 2000, under constitutional provisions made in the process of devolution. Set up at the Prime Minister's request, it followed Blair's announcement of a commitment to raise health spending to the European average. In its first year, the JMC(H) met in Cardiff and then in London and Edinburgh. But it has since fallen into disuse, seeming to have served only as a mechanism for coordinating Labour health policy across the territory of the United Kingdom rather than for the reciprocal benefit of those charged with executive responsibilities for health policy as such (Woods 2002).

Public and Private

For all that the NHS has changed in the sixty years since its inception, it continues to dominate British health care. It accounts for 83 percent of all U.K. health care spending (OECD 2005), while 94 percent of that continues to come from public sources. The share of private health insurance is static at around 11 percent, with a further 3.5 percent paid ad hoc by patients in cash ("out-of-pocket spending") (Oliver 2005). What is distinctive about U.K. private insurance is its very basic supplementary role. When health care is funded by general taxation, it is effectively impossible not to pay for it (however indirectly). The simple residence requirement, moreover, entitles one to the care it provides. Many of those with private insurance coverage also use NHS services. Voluntary and commercial health insurance buys off what might be some of public health care's most demanding users (just as private provision lends one of its more demanding interest groups, hospital specialists, opportunities to increase their earnings; see discussion later in this chapter). The political importance of this private financing of private provision cannot be overlooked in any account of health care in the United Kingdom. At the same time, it should not be overstated.

The central government largely determines the funding available to the NHS. This funding thus competes with other claims on public expenditure (such as education, defense, or social security) in negotiation with the Treasury. The DoH allocates finances on a weighted per-capita basis to Strategic Health Authorities and Primary Care Trusts. These are in theory "cash-limited"; the services they provide are constrained (or expanded) by the budgets they receive.

Such funding mechanisms have several advantages: a degree of equity and social solidarity, low administrative costs, and an effective constraint on overall health spending (Robinson, Evans, and Exworthy 1994). Indeed, in responding to a Treasury review of resource requirements for the NHS in 2002 (Wanless 2002), then-Chancellor Gordon Brown committed the government to continuing its tax funding. However, critics claim a lack of transparency and lower levels of service than desirable. When demand for health care exceeds supply, the NHS uses various rationing devices. The most visible is making patients wait for treatment, notably for elective hospital procedures.

In recognition of these problems and partly in response to unfavorable comparisons with other countries, Prime Minister Tony Blair in January 2000 remarkably committed his government to matching European levels of spending on health. He promised that levels of spending on health care in the United Kingdom would reach 9 percent of GDP by 2008. As of 2007, increased investment has indeed been flowing into the NHS. On the other hand, the money available for new services has been effectively limited by pay increases and other pressures (King's Fund 2005; House of Commons 2007a).

At the same time, however, the government began to use the private sector for provision in such a way as to call into question the public nature of the NHS. The signal expression of this shift was the "concordat" between the government and the Independent Healthcare Association in 2000, which allowed health purchasers to contract with private and voluntary providers in order to reduce waiting times for elective surgery (DoH 2000a).

The private finance initiative (PFI), initiated by a Conservative government in 1992 but continued under Labour, is a way of raising private capital for NHS building projects. Under this scheme, the NHS enters into a long-term contract (usually thirty years) with a private company that builds a facility and leases it back to the NHS. In this way, the government avoids current budget expenditure and secures new buildings relatively quickly. As many of its buildings are older than the NHS itself, DoH set a renovation program in motion to provide one hundred new hospitals by 2010. The PFI hospital has a primary care equivalent in the Local Improvement Finance Trust (LIFT), a public-private partnership to develop facilities that primary care providers can lease. However, while many of the assumptions used to compare the public and private sectors have been questioned (Pollock 2003), assessment of early PFI schemes suggest that they have cut bed numbers and delivered poor-quality buildings (King's Fund 2005).

Meanwhile, to reduce waiting times to a maximum of eighteen weeks, the government stated that 15 percent of operations and tests in England must be carried out in the private sector by 2008 (DoH 2004a). To meet growing NHS demands, private providers have expanded their capacity (although their staff usually have dual contracts with the NHS). For example, private investors have funded new Diagnostic and Treatment Centres. Many of these providers have their base outside the United Kingdom, including Capio (Sweden), UnitedHealth (United States), and Kaiser Permanente (United States). In England, the DoH seems to consider the expansion of the private sector as a goal in itself. The rhetoric emphasizes market "contestability" on the assumption that private supply will stimulate improvements in the NHS that the internal market did not.

Similarly, the NHS draws on a professional labor market that is increasingly international. For many years, the United Kingdom trained fewer doctors than it needed, relying on migration of qualified staff from abroad. In the 1960s and 1970s, most immigrant doctors came from the Indian subcontinent. As these doctors approach retirement, the DoH aims to address the prospective shortage by recruitment from Europe (enabled by the mutual recognition of qualifications by the European Union) and the establishment of four more medical schools in the United Kingdom (DoH 2001a). The international recruitment of nurses from countries such as South Africa and the Philippines has prompted considerable criticism for undermining, it is claimed, those countries' capacity to operate their own health services.

In these different ways, market relations have intensified within what remains the public framework of the NHS. As a corollary, the government has placed the concept of "patient choice" at the rhetorical center of health policy development in England (DoH 2000b; Greener 2003). The policy promotes a more patient-responsive health service and anticipates reduced waiting times from greater competition between providers. It requires that patients referred for elective surgery be offered a choice of four or five providers, one of which must be private or commercial. With all the rhetoric of market competition, however, these different options do not have direct financial consequence for patients.

NHS traditionally placed little emphasis on the notion of "choice" (excepting choice of GPs). Its infrastructure was geared more to the needs of providers than patients. Policy makers have hesitated to change this arrangement, fearing that increased choice will generate more inequality in access to care (Exworthy and Peckham 2006). However, both they and the public have become aware that other countries, including those with tax-funded health systems, offer patients greater choice of professional services than the United Kingdom (Health Policy Monitor 2005c). Current initiatives promote patient participation in decision making. They aim as well to increase access to a wider range of services in primary care, greater variety in the ways prescriptions are obtained, choice of hospital, and choice of treatment in maternity care and end-of-life care (Health Policy Monitor 2005c). These policies have provoked some skepticism about the willingness of patients to travel to distant providers (Exworthy and Peckham 2006). To bolster increased choice, the NHS has given financial incentives to providers, including payment-by-results.

The appeals to the language of choice have also been accelerated in the NHS by external factors. The European Court of Justice (ECJ), for example, has ruled that patients in Europe may travel to other E.U. countries for treatment without prior authorization from their domestic insurer or provider (in England, the PCT). Although it is likely that the numbers of patients using this system will remain small (Exworthy, Kanavos, and Khondoker 2001), the ruling amplified the message that patients can and will travel further afield for treatment.

Government and Medicine

When formed, the combination of centrally controlled funding and local professional autonomy can be said to have made the NHS an arena of "private government" (Heclo and Wildavsky 1974). The advantage to government lay in securing an electorally popular service that has long been cherished by the overwhelming majority of the British public. At the same time, the medical profession obtained the resources as well as considerable professional freedom to deliver such services. Klein (1990) characterized this arrangement as the "politics of the double bed." The growing emphasis on management in the NHS reflects both managerialism in all areas of social and public life, and the specific problems of delivering increasingly sophisticated health services in the 1980s and 1990s under perceived provider capture. This 'managerial turn' inevitably meant that the original settlement between the state and the medical profession would be revisited. The process has been slow and subtle, and consequent change for the most part incremental but nonetheless significant.

In most countries, what we think of as the health care system is a way of paying doctors and hospitals. The NHS is both payer and provider—and employer of doctors. This relationship means that the most immediate and explicit expression of the relationship between doctors and government, and their most frequent point of conflict, is the doctor's contract of employment. The contract defines how doctors are to be paid and for what, and sets other conditions of employment such as working hours and opportunities to work privately. Changes to the contract are made not only for fiscal and administrative reasons, but also to induce changes in physicians' behavior. Contracts not only determine "who gets what, when and how" in the NHS but also define meanings and motivations. They shape the way the NHS is understood by those doctors who work for it. Changes to their terms of employment are embedded in an increasingly elaborate discourse of managerialism.

In 1948, the consultant contract was a way to attract doctors to join the nascent NHS. In addition to their NHS salary, consultants could continue private practice in NHS "pay beds"; they also benefited from a lucrative merit bonus system (awarded by doctors to colleagues). In 1974, arguing that opportunities for private practice encouraged doctors to keep waiting lists, the then Labour government sought unsuccessfully to end consultants' use of pay beds. In 1990, the (Conservative) government introduced "job plans" to enable managers to keep track of consultants' private practice. Successive efforts to revise the contract focused on the amount of private practice that consultants are allowed to undertake within their NHS contract. By and large, doctors have been able to maintain the right to practice privately as integral to their autonomy. But the 2004 consultant contract included a significant rise in their salary in return for greater clarity and specificity about their time on NHS activities.

Meanwhile, the advent of the clinical director, like the fundholder in general practice, illustrates the extent to which doctors have themselves assumed managerial functions (Causer and Exworthy 1999). The key element of clinical governance is the extent to which doctors' performance is subject to external scrutiny. Clinical audit, backed by a raft of inspections and regulatory agencies, has made doctors' work more transparent to managers and, in turn, to outside agents (Power 1997). For example, "star ratings" awarded to Trusts in England by the Healthcare Commission made information about the combined performance of doctors and managers, however crudely measured, available to the wider public. The new "annual health check" is also available to the public and comprises a "weak/fair/good/excellent" scale to service quality and the use of resources. Foundation Trust performance is gauged by an independent regulator (Monitor) according to the following headings: patient responsiveness, clinical standards, leadership and management, commitment and support of staff, partnership working and stakeholder support, and financial support (Health Policy Monitor 2005b).

Similar processes are evident in primary care, which has become the principal vehicle of the government's modernization of the NHS. The original GP contract served to ensure that all patients could be registered with a GP who would provide twenty-four-hour care for them. But it left the GP organizationally independent and for a long time outside the purview of health service managers (Peckham and Exworthy 2003). In 1990, a new contract specified the terms of employment in more detail. It was more managerial in its mode and aims, requiring GPs to produce annual reports and conduct needs assessments of their patients. The contract offered payments to meet targets for specific procedures such as cervical cytology and immunizations. The revised contract implemented in 2004 was made with a practice, not with an individual practitioner. GPs must now specify more precisely the range and quality of services they will provide. Of equal importance, they no longer are responsible for comprehensive access 24/7. They can relinquish their responsibility for out-of-hours coverage. This reduces their own pay but leaves the NHS to finance more expensive deputizing services. Moreover, they now receive additional payments (which may comprise up to 30 percent of their income) linked to performance. A "Quality and Outcomes Framework" (QOF), which consists of 136 specified clinical, organizational, and "patient experience" factors is the vehicle for this assessment. The government underestimated the financial consequences of QOF, as many practices performed better than expected on different indicators and accordingly received higher financial rewards (Kmietowicz 2006; Maynard and Street 2006).

Primary care (including both general practice and community health services) has often been seen as the "poor relation" in the NHS, lacking the clinical authority and financial import of the hospital. Given its strict referral system, an NHS patient's first and often only contact with the NHS is with primary care services. The reform of primary care has sought to integrate it more fully into the NHS as well as use it as a lever to influence change elsewhere in the NHS (mainly hospitals) (Flynn 1997). One of the clearest markers of this is the extent to which GPs have begun to ask for specialist consultations for their patients outside the hospital.

The DoH initially regarded general practice fundholding as a marginal element in the reforms of the early 1990s. It counted for only about 20 percent of the budget of participating GPs, covering mainly the costs of elective surgery (with the remainder of the budget spent on their behalf by Health Authorities). Yet GPs' contracting power began to make hospitals more responsive to patient needs in ways that PCGs and PCTs were later to emulate. It prompted Health Authorities to create local mechanisms to address the concerns of non-fundholders (Exworthy 1993). The principal criticism of the scheme was that it provided better access to patients of fundholding practices than others, thus formalizing a two-tiered, inequitable service.

The new Labour government addressed the equity issue in a way that furthered what might be described as the corporatization of primary care (Smith and Walshe 2004). In 1998, all GPs were included in new Primary Care Groups, which later (2002) became Primary Care Trusts. Rather than individual GP practices holding purchasing functions, the PCG/T was to do so on behalf of a group of GPs in a locality—and with more explicit financial constraints and performance incentives. They also included nurses, midwives, health visitors, and sometimes social workers. Chief executives head the PCTs (the first time such a position had been established in primary care), though GPs have retained key decision-making positions in these new organizations. PCTs have begun to experiment with new organizational and service arrangements, prompted partly by change and innovation elsewhere. These include the telephone service NHS Direct and immediate access, walk-in facilities in city centers as well as the new independent providers in both hospital and primary care. At the same time, however, the PCTs risk becoming more remote from their constituent GPs and less responsive to local needs. In April 2005, the government introduced yet again a new set of purchasing mechanisms for GPs called "practice-based commissioning." Practices receive a budget (based on a weighted capitation basis) to commission services from other providers. This measure was an attempt to continue to engage the agents most likely to sponsor clinical and organizational improvements as well as to ensure local responsiveness. While constrained by a skill shortage and the limited commissioning power of practices, this move appeared to many as a return to fundholding (Health Policy Monitor 2005d; House of Commons 2006).

INFORMATION TECHNOLOGY

Meanwhile, by investing in the development of the electronic medical record, the government sought to intervene in communications among doctors and between doctors and administrators. Information technology (IT) policy in the NHS had two principal elements: the computerization of the medical record and the construction of an electronic communications network, or intranet. Taken together, they constitute a notable aspect of organizational integration, or state building, that enrolls the profession (Freeman 2002a).

While the introduction of general management increased the demand for service-based information within the NHS, a new Information Management and Technology Strategy published in 1992 recognized that the internal market in turn required a new intensity of data collection and processing. At the same time, the assumption was that more detailed and more comparable information would improve the capacity for clinical audit. It would help government assess the performance of providers, both individual and institutional. The government's IT strategy envisaged common classification and coding of clinical data, a dedicated network of administrative registers, and the introduction of a new NHS number for patients (Keen 1994a, 1994b). The purpose of the new number was to make data computer-compatible, to improve its accuracy and accessibility, and to enable linkage between records kept at different sites. The incoming Labour administration issued a new information strategy statement, *Information for Health,* in 1998 (NHS Executive 1998). Playing again on the theme of modernization, it emphasized the benefits of health service information. It promised to develop appropriate infrastructure, including software and network systems (by now known as NHSnet). A new National Health Service Information Authority was formed in April 1999. From October 1, 2000, GP terms of service were amended to remove the obligation on general practitioners to keep paper records and to permit them to rely solely on electronic forms (NHS Executive 2000). The progress in NHS IT, it must be noted, has been poor. The Public Accounts Committee (of the Westminster Parliament) identified four key shortcomings of the national program, including implementation delays, shortcomings in delivery, poor engagement with clinicians, and uncertainty about rising costs (House of Commons 2007b, 3–4).

Computer networks aim to overcome divisions between specialist and generalist, community-based and hospital-based provision, payer and provider, and health care and social care. NHS documents continue to reiterate the original ambition to provide health care "from cradle to grave," an antique expression alternating with its contemporary equivalent, "seamless care." Crucially, however, integration depends on standardization. Successful communication depends on a common language. Network-based communication in health care requires the common coding and classification of professional activity, as well as a standard representation of the patient (the patient number or "permanent patient identifier"). Both therapeutic codes and patient numbers are embedded in—carried by—the electronic medical record. Meanwhile, the computerized record decreases the control of patient information by the individual physician while increasing control of it by the organization of which she or he is a part. These related processes of separation and standardization make the medical encounter (what the record is a record of) more amenable to the panoptic control of government (Exworthy et al. 2003).

Health Policy Learning in the NHS

One of the principal effects of the political and managerial activity we have described in this chapter has been what we might call a self-conscious NHS. Like other organizations large and small, public and commercial, the National Health Service is an organization concerned with the measurement and regulation of its own performance. One effect of management is to produce information that requires more management. Just as doctors lack the information to compare their own practices with those of their peers, so too do hospitals and groups of providers, as well as much larger entities such as regions and the different countries of England, Scotland, Wales, and Northern Ireland.

The salience of health policy debates across countries and the internationalization of news media, as well as research and debate in academic and professional networks, mean that it is now difficult for health policy makers in any one jurisdiction not to know something about what is going on in others. But the quality of that information and the sophistication with which it is understood and used vary widely.[4]

Cross-national exchange at the parliamentary and ministerial level is increasingly common. Early in 2002, for example, Alan Milburn and Bernard Kouchner, then health ministers for England and France, respectively, met to discuss performance measurement and patient choice as well as issues relating to cross-border health care. In 2000, the House of Commons Health Committee visited Cuba in preparing its report on public health (House of Commons Health Select Committee 2001). The National Audit Office (NAO) produced a compendium of *International Health Comparisons* in response to interest expressed by members of the Committee of Public Accounts in 2003 (NAO 2003), while the Department of Health's research division invited bids for an "on-call" facility for international health care comparisons at the end of 2004. Similarly, cross-national "learning" sometimes becomes the stuff of party politics. The Conservative opposition has shown interest in Australia (Hall and Maynard 2005), as it did before in France.

As is frequently observed, however, foreign experience often falls victim to the selective perception of domestic policy makers. Foreign evidence is used instrumentally, as "ammunition" (O'Neill 2000) in domestic "policy warfare" (Marmor and Plowden 1991). What are taken as policy "lessons" are derived from comparison that is inappropriate, pays little attention to evidence and evaluation, and ignores the particular needs and requirements of different policy contexts (see the Introduction to this volume). A particular British failing is the inability to distinguish between social and private or commercial insurance (McKee 2001; Dixon and Mossialos 2002).

Where British health policy discussion addresses foreign models, U.S. experience dominates. This influence extends to other areas of social policy, such as welfare-to-work initiatives and penal policy, and may be explained by a mixture of ideological convergence, notably among certain individuals and some think tanks, and the opportunity presented by a common language (Dolowitz, Greenwold, and Marsh 1999). In health care, Alain Enthoven's contribution to the reconfiguration of the NHS in the second and third Thatcher administrations—leading to the introduction of the internal market in 1991 (Enthoven 1985, 1991)—remains a point of departure, though the significance of that contribution is itself debated (Ham 2000). And despite routine skepticism and major differences between the two countries, U.S.–U.K. comparison continues, reemerging periodically in policy debate. The most vigorous recent exchange has been over the putative lessons for the United States to be drawn from Kaiser Permanente, which prompted DoH and King's Fund visits to California in 2002 and 2003 (Feachem, Sekhri, and White 2002; Donaldson and Ruta 2005; Ham 2005). There has also been rising interest in the Veterans Health Administration as a more suitable comparison for the NHS (Oliver 2007). Though the concern is mostly with funding mechanisms and their relationship to quality and productivity (Quam and Smith 2005), exchange goes on in other areas such as ethnic minority health, too, in more low-key but perhaps no less significant ways (Bhopal 1998; Exworthy and Washington 2006). This policy traffic tends to be one-way, from the United States to the United Kingdom, though some U.S. commentators, such as Donald Berwick and Barbara Starfield, have been expressly positive about NHS modernization and primary care, respectively (Berwick 2002, 2004; Berwick and Leatherman 2006; Starfield 2005).

Meanwhile, in general terms, the availability of cross-national data and the prominence of international debate about it make it difficult for major review and reform not to consider the example and experience of other countries. Such learning does not always make for substantive policy change, though it invariably changes the terms of debate. Cross-national comparison, for example, was a key part of the argument for Chancellor Gordon Brown's use of the Wanless Review to reject alternative funding arrangements for the NHS. When Wanless reported in 2002, it was in the course of a speech to the Social Market Foundation that Brown discovered an ambition to make the NHS—perhaps the paradigmatic example of a tax-funded system—the "best insurance policy in the world."[5]

We began by suggesting that we might best understand the NHS by its history, identifying and tracing the principal axes around which it revolves. We conclude by suggesting we might better understand both it and its history by understanding the way it learns.

Health care systems, as they are formed and even in the early stages of their development, are shaped by exogenous forces, by governments and economic actors (and parties on their behalf), and by professions not yet committed to or defined by them. Across countries, in Europe at least, the overriding tendency over the hundred years from the 1880s to the 1980s has been to universalism (Freeman 2000). No advanced industrial country, apart from the United States, seriously questions this universality (the extent of coverage might be, but that minimum coverage should be available to all is not; Marmor, Okma, and Latham 2006). Even where countries allow individuals to exit the system, this privilege is extended only to those (the rich) deemed able to access health care in other ways.

In the United Kingdom, this process took a particular form. Among liberal democracies, the nationalization or public incorporation of health care proceeded further here than elsewhere. Its core characteristic—the guarantee of universal access paid for by general taxation—seems politically irreversible, both on financial and on electoral grounds. Once assumed, public responsibility is difficult to renounce (Pierson 1994).

As systems mature, path dependence sets in. This does not mean that the system cannot change. In many ways, the NHS has changed more radically

over the last fifty years and remains more susceptible to government direction than almost any other system. But it does mean that it is more likely to
change in particular ways. The system continues to be driven by endogenous
processes: the politics of the NHS appear to be built-in, or perhaps gene-
tically coded, as the service confronts problems it has itself posed.

The engine of this process is management, sometimes cast as "modernization." The NHS is now characterized by an increasing variety of internal actors attempting to steer the system and its component parts on the basis of
information about its inputs, outputs, and outcomes, as well as about the
processes that translate from one to the other. Managers and management
have served different purposes, from breaking the institutional stalemate of
"consensus management" to becoming agents of the center, scapegoats of
system failures, and later market entrepreneurs (Harrison 1988). One of the
reasons management techniques are now so ubiquitous in health care is that
they serve the interests of at least some local administrators and at least
some professional leaders; management now acts in and not simply on the
system.

In terms of the political dynamics we have outlined here, modernization-
through-management appears to be a way of brokering ambiguous relationships between center and locality, public and private, government and
medicine. It seeks to offer both central direction and local autonomy, both
public accountability and private efficiency, both minimum standards and professional excellence. Sometimes these various tensions are resolved, sometimes
exposed and exacerbated; invariably, the terms of debate they set are repro-
duced. And this means, in turn, that modernization is likely both to accelerate
and never to be completed (Freeman 2002b).

If we were to describe the "learning style" of the NHS on this basis, it
would be as an organization that is introspective, driven, almost obsessive.
However, note that both general management and the internal market, as
well as more specific managerial instruments such as target setting and performance ratings, were part of a wider trend in the United Kingdom (and elsewhere) in the 1980s and 1990s toward new public management (Le Grand
and Bartlett 1993; Ferlie et al. 1996; Exworthy and Halford 1999). The assumption is that for an organization to appear as functional and accessible to
the public, it must look something like a shop. The shop may be intrinsic to
our ideas of the market, choice, and quality, but it is also increasingly highly
managed. What increased management means in health care is that the corner
shop that was general practice has become a much larger primary care outlet,
while arrangements negotiated with commercial and other providers are
much like franchising, both in conception and in effect.

This sort of cross-sectoral isomorphism has various sources. Some of them are specific, such as the government's use of management consultants (Leys 1999; Saint-Martin 2001), and some are more general, such as the training managers in all sorts of organizational environments now undertake, or the "common sense of the age" in which the managerialization of the NHS appears to make sense simply because it is familiar. When NHS decision makers look abroad, they do so only with any real intensity to the United States, not just because they speak English and not really out of any ideological conviction but because that is where the management of health care is even further advanced.

Notes

The authors of this chapter are glad to acknowledge the comment and criticism made by the co-editors of the volume, as well as the discussion of it that took place in the *jour fixe* on Health Care Systems Research at the University of Bremen.

1. At the end of 2004, the government decided to reduce (from thirty-eight to twenty) the number of arm's-length bodies linked to the DoH, most of which relate to regulation, inspection, information gathering, and innovation (Health Policy Monitor 2005a). In doing so, it expects to save £500 million by 2007–08.

2. The DH Policy Collaborative: http://www.dh.gov.uk/en/Publicationsandstatistics/Lettersandcirculars/Dearcolleagueletters/DH_4006367, accessed 11 December, 2008.

3. Organizational learning, of course, is often prompted by failure. While CHI held institutional responsibility for investigating system breakdown (CHI 2004), the DoH convened an expert group to reflect on the possibilities of learning from adverse events (DoH 2000c, 2001b), followed by similar reflection on serious case reviews in child protection (Sinclair and Bullock 2002) and medication safety (DoH 2004b). Forming a backdrop to these efforts was a series of major inquiries into the failings of children's heart surgery in Bristol, pathology services in Liverpool, and the GP Harold Shipman, among others (Walshe and Higgins 2002; Walshe 2003).

4. There are surprisingly few treatments of health policy in the burgeoning literature on cross-national policy transfer and learning (see the Introduction to this volume). Ham and colleagues show perhaps the most explicit interest in health policy literature on the United Kingdom (1997a, Ham 1997b), though the nature and process of that learning even here is more or less taken for granted.

5. HM Treasury (UK): speeches: http://www.hm-treasury.gov.uk/935.htm, accessed 11 December 2008.

Further Readings

Klein (2006) is the most engaging political history of the NHS, but see also Webster (1998). Ham (2004) provides the most effective introduction to policy, while Mohan (1995) focuses on geographical aspects. Gray and

Harrison (2004) and Salter (2004) provide the fullest recent accounts of medical professional regulation. Oliver (2005) provides a useful normative assessment of recent change in the NHS in terms of its founding principles. The Department of Health is at http://www.dh.gov.uk/Home/fs/en and the NHS at http://www.nhs.uk.

References

Alvarez-Rosete, A., G. Bevan, N. Mays, and J. Dixon. 2005. Effect of diverging policy across the NHS. *British Medical Journal,* 331: 946–50.

Berwick, D. M. 2002. The HSJ interview: Don Berwick; A case of US and them. By Paul Dempsey. *Health Service Journal* 113 (5850): 20–21.

Berwick, D. M. 2004. The improvement horse race: Bet on the UK. *Quality and Safety in Health Care,* 13: 407–9.

Berwick, D., and S. Leatherman. 2006. Steadying the NHS. *British Medical Journal,* 333: 254–55.

Bhopal, R. 1998. Spectre of racism in health and health care: Lessons from history and the United States. *British Medical Journal,* 316: 1970–73.

Causer, G., and M. Exworthy. 1999. Professionals as managers across the public sector. In *Professionals and the new managerialism in the public sector,* ed. M. Exworthy and S. Halford. Buckingham, UK: Open University Press.

CHI. *See* Commission for Health Improvement.

Commission for Health Improvement. 2004. *Lessons from CHI investigations 2000–2003.* London: Commission for Health Improvement.

Davies, H. T. O., and S. M. Nutley. 2000. Developing learning organizations in the new NHS. *British Medical Journal,* 320: 998–1001.

Day, P., and R. Klein. 1997. *Steering but not rowing? The transformation of the Department of Health.* Bristol, UK: Policy Press.

Department of Health. 1997. *The new NHS: Modern. Dependable.* Cm 3807. London: Stationery Office.

Department of Health. 2000a. *For the benefit of patients. A concordat with the private and voluntary health care provider sector.* London: Department of Health.

Department of Health. 2000b. *The NHS plan: A plan for investment, a plan for reform.* Cm 4818-I. London: Stationery Office.

Department of Health. 2000c. *An organization with a memory: Report of an expert group on learning from adverse events in the NHS.* London: Stationery Office.

Department of Health. 2001a. Press release 0164, March 30.

Department of Health. 2001b. *Building a safer NHS for patients: Implementing an organization with a memory.* London: Department of Health.

Department of Health. 2004a. *The NHS improvement plan: Putting people at the heart of public services.* Cm 6268. London: Stationery Office.

Department of Health. 2004b. *Building a safer NHS for patients: Improving medication safety; A report by the Chief Pharmaceutical Officer.* London: Department of Health.

Dixon, A., and E. Mossialos. 2002. Social insurance: Not much to write home about? *Health Service Journal* 112 (5789): 24–26.

DoH. *See* Department of Health.

Dolowitz, D., S. Greenwold, and D. Marsh. 1999. Policy transfer: Something old, something new, something borrowed, but why red, white and blue? *Parliamentary Affairs* 52 (4): 719–30.

Donaldson, C., and D. Ruta. 2005. Should the NHS follow the American way? *British Medical Journal,* 331: 1328–30.

Elliott, H., and J. Popay. 2000. How are policy makers using evidence? Models of research utilisation and local NHS policy making. *Journal of Epidemiology and Community Health,* 54: 461–68.

Enthoven, A. C. 1985. *Reflections on the management of the National Health Service.* London: Nuffield Provincial Hospitals Trust.

Enthoven, A. C. 1991. Internal market reform of the British National Health Service. *Health Affairs* 10 (3): 60–70.

Exworthy, M. 1993. A review of recent structural changes to District Health Authorities as purchasing organizations. *Environment and Planning C: Government and Policy,* 11: 279–89.

Exworthy, M. 1998. Localism in the NHS quasi-market. *Environment and Planning C: Government and Policy,* 16: 449–62.

Exworthy, M. 2001. Primary care in the UK: Understanding the dynamics of devolution. *Health and Social Care in the Community* 9 (5): 266–78.

Exworthy, M., and S. Halford, eds. 1999. *Professionals and the new managerialism in the public sector.* Buckingham, UK: Open University Press.

Exworthy, M., P. Kanavos, and F. Khondoker. 2001. *Cross-border patient flows for health-care in Europe.* Report for the Department of Health, vols. 1 and 2. Final report, December. London: LSE Health.

Exworthy, M., and S. Peckham. 2006. Access, choice and travel: Implications for health policy. *Social Policy and Administration* 40 (3): 267–87.

Exworthy, M., M. Powell, and J. Mohan. 1999. The NHS: Quasi-market, quasi-hierarchy and quasi-network? *Public Money and Management* 19 (4): 15–22.

Exworthy, M., and A. E. Washington. 2006. Organizational strategies to tackle health-care disparities in the US. *Health Services Management Research,* 19: 44–51.

Exworthy, M., E. K. Wilkinson, A. McColl, P. Roderick, H. Smith, M. Moore, and J. Gabbay. 2003. The role of performance indicators in changing the autonomy of the general practice profession in the UK. *Social Science and Medicine,* 56: 1493–1504.

Feachem, R. G. A., N. K. Sekhri, and K. L. White. 2002. Getting more for their dollar: A comparison of the NHS with California's Kaiser Permanente [with commentaries by J. Dixon, D. M. Berwick, A. C. Enthoven]. *British Medical Journal,* 324: 135–43.

Ferlie, E., L. Ashburner, L. Fitzgerald, and A. Pettigrew. 1996. *New public management in action.* Oxford: Oxford University Press.

Flynn, N. 1997. *Public sector management.* Hemel Hempstead, UK: Harvester Wheatsheaf.

Freeman, R. 2000. *The politics of health in Europe.* Manchester, UK: Manchester University Press.

Freeman, R. 2002a. The health care state in the information age. *Public Administration* 80 (4): 751–67.

Freeman, R. 2002b. Following "fads and fashions." *British Journal of Health Care Management* 8 (2): 69–70.

Freeman, R. 2007. Social democracy, uncertainty and health in Scotland. In *Scottish social democracy: New ideas and progressive policy,* ed. M. Keating. Brussels: Presses Interuniversitaires Européennes.

Freeman, R., and K. Woods. 2002. Learning from devolution: UK policy since 1999. *British Journal of Health Care Management* 8 (12): 462–66.

Gray, A. G., and S. Harrison, eds. 2004. *Governing medicine: Theory and practice.* Buckingham, UK: Open University Press.

Greener, I. 2003. Who choosing what? The evolution of the use of "choice" in the NHS, and its implications for New Labour. *Social Policy Review,* 15: 49–67.

Greer, S. L. 2004. *Territorial politics and health policy: UK health policy in comparative perspective.* Manchester, UK: Manchester University Press.

Hall, J., and A. Maynard. 2005. Healthcare lessons from Australia: What can Michael Howard learn from John Howard? *British Medical Journal,* 330: 357–59.

Ham, C., ed. 1997a. *Health care reform: Learning from international experience.* Buckingham, UK: Open University Press.

Ham, C. 1997b. Priority setting in health care: Learning from international experience. *Health Policy,* 42: 49–66.

Ham, C. 2000. *The politics of NHS reform 1988–97.* London: King's Fund.

Ham, C. 2004. *Health policy in Britain: The politics and organization of the National Health Service.* 5th ed. Basingstoke, UK: Palgrave Macmillan.

Ham, C. 2005. Lost in translation? Health systems in the US and the UK. *Social Policy and Administration* 39 (2): 192–209.

Harrison, S. 1988. *Managing the National Health Service: Shifting the frontier.* London: Chapman and Hall.

Harrison, S. 1999. Clinical autonomy and health policy: Past and future. In *Professionals and the new managerialism in the public sector,* eds. M. Exworthy and S. Halford. Buckingham, UK: Open University Press.

Health Policy Monitor. 2005a. Cutting bureaucracy in the NHS. http://www.health-policy-monitor.org.

Health Policy Monitor. 2005b. New Foundation Trusts. http://www.health-policy-monitor.org.

Health Policy Monitor. 2005c. Choice and responsiveness in the English NHS. http://www.health-policy-monitor.org.

Health Policy Monitor. 2005d. Empowering GPs: A return to fundholding. http://www.health-policy-monitor.org.

Heclo, H., and A. Wildavsky. 1974. *The private government of public money.* Basingstoke, UK: Macmillan.

Holliday, I. 1995. *The NHS transformed.* Manchester, UK: Baseline.

House of Commons Committee of Public Accounts. 2007a. *Financial management in the NHS: Seventeenth report of session 2006–2007.* HC361. London: Stationery Office.

House of Commons Committee of Public Accounts. 2007b. *The Department of Health: The national programme for IT in the NHS; Twentieth report of session 2006–2007.* HC390. London: Stationery Office.

House of Commons Health Select Committee. 2001. *Second report 2000–2001.* London: Stationery Office. http://www.parliament.the-stationery-office.co.uk/pa/cm200001/cmselect/cmhealth/30/3007.htm.

House of Commons Health Select Committee. 2006. *Changes to Primary Care Trusts: Second report of session 2005–2006.* HC646. London: Stationery Office.

Iles, V., and K. Sutherland. 2001. *Organizational change: A review for health care managers, professionals and researchers.* London: National Co-ordinating Centre for NHS Service Delivery and Organisation R&D, London School of Hygiene and Tropical Medicine.

Innvaer, S., G. Vist, M. Trommald, and A. Oxman. 2002. Health policy makers' perceptions of their use of evidence: A systematic review. *Journal of Health Services Research and Policy* 7 (4): 239–44.

Jervis, P., and W. Plowden. 2003. *The impact of political devolution on the UK's health services.* London: Nuffield Trust.

Keen, J. 1994a. Information policy in the National Health Service. In *Information management in health services,* ed. J. Keen. Buckingham, UK: Open University Press.

Keen, J. 1994b. Should the National Health Service have an information strategy? *Public Administration,* 72: 33–53.

King's Fund. 2005. *An independent audit of the NHS under Labour, 1997–2005.* London: King's Fund.

Klein, R. 1990. The state and the profession: The politics of the double bed. *British Medical Journal,* 301: 700–702.

Klein, R. 2006. *The new politics of the NHS.* 5th ed. Oxford: Radcliffe Publishing.

Kmietowicz, Z. 2006. GP services improve on last year. *British Medical Journal,* no. 333: 721.

Koeck, C. M. 1998. As others see us: Views from abroad; A rational bureaucracy in a civilised society. *British Medical Journal,* 317: 48–49.

Le Grand, J., and W. Bartlett, eds. 1993. *Quasi-markets and social policy.* London: Macmillan.

Le Grand, J., N. Mays, and J. Mulligan, eds. 1998. *Learning from the NHS internal market.* London: King's Fund.

Le Grand, J., and R. Robinson, eds. 1994. *Evaluating the NHS reforms.* London: King's Fund.

Leys, C. 1999. Intellectual mercenaries and the public interest: Management consultancies and the NHS. *Policy and Politics* 27 (4): 447–65.

Marmor, T. R., K. G. H. Okma, and S. R. Latham. 2006. Values, institutions and health politics: Comparative perspectives. In *Soziologie der Gesundheit,* ed. C. Wendt and C. Wolf. Sonderheft der Kölner Zeitschrift. Wiesbaden, Germany: VS-Verlag.

Marmor, T. R., and W. Plowden. 1991. Rhetoric and reality in the international jet stream: The export to Britain from America of questionable ideas. *Journal of Health Politics, Policy and Law* 16 (4): 807–12.

Maynard, A., and A. Street. 2006. Seven years of feast, seven years of famine: Boom to bust in the NHS? *British Medical Journal*, no. 332: 906–8.

McKee, M. 2001. Insurance policy for NHS. *The Guardian*. November 26. http://www.guardian.co.uk/letters/story/0,,605908,00.html.

Mohan, J. 1995. *A National Health Service?* Basingstoke, UK: Macmillan.

NAO. *See* National Audit Office.

National Audit Office. 2003. *International health comparisons: A compendium of published information on healthcare systems, the provision of healthcare and health achievement in 10 countries*. London: NAO. http://www.nao.org.uk/publications/Int_Health_Comp.pdf.

National Health Service Management Inquiry. 1983. *Report*. London: Department of Health and Social Security.

NHS Executive. 1998. *Information for health: An information strategy for the modern NHS 1998–2005; A national strategy for local implementation*. Leeds, UK: Department of Health.

NHS Executive. 2000. *Electronic patient medical records in primary care: Changes to the GP terms of service*. PC-01/10/00. Leeds, UK: Department of Health.

OECD. *See* Organisation for Economic Co-operation and Development.

Oliver, A. 2005. The English National Health Service: 1979–2005. *Health Economics* 14 (S1): 75–99.

Oliver, A. 2007. The Veterans Health Administration: An American success story. *Milbank Quarterly* 85 (1): 5–35.

O'Neill, F. 2000. Health: The "internal market" and reform of the National Health Service. In *Policy transfer and British social policy*, ed. D. Dolowitz. Buckingham, UK: Open University Press.

Organisation for Economic Co-operation and Development. 2005. *Society at a glance: OECD social indicators*. Paris: OECD.

Peckham, S., and M. Exworthy. 2003. *Primary care in the UK: Policy, organization and management*. Basingstoke, UK: Palgrave.

Pierson, P. 1994. *Dismantling the welfare state: Reagan, Thatcher and the politics of retrenchment*. Cambridge: Cambridge University Press.

Pollitt, C., J. Caulfield, A. Smullen, and C. Talbot. 2004. *Agencies: How governments do things through semi-autonomous organizations*. Basingstoke, UK: Palgrave Macmillan.

Pollock, A. 2003. *NHS plc: The privatisation of our health care*. London: Verso.

Powell, M. 1998. In what sense a National Health Service? *Public Policy and Administration* 13 (3): 56–69.

Power, M. 1997. *The audit society*. Oxford: Oxford University Press.

Quam, L., and R. Smith. 2005. What can the UK and US health policy systems learn from each other? *British Medical Journal*, 330: 530–33.

Rivett, G. 2005. NHS history. http://nhshistory.net/organisation_and_finance.htm.

Robinson, R., D. Evans, and M. Exworthy. 1994. *Health and the economy*. Birmingham, UK: National Association of Health Authorities and Trusts.

Saint-Martin, D. 2001. *Building the new managerialist state*. Oxford: Oxford University Press.

Salter, B. 2004. *The new politics of medicine*. Basingstoke, UK: Palgrave Macmillan.

Saltman, R., and C. von Otter. 1992. *Planned markets in healthcare*. Buckingham, UK: Open University Press.

Secretary of State for Health. 1998. *A first class service: Quality in the new NHS*. London: Department of Health.

Sinclair, R., and R. Bullock. 2002. *Learning from past experience: A review of serious case reviews*. London: Department of Health.

Smith, J., and K. Walshe. 2004. Big business: The corporatization of primary care in the UK and the USA. *Public Money and Management* 24 (2): 87–96.

Starfield, B. 2005. Why is the grass greener? *British Medical Journal*, 330: 727–29.

Walshe, K. 2003. *Inquiries: Learning from failure in the NHS?* London: Nuffield Trust.

Walshe, K., and J. Higgins. 2002. The use and impact of inquiries in the NHS. *British Medical Journal*, 325: 895–900.

Wanless, D. 2002. *Our future health: Taking a long-term view*. London: HM Treasury.

Webster, C. 1998. *The National Health Service: A political history*. Oxford: Oxford University Press.

Woods, K. J. 2002. Health policy and the NHS in the UK 1997–2002. In *Devolution in practice: Public policy differences within the UK*, ed. J. Adams and P. Robinson. London: Institute for Public Policy Research.

Woods, K. J. 2004. Political devolution and the health services in Great Britain. *International Journal of Health Services*, 34: 323–39.

7

Primary Care and Health Reform
Concepts, Confusions, and Clarifications

JOSEPH WHITE AND THEODORE R. MARMOR

The national health care arrangements emphasized in this book—of Germany, the Netherlands, Canada, the United States, and the United Kingdom—undeniably differ in the structure of their governing institutions, the ways they finance and contract medical care, and in subtle cultural forms. The earlier chapters demonstrate these differences. Yet, it is also the case that in the period since the stagflation of the 1970s, the repertoire of proposed "health reforms" seemed quite similar across these and other wealthy democracies. At the level of discourse, one of the most sacred cows of Western health policy, the topic of primary care—and the slogan of "primary care–led reform"—provides striking evidence of cross-national parallels. Yet, at the same time, primary care turns out to be a highly varied notion. Reforms heralded as instances of it turn out to be, depending on one's taste, charmingly different or stunningly confusing.

When the Four Country Conference met to discuss primary care in 1997, the participants found that it was easier to define what primary care reform was meant to displace (specialist and hospital care, medical care that could be avoided by prevention, or uncoordinated health services) than what it was supposed to be. It also appeared that a greater emphasis on primary care tended to have far greater support among policy analysts and system managers than among patients or citizens and health care providers. Although advocacy positions for such "reforms" thus were related to disciplinary and positional biases, the discussion also revealed that there were differences in emphases across countries, and that reflected the fact that in practice, primary care (by some definitions) played a more important role in some countries than in others.

This chapter discusses, in three parts, the myths and realities of what has come to be known as "primary care reform." The first section addresses the various conceptual versions of what counts as "primary." That in turn shapes what is thought to be primary care, and hence primary care reform. The second section shows the variation, as well as some similarities, in the discussion and practice among the five countries in our comparisons. The third section summarizes the patterns of *reform advocacy* and *system practice,* and the relationship between those very different phenomena. We argue that, in spite of the conceptual ambiguities, the topic of primary care reveals two interesting patterns. The first is that "primary care" is a highly elastic term with many denotations but a positive connotation. Reforms said to emphasize primary care differ substantively across countries because of different policy inheritances. The very vagueness of the concept allows it to be used in different ways, but those ways do have a basis in system reality. The second is that the advocacy for primary care is consistently far more popular among health policy analysts than with the public and medical providers. Because analysts generate policy proposals (seeing cost savings and longer-term health benefits), but patients and providers (actually experiencing restraints) must accept and implement them, this popularity difference helps explain why proposals, but not implementation, tend to be common.

The conceptual issues about primary care as a reform concern illustrate the contention of the book's Introduction that confusion, more than clarity, dominates the international transfer of broad policy reform ideas in the health sector. Had we concentrated on concepts such as "managed competition," "integrated delivery system reform," or "stewardship in health care reform," we most likely would have had comparable illustrations.

Conceptual Preliminaries

Anything to which the term "primary" is applied presents a puzzle because the term has many, quite different meanings. So, for instance, primary means "important" when used in expressions such as the following: "The primary cause of poor maintenance in rent-controlled apartments is the restriction on what the income owners can earn on their property investments." The claim may be true, false, or hard to evaluate, but the meaning of primary is clear. A variant of that meaning in the health literature shows up when commentators assert that nonmedical care factors—such as income inequality, social distance, or the conditions of work—are "primary" and that the availability of medical care is "secondary" in explaining the health status of populations. Or claims that prevention is "primary" imply that it contributes more to health status than care once patients are sick.

Quite different is the use of "primary" in terms of a sequence of events. The first thing to do or the first place to visit is "primary" in this formulation. When employed in medical care, this term can refer, as is common in the United States, to the emergency room as the first point of contact for families without regular access to a physician, visiting nurse, or health clinic. Or it can simply refer to the health professional one usually visits first, one's "primary provider" in the jargon. Finally and still different, "primary" refers to the lowest level of complexity of a medical setting or of medical personnel. Primary versus secondary (and tertiary) care employs distinctions that parallel the offices of general practitioners, community hospitals, and more complex academic or specialized "health centers."

As we shall see later in this chapter, these conceptual distinctions are crucial for understanding what is at stake, not simply for intellectual neatness. For decades now, appeals to something termed "primary care" carried presumptions that de-emphasizing access to or reliance on hospitals and specialist physicians would be a good thing.[1] But it is by no means clear (a) what that entailed about reform in the world beyond or before hospitals and specialist physicians and (b) what the evidence was that would support any of the various reforms made in the name of the primary care.

In the United States, as elsewhere, the calls for primary care reform have been as persistent as they have been confusing about what they entail. The scope of hopes associated with primary care aspirations is amazingly large. To see that clearly, consider the difference between primary care understood as what general practitioners do or the first point of contact for patients with the following excerpt from an article in *Health Affairs*. "Primary care," we are urged to believe, "stands at the center of medical systems," a claim that is false empirically and contentious normatively when using the following definition: "[The] key functions include providing an entry point, delivering core medical and preventive care, and helping patients coordinate and integrate care. When working well, each of these dimensions is instrumental in improving health outcomes and cost performance" (Schoen et al. 2004, 487).

What is clear in this statement is that primary care is both an aspiration of performance and a stipulation of what counts as the important criteria. Its usefulness as a way of understanding what is done in practice is greatly limited by this conflation. Indeed, what is one to make of the claim that "differing performance levels [on these very broad dimensions] highlight the potential for improvement and cross-national learning" (Schoen et al. 2004, 487)? Are there any systems that do not "provide an entry point?" Is it really patients who are expected to "coordinate and integrate care?"

To advocates, greater emphasis on primary care—and less on secondary and tertiary care—promises both reductions of cost and improvements in the quality of their nation's health and health care. Such primary care growth might be less expensive because it reduces high-tech, capital-intensive interventions by medical specialists. Good primary care would, for some, surely lead to earlier detection of and (even) prevention of serious illness. A physician responsible for the whole person (for example, "patient-centered" primary care) might be better at coordinating care than multiple specialists treating separate organ systems. In still other visions, primary care includes long-lasting relationships between patients and clinics of providers (both physicians and nonphysicians), arrangements that promise improved prevention not just for individuals but for the community as a whole. As Fitzhugh Mullan writes, "Many proponents of primary care have seen the primary care movement as a battle for the soul of medicine—medicine that had become a balkanized land of technologies and specialists" (Mullan 1998).

These varied notions of possible improvement thus appeal to standard criticisms of traditional medical care by modern economists and public health leaders alike. Both groups argue that savings may be made if services are more efficiently integrated or if there is substitution of less expensive for more expensive medical personnel. Primary care physicians, in this view, are the potential "managers" of an inefficient, unmanaged system. Quality improvements would be served better by shifting emphasis from the "medical model" of mechanistic response to disease to a "wellness model" founded on health and the whole person. Hence two visions complement each other in a negative sense. Both the primary care and the wellness enthusiasts regard highly specialized medicine and its hospital-dominated world with skepticism. Yet, as Mullan notes, the two visions represent very different worldviews: the former one of "industrial efficiency" and the latter one of "social justice" (Mullan 1998, 121).

The continual emphasis on controlling the costs of medical care has prompted contemporary promotion of what passes in each setting as primary care. This approach has been apparent in efforts to restrain hospital use in the United States, to entice Quebec citizens into community health centers, and in frequent efforts to revise fee schedules (and capitation rates) at the expense of specialists in a number of national settings. Finally, concerns about the costs of modern medicine have prompted proposals to have primary care providers or organizations bear financial risk for the costs of other medical services.

We turn now to national experiences.

Findings from the Field: Primary Care Discourse and Realities in Five Countries

The background of widespread but loosely defined appeals to primary care reform was part of what was startling in our conference discussions of this topic. Presenter after presenter employed, it turned out, somewhat different definitions of primary care. And, in addition, they relied on quite different grounds for either supporting or questioning this line of reform thinking.

For instance, it was not at all clear who is the "primary care provider" in discussions of national practice. Many gynecologists, responding to market pressures in the United States, were claiming to be their patients' "primary care" provider. Gynecologists would not qualify for the role if one presumes a primary physician is a professional whose general knowledge is sufficient for a first examination of any patient with any symptom and whose further task is to determine whether specialist care is required and to which specialist the patient should be referred (the gatekeeper model). Yet, in other respects it is quite plausible to regard a gynecologist as a woman's primary physician. Gynecologists may see their patients much more often than any other doctor. Regular gynecological checkups, as with pap smears, are more likely to be funded by insurance than periodic, asymptomatic checkups, at least in the United States. In any case, women may attend to the former more regularly, which comports with the concept of primary as the first point of contact. Moreover, the gynecologist may, because of regular checkups, be much more aware of the patient's state of mind, the "whole person" in the jargon of the primary care field. Similar problems arise in connection with chronically ill patients. Patients with a serious chronic condition are likely to consider the specialist who regularly treats their condition as their primary provider, no matter what health policy experts might think.

Thus it is clear that countries or experts differ in whom they see as a provider of primary care. But equally, there are striking differences in what categories of services are understood as "primary care." Table 7.1 summarizes what was included within the national label of primary care.

This diversity illustrates one of the main benefits of a cross-national perspective: namely, clarifying what it is that a topic means in one setting by contrast with similar and very different formulations elsewhere. But, while

Table 7.1 Services under primary care, by country

Health service seen as primary care	U.S.	Canada	Germany	Netherlands	U.K.
Ob/Gyn	Yes	No	No	No	No
General Internist	Yes	No	Yes	No	No
GP/Family doctor	Yes	Yes	Yes	Sometimes	Yes
Prescription drugs	Yes			No	No
Allied health professionals	No	No	Yes	Yes	No
Home care (nursing, home help)	No	No	Yes	Yes	No
Related social care	No	No	Yes	Yes	No

Source: *Four Country Conference: Primary health care.* 1997. Conference Report. Boppard, Germany, June 5–8.

clarifying, the diverse notions of primary care and its relation to health reform are a source of complexity as well.

It is possible, of course, to stipulate a definition and then use it for analytical purposes. Macinko, Starfield, and Shi (2003) compared eighteen countries to establish the "strength" of their "primary care systems" and then related the results to some health care outcomes. Some of their variables, for example, whether patients must be on a given primary care practice's "list" or whether the "primary" practice keeps the gate to other care, concern care delivery. Others, such as whether the primary care practice keeps "community-based data" or involves "community members in primary-care management or priority-setting," tap the ideology of preference for "community" and public health over individual care. Still other variables relate more to features of distribution and redistribution, more to the system as a whole than to primary care per se (Macinko, Starfield, and Shi 2003, 840–41).[2] Using this scale, they reported that out of eighteen OECD nations, the United Kingdom had the highest performance for primary care policy in 1995; the Netherlands was fourth; Canada, ninth; the United States, fifteenth; and Germany, sixteenth (845).[3]

GERMANY AND "LIP SERVICE"

In Germany, for instance, Schwartz reported decades of "lip service" about "strengthening . . . the primary care sector." That notion includes the practice of gatekeeping family doctors, to help reduce the volume of specialist and hospital care. As in other countries, primary care in Germany has grown less than other medical care. That sector, understood mainly as the care given by family practitioners (general practitioners), he noted, had decreased from over 50 percent of all "office-based physicians . . . in 1975 to less than 40% in 1996." The report from Germany, then, revealed a "schism between rhetoric [of reform and growth of the sector] and reality" (Schwartz 1997).

The reality of this primary care gap gave a distinctive shape to German policy debates. It affected disputes about the role of pharmacists, concerns about continuity of care in the face of 1996 legislation for a social insurance form of long-term care financing, and efforts by sickness funds to give family physicians (the *Hausarzt* idea) some form of gatekeeping role. Both noncooperation by physician organizations and the public's disinterest led to the demise of the latter. What Schwartz describes as a "public health oriented view of primary health care [that] includes broader determinants of health" barely made it to the bargaining table. The health reform law of 1988 also supported "broad non-medical health promotion activities" by the sickness funds, but those terms were "abruptly stopped" by the third "wave" of health reform legislation in 1996 (Schwartz 1997, 78).

In each area, the issue in the German debate was not only conceptual but a matter of professional "turf." The dominant model treats the care by general practitioners, general internists, and pediatricians in single or small-group practices (*Hausärzte*) as appropriate. The physician associations use these understandings as a base for their bargaining with sick funds over payments. This practice has prompted controversy over "the role of gynecologists and, for the elderly—the ophthalmologists." The most prominent turf factor was (and still is) that the specialists dominate the physicians' associations, and therefore these associations had (and have) little interest in reforms that would create separate funds for "primary" care, however defined, let alone give one (smaller) group of physicians gatekeeping power over the other (larger) group. In this regard, Germany differs greatly from its smaller neighbor the Netherlands, in which patients have accepted the gatekeeping role of their GPs for decades.

The picture that emerged from the discussion was one of long-standing criticism of the German model by reformers and persistent difficulties in making substantial changes in German practice. For instance, in the late 1980s, the Advisory Council for Concerted Action in Health Care published a number of studies critical of the status quo. The critique focused on the high "volume of services" in the sector, "diagnostic overload," the overemphasis on somatic symptoms of ill-health, and the absence of a "preventive orientation." In content, the diagnosis was familiar to the public health community. But the criticism extended to another area as well: namely, the widespread shopping for specialist physicians, thus bypassing their family physicians as gatekeepers. What is striking about the German developments is not the diagnosis but the organizational history of reform. The reform movement was dominated by experts and reflected neither citizen preoccupations nor general support in the physician community (Schwartz 1997).

"[Reform] recommendations . . . reflected mainly the views of experts and the results of administrative data analysis and interpretation, but did not necessarily reflect the need or visions of consumers or patient groups or organizations. The few user oriented studies showed no significant demand for major health reform." There was some demand for integration: "self-help organizations of chronic sick patients . . . [promoted] new problem-oriented forms of care integrating preventive, curative, rehabilitative and long-term care elements of 'primary care' " (80). This too would have required change in power relations within the medical profession and did not clearly offer savings. Meanwhile, public preferences were revealed nicely when the introduction of an electronic "patient card" in 1994, which made self-referral to specialists easier, "produced within one year . . . an enormous increase of direct patient contacts with specialist practices without formal referrals" (81). Given the opportunity to avoid a gatekeeper, people took it.

Despite elite advocacy for a greater role for primary care, events if anything actually strengthened the dominance of specialist care. While physician organizations opposed a greater role for their primary care minority and the public was at most indifferent, even sickness fund and political leaders were "at best" doubtful backers of primary-care-led reform. In short, Germany was unlikely to change in the direction of an "integrated, community approach" to care. Nor would it move to "greater integration of preventive, curative, rehabilitative, and long-term care" or "even a gatekeeping role" with significant power (82).

In the ensuing years, primary care has not been a major theme of the German health policy debate, although time and again reformers tried to push it onto the agenda (see Chapter 4). We can speculate that there are two main reasons. First, other health policy challenges seemed more pressing—ranging from reform of the financing system (a modest move from payroll finance to general revenues) to implementing the new long-term care entitlement, to dealing with the consequences of increased choice among sickness funds. Second, the German system already had powerful measures to control physician service costs.[4]

From simply looking at a map or at a bit of history (the Dutch health insurance system was substantially structured by the German occupiers in 1941), one might expect the Dutch situation to be similar to Germany's. Yet the conference discussion led Martin Pfaff to ask why it was that in "two countries—the Netherlands and Germany—which have roughly similar health care systems, primary care plans [have] such a different role in practice to-day?" Not only does primary care play a different and weightier role in the Netherlands, but there is "seemingly . . . no real conflict between the primary care physicians [general practitioners] and the specialists. How come?" (Pfaff 1997, 15).

DUTCH SUCCESS AND DISCONTENT

This question provides a useful transition to the findings about primary care practice in the Netherlands. The initial point to emphasize is the need for an accurate understanding of the realities of Dutch general practice. Primary care there usually includes what family doctors do, and while they do much of what counts as medical care in the Netherlands, home care also fits under the "primary care" label. Patients with social insurance (until 2006, 65 percent of the population) must be listed with a practice, and so are committed to that practice. They need a referral to access specialists and hospitals. Dutch GPs generally act as physicians and gatekeepers to specialist medical care for an entire family.[5] They also can use institutional diagnostic facilities (so they do not have to hand off patients to specialists for that purpose). Moreover, Dutch GPs have their own strong and effective lobby (unlike German GPs).[6]

For those Dutch citizens compulsorily enrolled in social health insurance (and, as of January 2006, all Dutch citizens—see Chapter 5), Dutch general practitioners received a mix of capitation fees, fees for service, plus additional payments for specific activities. There were in 1997 about twice as many general practitioners as specialists. Moreover, the range of services listed as primary care includes home care, physical therapy, and other nonmedical services. In short, the Netherlands were close to the kind of model that primary care advocates in other countries sought to achieve.

Why there has been this difference, the comparative puzzle, is heightened by common features between Germany and the Netherlands. These two continental nations share a number of crucial characteristics, including dependence on social insurance for the bulk of their populations, multiparty coalitions as a persistent feature of governance in the postwar world and—until recently (see Chapter 5)—a tradition of social policy commitments by Christian Democratic parties that largely parallel the welfare state commitments of their Social Democratic counterparts. Without attempting a detailed answer, what is clear is that once the general practitioner–specialist split was established in the Netherlands and the payment system organized around capitation for the former, the terms of competition and cooperation sharply distinguished Dutch practice from what was prompted by the division of labor (and remuneration) in Germany. Earlier in the twentieth century, the GP and specialist sectors were separated in the Netherlands but not in Germany; that in turn led to organizational structures that rigidified and reinforced the distinction. Generally, Dutch patients accept that their GPs exercise restraint in their referral patterns, even though they face no financial risk from referrals. Generally, patients trust their GP; apart from some more mobile urban groups, most families stay with their doctor. GPs take their gatekeeping seriously and believe they will lose their strong position in the system if they just become referral mills. In the 1990s, Dutch GPs were successful in bargaining: By the early 2000s, their incomes ranked highest in Europe (OECD 2006).

Somehow, this presumption does not appear to have given Dutch policy elites any less interest in health care reform than was the case in other countries. Indeed, they still worry about coordination and efficiency. Instead of believing their successful gatekeeping was assuring system efficiency, Dutch policy makers in the mid-1980s set off on a so-far unfulfilled quest to "increase the efficiency of the health-care system" through "a growing attention to the role of incentives" and so "market-oriented reforms" (Schut and Van de Ven 2005, S62). While the reform efforts sought to increase the role of health insurers, government did not give up its reliance on the payment structure. Dutch policy makers did favor primary care in that they squeezed specialists' fees more tightly than GPs' payments. In 1995, for example, they put specialist incomes within hospital global budgets. This policy drastically reduced incentives for production by specialists, waiting times increased, and in 2001 policy makers reinstated fees for specialist services.[7] Interestingly, the Dutch, having already created the gatekeeping role, did not associate it per se with competition—unlike, as we shall see, the Americans.

Dutch patients, while mainly accepting the gatekeeper role because it was the status quo, started to become restive. "With the ongoing introduction of new medical technologies and pharmaceuticals which improve the quality of life and lengthen the life expectation itself, and a more demanding role of the patient, the position of a gatekeeper is under fire. Patients in Holland claim more and more their 'rights' " (Hendriks 1997, 87). The Netherlands therefore resembles Germany in one way: Gatekeeping was more popular with policy makers than the public. It is different in that, being the status quo, it was accepted by the medical profession (especially the dominant primary care providers). And also because it was the status quo, it was not seen by elites as a solution to the system's problems.

The discussion of what counted as primary care reform in the United States, Canada, and the United Kingdom reiterated what we have noted in the

German-Dutch contrast. In Canada, where general practitioners are nearly as common as in the Netherlands but capitation and practice listing are not, the scope of reform ideas is much broader. In the United States, where general practitioners and family doctors have been a smaller (and decreasing) proportion of the physician population, primary care reform ideas widen even more, as we shall see. In the National Health Service of the United Kingdom, the general practitioner remains the gatekeeper to the hospital and specialist services, but general practice has seen constant change since the 1980s.

CANADA: GERMANY LIGHT

For Canada, according to our conference informant and other sources, the reform ideal of primary care was widely shared as an objective by experts, royal commission reports, and a considerable number of political leaders. The call was "heard throughout much of Canada . . . and [meant] multidisciplinary teams to provide care to a defined (rostered) population." That vision included capitation funding, as opposed to traditional fee-for-service remuneration for general practice doctors (Schurman 1997).[8]

Beyond this policy-maker interest in primary care as a means to capitation, however, lurked many diverse views. In some provinces "primary care" referred to emphasis on prevention and the nonmedical determinants of health; in others, not. And in all cases the patients and providers were less enamored of the goal, whatever its details might be. A 1995 report by the Advisory Committee on Health Services, which called for primary care organizations with rostered patients and capitation, met "a storm of protest from physicians from across the country and some concern by consumers" (Schurman 1997, 71).[9] While physicians objected to capitation and bearing risk, some patient groups worried that sicker patients would be avoided by providers whose payments were limited to a capitated amount (72).

In the face of this opposition, the provincial health ministers punted and called for more study. Ontario provided a good example of what happens when the physicians and public are involved in the policy initiatives. First, it set up pilot programs. Ontario's Primary Care Implementation Steering Committee produced a report that defined primary care basically as first contact and then emphasized relatively unexceptionable goals for pilots (improved access, coordination, preventive care initiatives) while downplaying the controversial measures such as capitation and rostering. Communication between primary care providers and specialists was to be improved through measures such as written consultation reports; patients should learn to go to physicians instead of the emergency room; there should be less duplication of diagnostic testing and more use of information technology (Primary Care Implementation Steering Committee 1997).

While the ideal vision of primary care receded, actual Canadian practice—the strict spending restraints of the mid-1990s—revealed an interesting reality. As budget cutting shut down institutions in Ontario, 250 hospitals in Toronto were combined into about 70. And it turned out that those institutions had been providing a lot of the care for people—physical therapy, psychiatric care, and nutritional advice. Suddenly the family practitioners had much less left to coordinate. Ironically, for primary care to be effective in coordinating and referring, there has to be a substantial further system. If primary care means GPs replacing all other providers, there is no conflict. But if the vision requires coordination, then cutting the rest of the system may worsen "primary care," not improve it.

THE UNITED KINGDOM AND THE LIMITS OF PRIMARY CARE

If, as Macinko, Starfield and Shi (2003) argue, the United Kingdom in 1997 was the closest approximation to the primary care ideal, what kind of primary care reform agenda could exist? One answer is that the agenda could consist of discussions about marginal change. In the United Kingdom, the appeal to primary care varied from the first contact idea to what happened in general practice. In first contact terms, telephone calls at all hours increasingly came to the foreground for attention and policy change. So, NHSDirect, the twenty-four-hour service funded nationally, was a major change given great prominence in the United Kingdom. So-called comprehensive services received much less attention.

Yet, in the late 1990s, the British primary care reform agenda was dominated by the more significant issues about implementation of GP fundholding. The organization of the NHS did require referrals by GPs in order to access specialists (consultants, in British terms). Yet strict controls on the number of consultants substantially constrained access anyway. Moreover, the use of sessional fees to pay physician services in hospitals gave consultants little incentive to provide services. As a result, the policy problem in the United Kingdom was not how to get GPs to keep patients away from specialists, but how to get specialists to respond to GPs (and patients). Fundholding started in 1991. It was part of the late-1980s NHS reforms initiated by Prime Minister Margaret Thatcher. It allowed GP practices (above a certain size) to contract with consultants to provide a portion of services. The fact that consultants had to satisfy GPs in order to receive contracts and that the contracts provided some income above the sessional fees in the hospitals appeared to make consultants more responsive. In essence, fundholding gave general practices more power.

Yet fundholding raised concerns about potential inequalities and competition between fundholding and other GP practices. It also had only marginal impact on the basic problem of inefficiency (from one view) or insufficiency (from another) of secondary and tertiary services. Moreover, having fundholders "commission" some services while most other services were commissioned by District Health Authorities contradicted the desire for greater coordination. Hence in 1997 the Labour party took office determined to change the system.[10]

The new Labour government replaced the fundholding (and nonfundholding) GP practices with a system of Primary Care Trusts. These local organizations include all GPs in the area as well as other providers such as nurses and health visitors, but not the hospitals and consultants. Primary Care Trusts then contract for most other services; hence, in theory, GPs have a substantial voice in the contracts with consultants and hospitals.[11] Given perceived shortages of hospital and consultant capacity, however, any hopes that GPs could shape services in their local areas through contracting were likely to be thwarted. Choice requires choices.

Moreover, public opinion was not focused on primary care but on shortages of other services. Public discontent resulted not only from continued long waiting lists but also, in the revealing words of the prime minister's health policy adviser, from "a growing tendency of the British media to substitute its long-standing stereotype of the NHS ('good') versus the US health system ('bad'), with an equally polemical comparison of the NHS ('bad') with continental Europe ('good')" (Stevens 2004). The contrast showed that France and Germany had universal care but few if any waiting lists. In response, after a few years the government decided to raise total U.K. health spending from the 6.8 percent of GDP in 1997 to a goal of 9.4 percent of GDP in 2007–08. It promised to match European levels of spending, using the money mainly to dramatically increase the supply of health professionals, increase salaries, and modernize infrastructure (Stevens 2004, 38–39; Oliver 2005, S80).[12]

Hence the nation that ostensibly had the strongest primary care system was forced, by public discontent, to pursue a reform agenda directly opposite to the negative logic of the primary care advocates. The goal was to spend more money and thereby expand access to specialist and hospital services. At the same time, some health policy makers wished to redirect medical practice to emphasize preventive measures such as "early detection and systematic management of hypertension, cholesterol, diabetes, and mental ill health." Capitation per se creates no incentives to GPs to provide such services, so "the new GP contract . . . made available generous fee-for-service rewards to provide a range of services to the chronically ill" (Maynard 2005, 256). In essence, capitation and GP rostering were not producing the right practice patterns. They created a mix of central regulations (such as outcome targets for particular conditions) and centrally defined incentives (extra fees for favored services) in order to reshape practice (Maynard 2005; Oliver 2005).[13] These policies reflected the fact that critics of the medical profession did not perceive GP behavior as any better grounded in evidence than the practice of any other physicians.

British reforms therefore reflected a confusing mix of theories. Beginning from a point at which primary care's place in the system approximated the form and role desired by primary care advocates, governments gave primary care providers (that is, GPs), in various forms, an even larger voice in directing the system. Yet, since the major public concern was insufficient access to other levels of care, increasing GPs' influence did not solve the problem. Eventually the government responded by deciding to increase supply of secondary and tertiary care. At the same time, the relatively coordinated and systematic system of GPs, with gatekeeping and some organization into larger practices with ancillary providers, did not satisfy critics who believed medical care per se was overemphasized at the expense of nonmedical measures such as "nutrition and education of child-bearing women and the young" (Maynard 2005, S261).

Hence British developments illustrate, first, that the different dimensions of primary care advocacy do not necessarily fit together well. Primary care can be emphasized relative to secondary care, yet that in itself does not lead to an emphasis on public health concerns. The British events further support tentative indications from Canada that coordination of medicine through the primary care system requires that there be enough secondary and tertiary care available to give the GPs flexibility to coordinate. In practice, cost control in the United Kingdom appears to have been most strongly related not to the gatekeeper role of primary care but to the strict restrictions on supply of secondary and tertiary care (and the use of capitation, budgets, salaries, and other financial controls). Attempts to increase value for money through competitive reform were not sufficient, and eventually the government responded to public pressure by pledging to increase supply of all services through spending a lot more money.[14]

The British, however, did not try one other theory about how to both control costs and increase efficiency through an emphasis on primary care: making primary care physicians bear risk for the costs of other care. Nor did the Canadians, Germans, or Dutch. Only the American private sector tested that theory.

THE UNITED STATES: PRIMARY CARE AT RISK

In the mid-1990s, a wide range of definitions of primary care and presumed contributions of primary care were current in the U.S. health policy community. The Institute of Medicine's (IOM) attempt to define primary care in 1994 combined vagueness with breadth: "the provision of integrated, accessible health care services by clinicians who are accountable for addressing a large number of personal health care needs, developing a sustained partnership with patients, and practicing in the context of family and community" (Laetz 1997, 93). The IOM left the hard questions, such as who would do what to integrate how, never mind what "practicing in context" might be, to be answered later.

In the United States, increased emphasis on primary care clearly meant, to everyone concerned, decreased autonomy for specialists. The revolution in health insurance contracting generally (if inaccurately) known as "managed care" sought to decrease specialist autonomy in a variety of ways, two of which involved notions familiar in advocacy for primary care.[15]

The first of these was creation of large, integrated, multispecialty group practices such as the Permanente medical group of the Kaiser health plan. These groups would incorporate specialty services, with a lower proportion of specialists than was common in the rest of the U.S. health care system. The group's management would integrate care. Patients who received their services through the group would be confined to using that group's physicians; while the role of primary care physicians would be large compared to specialists, there would also be a greater than usual role for alternative caregivers such as nurse practitioners. Such groups would offer (in theory) all of the attributes that the IOM in 1978 referenced: "care that is accessible, comprehensive, coordinated, continuous, and accountable" (Laetz 1997, 93).

The second version of "managed care" that emphasized a version of "primary care" was to turn primary care physicians into risk-bearing gatekeepers. As in the United Kingdom, primary care physicians would control referrals for other services and be paid largely by capitation. Unlike in the United Kingdom or much of anywhere else, in the new American contracts of the mid-1990s primary care physicians' own incomes could be reduced (through "withholds") if their referrals were too expensive or be increased (through bonuses) if their referrals were unusually low. This form of gatekeeping was very different from how fundholding worked in the United Kingdom, for two reasons.[16] First, fundholding practices allocated a budget for referred care, but the incomes of the physicians in the practice were not affected by those decisions. (If they made more money, they had to reinvest it in the practice, not by increasing their own income.) Second, fundholding practices managed budgets on much larger patient bases than could be involved in the contracts that American primary care physicians made with insurance companies. Still, U.K. physicians did not face financial risk of certain very expensive treatments as they received separate payment. An American physician could have a contract for, say, one hundred patients, in which situation the total payment for that group could be greatly affected by random events (for example, whether one of that group developed a brain tumor, so highly expensive referrals).

The system of risk-bearing gatekeepers in health care in theory matched a hope that primary care physicians would serve a "general manager" role (Laetz 1997, 94). Yet this role was joined to extreme financial incentives to underserve—incentives that could also easily be perceived as unfair since physicians would be at financial risk due to factors over which they had little control. As a basic American health policy text summarizes, "Risk pools indexed to individual physician performance create the potential for massive swings in income, depending on a particular physician's 'success' at minimizing hospitalizations, referrals, and diagnostic tests—or at avoiding high-risk patients" (Bodenheimer and Grumbach 2005, 44).

Relative to the international experience, these two forms of managed care reflected the difference between a view of primary care that emphasized a gatekeeping role by independent GPs (as in the Netherlands) and a view that would call for larger, integrated practices (as, to some extent, in the United Kingdom for large fundholding practices and the health centers in some Swedish counties).[17] Yet the unique dimension of risk in the United States had two important implications. First, the health center (or large group practice) approach was inherently more stable because it spread the risk more widely. Second, each put the physicians and patients in an inherently adversarial relationship, in which sick patients would become economic burdens to their providers. As Deborah Stone (1999) would argue, the way "managed care" transformed relationships was at the core of the powerful "managed care backlash" of the late 1990s.

In Chapter 2, Joseph White explains much of what happened subsequently to 1997. In fact, the fully integrated delivery systems became a less important part of American health care, as their managers found that it was not so easy to manage risk while patients and employers preferred wider choice. The number of Americans in group or staff model HMOs (in which multispecialty group practices in essence sell insurance) declined from 1993 levels. As providers pushed back against the insurers and employers, they especially revolted against some of the risk-bearing contracts. Hence, while gatekeeping seemed to be continually increasing in 1997 in the United States, by 2001 insurers were backing off from both capitation and placing risk on physicians (St. Peter 1997; Strunk and Reschovsky 2002).[18]

In 1997, a series of events seemed to be favoring primary care providers over specialists. The elite consensus was reflected in common projections that the need for primary care providers would increase more than for specialists. Medical students seemed to be getting that message, too, as indicated by a major increase in the proportion of students choosing residencies in a primary care field. Seeking to maintain specialists' direct access to patients, the American Medical Association (AMA) even invented the concept of "principal care physicians," to emphasize that a specialist could be the first point of contact and coordinator of care for a person with a chronic condition in that specialty (Laetz 1997, 95, 102). Yet, as Chapter 2 shows, specialists regained the upper hand as they both found ways to increase their negotiating power (such as leaving multispecialty groups and forming single-specialty groups with large market share) and benefited from patient demand for direct access.[19] In short, the primary care revolution died with the managed care revolution.

Hence the United States represents a more complex and varied version of both the Canadian and German experiences. In each there was a lot of talk about increasing the role of primary care. In each country, what increasing the role of primary care actually meant was rather vague, better defined by what it was against (specialists and hospitals) than what it was for. In the United States, the much more decentralized and market-driven system allowed far more organizational change than in Canada and Germany. Yet the obstacles that blocked change in Canada and Germany emerged as both political (the "managed care backlash") and market (provider pushback and employee preferences) forces in the United States. By 2005, American health care appeared to have no more significant a role for primary care than it had in 1990. This statement appears true whether by primary care we mean the role of primary care physicians, the role of integrated delivery systems, emphasis on community health and prevention, or any other of the multiple definitions we have observed across and within countries.

Confusions and Patterns

The conceptual terrain of what is called primary care can be quite confusing. Is it a normative or empirical concern? Does "primary" mean first contact or most frequent contact? Does it mean integration or limitation, a focus on the "community" or "the whole individual," an emphasis on primary care physicians or integrated clinic practices? As we have seen, about all that can be said is that all visions of "primary care" as a good thing pose it in opposition to care by individual specialist physicians or within hospitals.

This definition can mean that advocacy for primary care within any country conflates a variety of measures that can have many different effects. In the United States, for example, the consequences of an integrated multispecialty practice would be much different from the consequences of placing risk on individual primary care physicians; yet each could be defined as "primary care" reform. When this diversity is taken into an international discussion, it becomes so obvious that it is hard to slide by and ignore.

In our review of both the 1997 Four Country Conference discussions and subsequent events in each country, we found that two patterns stood out. These patterns are discussed in the following section.

AGENDAS AND CIRCUMSTANCES

In Canada, Germany, and the United States, general practitioners (however trained) have limited roles as gatekeepers and are paid by fee-for-service.[20] Analysts and policy makers commonly define fee-for-service and levels of utilization as major causes of high costs. As cost controls dominate the policy process, "primary care reform" proposals largely involve attempts to shift toward capitation and gatekeeping—whether those reforms are proposed by government committees (Canada), a mix of government and sickness fund advocates (Germany), or mostly by private sector purchasers and insurers (the United States).

In the Netherlands and United Kingdom, general practitioners already serve as gatekeepers to much specialist care and are paid substantially by capitation. This arrangement does not mean they necessarily coordinate care effectively. It does mean that capitation and gatekeeping are not the usual goals of primary care reform. To some extent, then, the search for efficiency and savings is diverted from a focus on primary care to a broader advocacy of "competition." In the United Kingdom, that search involved attempts to change the role of primary care providers to increase the productivity of specialists. In the Netherlands, initiatives focused more on the payment scheme for specialists, without involving primary care providers. In each country also, there was elite advocacy for some form of greater integration of practice and emphasis on wellness or community health measures—the "community" side of the primary care ideology, rather than the "gatekeeping" side. In short, where one goal of the standard primary care vision is largely met, advocacy shifts to other goals, often with the same fervor and sense of urgency. Yet the British and Dutch experiences diverged due to another difference in conditions: Service shortages were arguably far worse in the

United Kingdom, caused by many years of fragility in public health spending, and so the political demand for more services eventually led to spending increases.

Hence the reform agendas differed substantially between the United Kingdom and the Netherlands, on one hand, and Canada, Germany, and the United States on the other. Different underlying conditions shaped both the dominant primary care reform ideology and the relative importance of primary care as a reform theme. It was present in all countries, but in somewhat different ways, and those differences reflected underlying national conditions even though the rhetoric was confusing everywhere.

WHO IS FOR "PRIMARY CARE" AS A REFORM METHOD?

In June 2005, one of this chapter's authors was in Tokyo and visited the Meiji shrine, a memorial to Emperor Meiji and his Empress. Outside this Shinto shrine were two gift shops, each selling good luck charms. The charm for general good health sold for ¥500 (¥=yen), but charms for protection against specific diseases, such as cancer, cost ¥1,000.

One could hardly find a better "market test" of the proposition that ordinary people tend to see specialized care as a higher priority than general care.

In Canada, Germany, and the United States, policy advocates sought to increase emphasis on primary care (variously defined) at the expense of specialty care for a variety of reasons, ranging from ideology to a search for cost control. In each case both patient and physician communities rejected these policies. The mechanisms differed, but the results were the same.

As Macinko, Starfield and Shi's (2003) analysis and our own discussions showed, health care delivery arrangements in the Netherlands and the United Kingdom involved a much greater role for gatekeeping primary care physicians. The public and physicians alike in each country appeared to be accepting this long-established status quo.

It surely had shaped the expectations of British GPs, as well as the political position of Dutch GPs. That meant there was little or no pressure from the physician community to undo the basic arrangements.[21]

Yet public acceptance of gatekeeping and rostering arrangements in no way indicated that patients (voters) had a deep commitment to the primary care role. Indeed, political rhetoric about "choice" in the Netherlands in the 1980s and 1990s led patients to begin to question referral requirements and rostering. Nor did the GP role seem to reflect any popular support for investing in "population health" or "community" at the expense of personal medical care in any country.[22] Most clearly, it did not reduce public interest in access to specialist services. Indeed, waiting lists for specialized care were the preeminent political issue for the U.K. health care system, and when waiting lists began to become a problem in the Netherlands, the government immediately adopted new payment arrangements that increased costs in order to reduce waits.

Hence, in different ways, all five countries' experience support the argument that health policy makers and analysts tend to be more attracted to "primary care" as a policy reform theme than are the physicians who operate systems and the voters who receive services. Perhaps this explains why primary care is such a common reform theme—it is easy to propose, but hard to define and equally difficult to implement any definition.

Notes

1. A 2005 review states, "In an effort to practice population-based medicine and to contain health expenditures, many health maintenance organizations, the Department of Veterans Affairs (VA), and the National Health Service in the United Kingdom have all attempted to shift the locus of care from specialty and inpatient settings to the primary care setting" (Fortney et al. 2005, 1423). The most prominent example in the international health policy community is the World Health Organization's Declaration of Alma-Ata: "primary care . . . is the first level of contact of individuals, the family, and community with the national health system bringing health care *as close as possible* to where people live and work, and constitutes *the first element* of a continuing health care process" (World Health Organization 1978). It is worth noting the conflation of the descriptive and the normative in this formulation, and the simultaneous embrace of first contact and closest setting as "primary."

2. Examples of policies that do not seem specific to primary care per se are specific national regulations of the distribution of primary care providers and facilities (such policies are unlikely to be confined only to primary care); the level of cost sharing (of which the authors disapprove, but cost sharing also is unlikely to be confined to primary care); and whether health care finance is progressive (they don't like payroll contributions). The study is interesting at a minimum for how it operationalizes the primary care ideology.

3. Note that this pattern was quite stable: The United Kingdom had been second in 1975; the Netherlands, third; Canada, tenth; Germany, fifteenth; and the United States, eighteenth. They credited the improvement (by their lights) in the U.S. score to the proliferation of HMOs.

4. While there had been some expectation that these measures would be weakened in 1998, in fact that did not occur. Instead, total remuneration for all Social Health Insurance physicians increased by only 15.2 percent from 1996–2001 (less than from 1990–1995), and remuneration per physician declined by 3.9 percent (Worz and Busse 2005).

5. These first three aspects are among the standards for strong primary care in the Macinko, Starfield, and Shi (2003) article.

6. These aspects are all emphasized in Hendriks (1997).

7. See the trends in Schut and Van de Ven (2005), table 1, S64.

8. In most Canadian provinces, the government insurance coverage for specialist fees was lower if the patient did not have a referral. Whether that arrangement actually saved money must be questioned. After all, if a patient self-referred, the provincial government would pay only one fee; if the patient did the right thing and went to a GP first, the provincial government would pay two fees. So, unless one can be sure that GPs would be quite unlikely to make referrals, having patients go through the GP to get a referral could well cost more. It is different if the GP is paid by capitation, so the visit to get a referral generates no extra fees.

9. The most telling comment was the title of a report by the British Columbia Medical Association: "Capitation: A Wolf in Sheep's Clothing?"

10. The discussion that follows is actually about the English National Health Service; because of devolution under the Labour government, reforms in Scotland, Wales, and Northern Ireland "are broadly similar to the English system, but differ in some of the details" (Oliver 2005, S95).

11. The extent of actual control by GPs remains obscure; see Oliver (2005).

12. The government was so convinced of the popularity of such an expansion and cost increase that it made raising taxes to pay for higher spending a campaign plank.

13. It is worth nothing that much the same discontent and initiatives also occurred in the Netherlands (see Chapter 5).

14. Whether increasing spending will work very well may be doubted, given that it is very hard to increase supply as quickly as the British will be increasing spending. Most likely, a lot of the money is simply being transformed into higher incomes within the medical system. See Maynard (2005) and Oliver (2005).

15. For more detail on the methods of cost control involved in "managed care," see White (1999). Besides the two methods described here, the third method to limit specialists' autonomy was third-party utilization review, such as requiring pre-approval for tests or hospitalizations. White's article explains some of the ways in which the term "managed care," as applied in the United States, is also misleading.

16. There was some transfer of risk for pharmaceutical expenses to physicians in Germany. But this was not concentrated on primary care physicians per se; any physician in the ambulatory care sector could, in these measures, have had income reduced due to excessive pharmacy costs. Some Canadian proposals imagined risk bearing, but they were not implemented.

17. Whether to require that patients receive primary care from "health centres with geographic responsibility" or to allow them to receive care from independent general practitioners was a contentious issue in Sweden during the 1990s (Anell 2005).

18. Aside from income concerns, one reason for physician resistance to capitation was that primary care physicians worried that they were being forced to practice beyond their competence (St. Peter et al. 1999).

19. In fact, even during the period when primary care physicians supposedly were gaining more of a role in the system, their incomes fell a bit more than those of specialists. This likely occurred because capitation was applied more broadly to primary care than specialty care (Reed and Ginsburg 2003).

20. While Macinko, Starfield and Shi (2003) consider Canada to be significantly different from the United States and Germany, and there is a limited gatekeeper role in Canada, the payment methods and ability for patients to directly access specialists in Canada make it more like the United States and Germany.

21. Pressures for higher payments within the basic structure were, of course, significant.

22. For a good summary of reasons why population health is likely not the primary goal of national health care systems, see Oliver (2005).

References

Anell, A. 2005. Swedish healthcare under pressure. *Health Economics* 14 (suppl. 1): S237–54.

Bodenheimer, T. S., and K. Grumbach. 2005. *Understanding health policy: A clinical approach*. 4th ed. New York: Lange Medical Books.

Fortney, J.C., D. E. Steffick, J. F. Burgess Jr., M. L. Maciejewski and L. A. Petersen. 2005. Are primary care services a substitute or complement for specialty and inpatient services? *Health Services Research* 40 (5): 1422–42.

Hendriks, J. 1997. Primary care in The Netherlands. In *Four Country Conference: Primary health care*, 90–107. Conference Report. Boppard, Germany, June 5–8.

Laetz, T. J. 1997. Primary care in the United States: New emphasis on an old concept. In *Four Country Conference: Primary health care*, 90–107. Conference Report. Boppard, Germany, June 5–8.

Macinko, J., B. Starfield, and L. Shi. 2003. The contribution of primary care sytems to health outcomes within Organisation for Economic Co-operation and Development (OECD) Countries, 1970–1998. *Health Services Research* 38 (3): 831–65.

Maynard, A. 2005. European health policy challenges. *Health Economics* 14 (suppl. 1): S255–63.

Mullan, F. 1998. The 'Mona Lisa' of health policy: Primary care at home and abroad. *Health Affairs* 17 (2): 118–26.

Oliver, A. 2005. The English National Health Service: 1979–2005. *Health Economics* 14 (suppl. 1): S75–99.

Organisation for Economic Co-operation and Development. 2006. *OECD Health Data 2006*. Health Reform Studies, Paris: OECD.

Pfaff, M. 1997. Concluding Remarks. In *Four Country Conference: Primary health care*, 13–16. Conference Report. Boppard, Germany, June 5–8.

Primary Care Implementation Steering Committee. 1997. Primary care reform goals, objectives, and targets. Manuscript. February 5.

Reed M., and P. B. Ginsburg. 2003. Behind the Times: Physician Income, 1995–99. Center for Studying Health System Change *Data Bulletin* 24 (March).

Schoen, C., R. Osborn, P. T. Huynh, M. Doty, K. Davis, K. Zapert, and J. Peugh. 2004. Primary care and health system performance: Adults' experiences in five countries. *Health Affairs*, Web Exclusive: w4–487–99, http://content.healthaffairs.org/cgi/content/full/hlthaff.w4.487/DC1.

Schurman, D. 1997. Primary care reform in Canada: Promise or reality? In *Four Country Conference: Primary health care,* 66–77. Conference Report. Boppard, Germany, June 5–8.

Schut, F. T., and W. P. Van de Ven. 2005. Rationing and competition in the Dutch health care system. *Health Economics* 14 (suppl. 1): S59–74.

Schwartz, F. W. 1997. Primary care and health care reform in Germany. In *Four Country Conference: Primary health care,* 78–83. Conference Report. Boppard, Germany, June 5–8.

St. Peter, R. F. 1997. Gatekeeping arrangements are in widespread use. Center for Studying Health System Change. *Data Bulletin* 7 (Fall).

St. Peter, R. F., M. C. Reed, P. Kemper, and D. Blumenthal. 1999. The scope of care expected of primary care physicians: Is it greater than it should be? Center for Studying Health Systems Change *Issue Brief* 24 (December).

Stevens, S. 2004. Reform strategies for the English NHS. *Health Affairs* 23 (3): 37–44.

Stone, D. A. 1999. Managed care and the second great transformation. *Journal of Health Politics, Policy and Law* 24 (5): 1213–18.

Strunk, B. C., and J. D. Reschovsky. 2002. Kinder and gentler: Physicians and managed care, 1997–2001. Center for Studying Health System Change *Tracking Report* 5 (November).

White, J. 1999. Targets and systems of health care cost control. *Journal of Health Politics, Policy and Law* 24 (4): 653–96.

World Health Organization. 1978. Declaration of Alma Ata, International Conference on Primary Health Care. Alma Ata, USSR, September 6–12. Accessed from http://www.who.int/hpr/NPH/docs/declaration_almaata.pdf on December 10, 2008.

Worz, M., and Busse R. 2005. Analysing the impact of health-care system change in the EU member states—Germany. *Health Economics* 14 (suppl. 1): S133–50.

8

Hospital Care in the United States, Canada, Germany, the United Kingdom, and the Netherlands

KIEKE G. H. OKMA AND MICHAEL B. DECTER

Hospitals in Western Europe have their historical roots in medieval institutions that provided shelter, food, and care for the sick, the homeless, the elderly, and the mentally deranged (De Swaan 1988). The institutions were funded and managed by monasteries, local communities, and charities. Over time, the roles and functions of hospitals gradually extended to include medical treatment, nursing and spiritual care, isolation of contagious disease, and education and research (Healy and McKee 2002). In the second half of the nineteenth century, the state showed growing interest in matters of public health and health care. The Poor Laws in the United Kingdom required local communities to take action and provide shelter for the growing numbers of homeless after the Industrial Revolution (De Swaan 1988; Timmins 1995). Publicly built systems for drinking water supply and sewerage removal reflected a growing awareness of the need for better hygiene, and state regulations of medical professionals protected both the profession and the public. At the beginning of the twentieth century, hospitals were still mostly places offering (long-term) nursing of poor patients and rehabilitation for tuberculosis and other contagious disease. Hospitals did not provide much in the way of real medical treatment, and richer patients paid physicians for home visits.

The role of hospitals changed dramatically after the Second World War. The discovery of penicillin and antibiotics and experience with seriously injured patients in wartime fueled rapid medical innovation and allowed for more invasive operations and new treatment (Healy and McKee 2002). The expansionary stage of modern medicine also caused a rapid rise in the costs of medical treatment, and fueled the need for expanding health insurance to cover larger segments of the population. The 1960s and 1970s saw the expansion of both public and private health insurance schemes to cover the costs of hospitalization and medical care in the industrialized world.

Several continental European countries including Austria, Belgium, France, and the Netherlands followed the German model that had started in 1883. It marked the first state-sponsored social health insurance when the German Chancellor Bismarck introduced mandatory sick fund membership for low-income wage earners. In the first half of the twentieth century, the scheme attracted much attention from abroad. It evoked a stream of cross-border traffic of government officials and expert committees to study the German experience. Gradually and often with much dispute over issues of redistribution and administration, other countries in Western Europe (and elsewhere) followed the German example and introduced one or more public schemes for income protection in case of illness, disability, unemployment, retirement, or death of the family breadwinner.

After the Second World War, the British National Health Service (NHS) became the second leading example for other countries (Klein 2001). The NHS expanded coverage to include the entire population. Based on the recommendations of Lord Beveridge (Timmons 1995), the NHS funding is largely tax-based. At the turn of the twenty-first century, these models of funding and administering health financing were still dominant in the health care of industrialized nations (OECD 1992, 1994, 2005). Over time, however, most if not all funding systems became hybrids, mixing elements of social health insurance with private insurance, general taxation, tax subsidies, and to a lesser extent, out-of-pocket payments by patients and voluntary contributions.

Public and private health insurance and general taxation thus became the main funding sources for health care in the Organisation for Economic Co-operation and Development (OECD) countries. With the advance of modern science and ample availability of funding for capital investment, hospitals became the centerpiece of modern medicine. They nowadays employ up to half of all physicians and three-quarters of nurses, and take up a substantial part of health care budgets (Healy and McKee 2002; OECD 2005). Teaching hospitals became the major places of training, and academic hospitals became the centers of medical research and advance treatment. In some countries—sometimes because of lack of alternatives—hospitals kept their functions as shelters and providers of respite care, nursing and long-term housing for frail and elderly patients. For example, some Canadian hospitals in remote places in the north of the country keep elderly patients in wintertime for longer periods of time than strictly needed for medical reasons. Likewise, the long average length of stay (LOS) in German hospitals at the end of the twentieth century reflected the shortage of nursing home capacity in that country. In contrast, U.S. hospitals face pressure from external payers to shift their patients out as soon as possible (a pressure that even evoked state legislation to protect patients against undue early dismissal; see Peterson 1999). For such reasons, the average length of stay varies widely between countries.

In all countries discussed in this volume, hospital capacity expanded rapidly in the three decades after the Second World War. Most societies saw that expansion (the "golden era of medicine") as part of the postwar reconstruction and development of the modern welfare state (Timmins 1995). Local communities proudly invested in new hospital buildings. Hospitals became the cathedrals of the modern age, with prominent buildings as visible symbols of modernity and important sources of employment in almost every town. But after the 1970s, the golden age of expansion turned into the age of accountability and cost control (Relman 1988). After the oil crises of the 1970s, with stagnating economic growth and high and persistent unemployment, the climate changed. The confluence of economic, demographic, and ideological factors led to three decades of almost continuous debate about the future of the welfare state. Fiscal and budgetary strain, changing understanding of the demographic transition in Western Europe, and changing views about the proper role of the state changed the stage for social policy (Altenstetter and Haywood 1991; Okma 1997; Ranade 1998).

Adding to the general erosion of status and authority of the state, church, and medical profession, there were two particular challenges to the dominant medical paradigm. Ivan Illich's *Medical Nemesis* (1973) eloquently questions the underlying assumptions and lack of solid scientific underpinning of medical decision making. Two decades later, the same criticism persisted (Skrabanek 1994). The second challenge came from "healthy policy" advocates who argued that health care is but one of the contributing factors to health. In doing so, they not only extended the definition of health, but also, the scope of health care and health policy. Canada's health minister Marc Lalonde framed the ideas about the "determinants of health" in his policy paper of 1974 (Lalonde 1974). The World Health Organization (WHO) became one of the carriers of the model (WHO 1978). All WHO member states embraced the "healthy policy stream" by signing the famous Alma-Ata declaration, but in the end, the stream looked more like a modest trickle rather than a major river sweeping existing institutions off their foundations (Okma 2002). Nonetheless, it added to the pressure to reassess the position of hospitals as the core of the medical system. Closely linked with that effort, more and more countries showed—at least on paper—interest in "primary care" as an alternative to inpatient care (another term with a striking lack of clarity about both its scope of activities and underlying assumptions; see Chapter 7). Supporters of the "economic stream" of health reform (Okma 2002) claimed that hospital services are, in fact, individual consumption goods and services and should be treated accordingly. This approach gained weight through the publications of the privatization unit of the World Bank (for example, Preker, Harding, and Travis 2000). And finally, empirical studies revealed considerable variations in medical treatment across institutions and across individual physicians, not explained by differences in patient mix (Wennberg 1973; Wennberg and Wennberg 2003). This finding led to efforts to standardize the measurement of activities (by "benchmarking" hospital activities and outcomes) and also to increase outside interference in the medical domain (Okma 2001).

Three decades of ideological debate, fiscal and budgetary strain in the face of ongoing medical innovation, and changing patient demands resulted in pressure on hospitals to improve their performance, increase accountability, and contain costs. Improved effectiveness of medical care reduced the need for extended hospital care. Hospital capacity decreased from 580 to 440 beds per 100,000 habitants in the OECD countries between 1980 and 1998. Shifts from inpatient care to outpatient care, day care, and treatment at home caused a drop in the average length of stay, from twelve to eight days (OECD 2005). While total hospital capacity decreased, both the number of admissions and the intensity of treatment (as reflected in the number of staff per bed and volume of advanced medical equipment) increased. The directions were similar, but the speed of change differed across nations. Another general trend was the rapid spread of modern management ideas and models borrowed from the corporate sector (Marmor 1998).

Thus, hospitals across countries face common pressures of changing ideology, shifting consumer demand, and financial and budgetary pressure. One of the interesting questions is whether such common pressure also led to similar policy directions and organizational change. This chapter addresses this question by looking at the experience of five industrialized countries: the United States, Canada, Germany, the Netherlands, and the United Kingdom. It starts with particular claims and expectations about the future of hospitals in the industrialized world due to common pressure. Four major "winds of change" affect hospitals everywhere: first, a shift in focus from individual health services to management of the health of populations; second, a consumer revolution that emphasizes quality, speed, affordability, appropriateness, and access of health care; third, a technological transformation based on silicon-chip and biotechnological innovations; and fourth, financial pressure from employers and governments driven by global competitive forces (Decter 1998, 2000; Decter et al. 2000). Those pressures, it was widely expected in the late 1990s, would lead to profound changes in the organization of hospitals and the position of hospital care in the medical systems of industrialized countries.

After presenting that general claim, the chapter turns to the actual experience of hospital development in the five countries. That experience reveals, indeed, many similar trends and developments. But, as we will see, there are also important differences in the speed and direction of change that cannot be explained by general factors. The chapter concludes with an effort to separate country-specific realities from generalized claims. It confronts those claims with developments that actually took place in those countries and presents other, competing explanations of change and nonchange. One important conclusion is that generalized claims never settle policy disputes. As the chapter shows, historical, cultural, and institutional factors influence the shaping and outcomes of social policy, and "windows of opportunity" (Kingdon 1984) for major change do not occur often. Next, it concludes that international comparison can benefit from not just looking at national health care systems, but rather at policy measures and programs in a more disaggregate way.

General Patterns of Change in Hospital Care: Claims and Realities

Hospitals are the most stable, visible, familiar, and durable institutions of modern health care systems (Decter 1998). Yet after nearly a century of gradual evolution and expansion, hospitals underwent a radical and rapid transformation in the last decade of the twentieth century. In less than ten years, the dominant role of the hospital has come under serious discussion. As functions and activities are undergoing a radical reappraisal, the institutions are radically transforming. Across industrialized nations, a remarkable and unprecedented phenomenon is under way—hospitals are closing and merging. Hundreds of hospitals across North America have shut down. Care has moved away from the hospital bed and patients spend less time in hospitals. Many surgical procedures take place in a doctor's office, in a day surgery center without beds, or in the outpatient department of a hospital. New drugs have eliminated entire classes of disease from hospitals.

However, hospitals are not disappearing. They are enduring as important institutions but are facing forces of new ideas, new technology, changing public expectations, and economic pressure. The four previously described, global "winds of change" are reshaping the way we think about health and the delivery of health care. These winds do not readily abate at national borders. Moore's Law (the power of computer chips doubles every eighteen months) will not be repealed in the near future. The silicon chip will continue to drive information technology, and its pace will likely accelerate in the near future and increasingly affect health care. The demand created by the baby boomer generation across industrialized countries presents a fierce challenge to health care orthodoxy. The demand of the boomers for informed consent and for rapid, high-quality and appropriate care is shaking health systems. Aging boomers will turn their attention increasingly to the demand of living longer in relatively good health. Yet a sizable share of citizens in each country will become frail, requiring substantial care to continue to live as independently as possible. Thus similar pressures on hospital systems will persist across industrialized countries.

Health managers and planners have tried to address those challenges by reshaping their services into lighter, more dollar-efficient, and better-quality health care delivery systems. Reformers have emphasized the need to move from an antiquated Ptolemaic idea of a health solar system in which the hospital was the all-powerful core, to a modern Copernican view where the rostered patient population is the new sun. But even without such full replacement from the center stage, the hospital faces growing competition from other forms and other settings of care. Not only its role and position in the overall health care system, but also the hospital's concept and operation are facing major change.

The modern North American hospital had its birth in Baltimore in the early twentieth century, when the board of trustees of Johns Hopkins hired a Canadian physician, William Osler. In turn, he hired a New York hotel manager as his chief administrative officer. The die was cast. The hospital organization would, for nearly a century, be conceived as a hotel where patients received medical treatment from doctors and care from nurses (Decter 1998). Twin realities shaped its character and organization. In the early days, labor costs were low. Indeed, the staff of many hospitals consisted of religious women who worked for the greater glory of God and room and board. The second reality was the model selected for the modern hospital—the hotel. Like a hotel, hospitals measured their performance by its occupancy, and its importance by the number of beds. The 1990s ushered in the most rapid and profound change since Dr. Osler.

Fiscal and budgetary pressures fueled relentless cost-cutting efforts of modern managers. Powerful forces of automatization and new medical technology favor ambulatory care settings. Combined, those forces led to a dramatic reduction in hospital capacity. For the first time in a century, a decade ended with fewer hospital beds than at its beginning in each industrialized country. Hospital closure, a hitherto rare phenomenon, has become—though locally still debated furiously—commonplace. The remaining hospitals are reshaping their role as managers of health services rather than managers of beds. Services, not beds, are the measure of performance of the modern hospital, as many treatments no longer require an overnight stay.

Large academic medical centers have become the secular cathedrals of our health care theology, but those cathedrals are crumbling. After three centuries of building and expanding hospitals, it is the reengineering of all, and the closure of some, hospitals that occupies the attention of health services managers across the industrialized world. If the old-style hospital was like a hotel in its organization, the modern hospital was like a grand department store in regard to the wide range of goods and services it offered. The emerging hospital of the new millennium owes more of its heritage to the shopping mall—a collection of boutique services in special niches. Typically, large general hospitals in major cities nowadays provide a narrower, more specialized range of services, and they are more likely to refer patients elsewhere for care they no longer offer. Hospital services are unbundling and shifting to ambulatory and home settings. The progress of modern medicine, the advance of minimally invasive surgery, and the advent of more robust home care services have all added to this shift.

Hospitals and their supporters cling to the status quo with extraordinary tenacity. However, the four "winds of change" will move the institution to a new place in health care. The likely outcomes of the next decade of evolution of the place and function of acute care hospitals can be summarized as follows: fewer hospitals subsumed into more complex, multisite health delivery organizations; fewer but on average, higher acuity patients in the inpatient settings; an acceleration of chip-driven information technology change and increased linkages among providers; a greater availability of consumer-usable information about quality and outcomes leading to more "shopping" by patients among providers; higher capital intensity, with displacement of less-skilled labor; narrower-focus specialty hospitals in some niche areas; and finally, more hospitals involved in a defined role within a "continuum of care" or disease management programs. Hospitals are unlikely to easily relinquish the affection of its main constituency: the public who considers the institutions as critically important elements in the local community. But they will take on a less-dominant position in the health care galaxy, and become more *primus inter pares*.

There are still many unsolved issues in this field. For example, as North America consolidates down from, at its heyday, nearly 10,000 individual hospitals into perhaps 2,000 to 3,000 health systems early in the twenty-first century, we may move closer to knowing how much they can improve the health of a particular population. We may also learn what are the best techniques for doing so and gain insight in the efficient scale of operation: How many people can be looked after effectively by a single system?

A decade after the framing of these expectations in the 1990s, there are different ways to assess the claims about the future of the modern hospital. First, by looking at the accuracy of the claims themselves: Did those general trends actually materialize? Does the evidence about the outcome of change processes in the industrialized world support such generalized claims? Second, by looking at possible competing alternative explanations of change and nonchange: What other factors played a role in the transformation of hospital care between the late 1970s and 2008? This chapter seeks answers by studying developments that took place in individual countries. The following sections analyze what happened during the last three decades in hospital care in the United States, Canada, Germany, the Netherlands, and the United Kingdom. That narrative will then serve as a descriptive base to take up the preceding questions in the last section of the chapter.

Hospital Care in the United States

The United States has the most "private" model of health care and hospital funding of all OECD countries. A large segment of the population has employment-based private health insurance offered and subsidized by employers (as well as by government tax subsidies). But public schemes play an important role, too (Marmor, Mashaw, and Harvey 1990). Medicare for the elderly, Medicaid for the poor, and the Veterans Health Administration are the main public schemes for specific population groups. For about 80 percent of the American population, public and private health insurance covers ambulatory and hospital-based medical costs, with varying rates of co-payments by patients (OECD 1994). However, decreasing numbers of Americans carry health insurance that fully reimburses the cost of hospitalization.

Similar to other OECD countries, most American hospitals started as not-for-profit institutions, owned and managed by local communities and charitable and religious organizations (Stevens 1971). In the last decades of the twentieth century, the number of new for-profit health facilities, as well as the number of conversions of nonprofits to for-profits has risen sharply. But still, by 2000, about 70 percent of all American hospitals were not-for-profit organizations (Sekhri 2000).

The majority of the medical specialists work in hospitals as self-employed professionals with hospital admittance privileges. During their training, junior doctors are usually employed by the hospital, as is the teaching staff in academic hospital centers. Family doctors, obstetrician-gynecologists, internists, and other medical specialists work as independent practitioners in solo or group practices. They can be part of one or more groups of physicians who have contracts with the government and private health insurers.

Hospitals negotiate with the federal Medicare Administration, with state Medicaid offices, and with a variety of insurance agencies over the payment and volume of their services. The rise of "managed care" and "health maintenance organizations" (HMOs)—organizations that basically combine the functions of health insurance and provision of health care (and that perhaps more accurately should bear the label of "managed cost organizations")—in the 1970s heralded an era of increased scrutiny and external interference in medical practice and hospital management by outside actors (Starr 1982; Peterson 1999). Ironically, one of the major grounds for the American Medical Association (AMA) to reject the proposals of the Clinton administration for universal health insurance in the early 1990s was the fear of undue government control over health care. By the end of the decade, HMOs were restraining the medical practice to a far greater degree than government regulators by selectively contracting with providers and by imposing detailed rules of pre-approval, detailed pricing for narrowly defined services, and other administrative rules. The "HMO backlash" of dissatisfied patients and frustrated health professionals alike prompted state governments to take action (Peterson 1999). Several states passed laws to restrain the restrainers and protect patients by setting rules for a guaranteed minimum length of stay in hospital after childbirth, safeguards for the continuity of providers, and the right of self-referral by patients (Sekhri 2000).

Another source of external scrutiny of hospital care originated in research findings of undue and unexplained variations in medical treatment across hospitals and physicians (Wennberg 1973, 2005). Other studies found that medical errors are much more common than generally believed, and that such errors are the source of many avoidable deaths of patients in hospitals (Kohn, Corrigan, and Donaldson 2000). Both the studies about practice variation and findings of widespread medical errors fueled the development of medical practice protocols or guidelines. At first, the medical profession saw those guidelines as a device to improve the quality (and transparency) of its own activities. But over time, the very existence of such protocols allowed outside actors to impose rules and restrictions and to interfere with medical practice. Similarly, benchmarking methods that initially offered individual practitioners, managers of health facilities, and medical schools measuring rods to compare their results to those of similar institutions became the instruments of funding agencies as the base for their payment. The carrot of professional-quality-improvement methods became the stick wielded by interfering outsiders (Okma 2001).

In the 1980s and 1990s, fiscal and budgetary strains led to freezes and sometimes cuts in hospital funding, as well as changes in payment methods by federal and state governments and private insurance. In the 1970s, most physicians received fees for their services and hospitals received fixed amounts per patient per day (per-diem payments). The next decade saw major change in contractual relations and payment methods of hospital care (Sekhri 2000). One important shift was the replacement of per-diem payment by prospective budgets and next by payment based on *diagnosis-related groups* (DRG-based payment).

Those changes in payment method implied not only a shift of financial risk from the third payer to the providers of health care, but also a shift in decision-making power from the medical professionals and hospital managers to health insurance. That trend is not unique to the United States. For example, in the early 1990s, U.K. fundholding general practitioners (GPs; see the section about the United Kingdom later in this chapter) received a fixed amount per registered patient (apart from additional payment for certain activities such as flu shots for elderly patients), regardless how many times a patient visited the doctor per year. But the GPs also faced restrictions as the administration of the U.K. National Health Service imposed many rules for administering a GP practice. Likewise, DRG-based payments (the model has spread rapidly across OECD countries since the mid-1990s) provide hospitals with a fixed amount per patient in a certain category, regardless how intensive the medical care for one particular patient may be in practice. In exchange, hospitals usually have to provide third payers with detailed information about their services. That increased transparency in itself allows for greater outside interference, for example, by imposing standardized lengths of stay (LOS) for certain conditions. Another consequence of the shift to the DRG payment model is that (American and other) hospitals have less opportunity to treat uninsured patients by charging others more.

The combination of technological innovation, organizational change, and new payment methods led to a sharp reduction of the average length of stay. Medical procedures require less and less time of after-surgery recovery, and more and more patients receive their treatments on an outpatient basis in hospitals or another ambulatory setting. In 2002, the average LOS in American hospitals was the lowest of all industrialized nations but because of higher intensity of treatment and higher incomes of health professionals, the costs were the highest (OECD 2005). This decline in average LOS aggravated existing problems of overcapacity, and in the 1970s and 1980s many small hospitals merged with others or closed down. Independent hospitals became part of larger groupings of hospitals and other health services under common governance, both in not-for-profit and for-profit organizations. At the same time, certain services moved away from the hospital setting. Groups of medical specialists started to offer specialized care in independent clinics, sometimes backed by private investors. A McKinsey 2004 study, however, noted that efforts to develop integrated delivery networks have not been very successful (Salfeld and Vaagen 2004). The study quotes patient resistance against closing down of facilities and high administrative costs of complex multilocation networks as the core problems. Thus, consolidation of hospital organizations and fragmentation of hospital services occurred side by side.

The external strains and organizational change created pressure for both physicians and hospital administrators. A recent survey found that U.S. managers were more likely to report a strong financial position, excellent facilities, resources available to expand or improve services, and shorter or no waiting times for elective care than their counterparts in New Zealand, Australia, Canada, or the United Kingdom. Nonetheless, there was a higher rate of dissatisfied hospital executives in the United States than elsewhere. "US hospitals operate within highly decentralized, competitive insurance and delivery systems in which revenues depend on volume and patient mix. US hospitals stand out for high costs (three times the OECD median cost per capita), low rates of hospital admission, and short average length of stay. Reimbursement incentives have encouraged and supported a migration of care to freestanding centers and the emergence of niche hospitals" (Blendon et al., as quoted in DesRoches et al. 2004).

In some well-reported cases, managers whose incomes and fringe benefits depended on the financial results of the organization engaged in outright fraud in order to boost the financial results. For example, in the case of Columbia HCA, managers whose annual bonus depended on financial results forced division heads to present unrealistically high profits. The latter responded to the pressure by forging the books when the actual results did not meet those standards. Similarly, in the *Tenet* case, four doctors who worked at a former Tenet Healthcare Corp. hospital agreed to pay $27.1 million to settle a federal investigation into claims that they performed unnecessary procedures (Bloomberg

News 2005). In 2003, Tenet established a $395 million fund for 750 people who had filed civil lawsuits against the company claiming that its physicians had performed unnecessary heart surgeries. In a separate case filed by federal prosecutors in San Diego, the company is awaiting a jury verdict over claims that a Tenet hospital offered illegal kickbacks to doctors.

Thus, in line with the predictions at the beginning of this section, technological change and external financial pressure have been major driving forces of change in American hospital care. However, even while the speed of change has picked up, its direction is not always clear or predictable. Like other OECD countries, total hospital capacity has shrunk following bed reductions, hospital mergers, and closures, and there has been a marked shift from inpatient care to ambulatory treatment. Hospitals have become more specialized and parts of specialized care have moved out of hospitals altogether.

HMOs and other health insurance agencies have taken steps to monitor health professionals and to increase the efficiency of hospital services, but with few exceptions, they do not seem to be paying much attention to broader issues of population health. As an example, a 2006 series of articles in the *New York Times* reported extensively on the diabetes epidemic in the city's population and the poor quality of health services that focus on treatment rather than prevention because health insurance usually does not reimburse preventive activities (Kleinfield 2006; Pérez-Peña 2006). Further, in spite of predictions of further shifts to for-profit medicine, the vast majority of American hospitals have remained not-for-profit.

One field where the high hopes and expectations of the early 1990s clearly failed to materialize is health information technology. Specialized journals, publications, and academic and trade meetings alike have emphasized information technology as a promising venue to improve quality and reduce costs. Ten years later, efforts to modernize and extend the administrative systems beyond the basic administration and billing have only been successful on a very modest scale.

Another field of concern is the modest progress in the improvement of the quality of health care services, loosely labeled as the "health care quality movement." This includes efforts to develop accreditation systems for hospitals, the framing of minimum standards for hospital care, and the activities of organizations such as the Physician Consortium for Performance Improvement (www.aha.org) or the Leapfrog group, an informal group of major employers that announced it would only contract health plans when they adhere to certain standards. Health care providers generally acknowledge the need to improve the transparency of their activities and to systematically report in order to comply with quality norms. But five years after the publication of *To Err is Human* (Kohn, Corrigan, and Donaldson 2000), there had been little if any progress in avoiding accidents or even patient deaths (Leape and Berwick 2005). Generally, studies show a slow pace of health information change within the medical profession.

Hospital Care in Canada

Until the 1970s, medical science, medical treatment, and the organization of medical care were very much alike in Canada and the United States. The levels and growth rates of health expenditures were almost the same. Health insurance and the organization of hospital care were very similar. There was mutual recognition of medical and nursing diplomas across the border. Since 1952, the two countries had a joint development of the curriculum for medical schools and a joint process of accrediting hospitals by the Joint Commission of Accreditation of Health Care Organizations. Like their American counterparts, most Canadian hospitals had their roots in voluntary and religious organizations (Boychuk 1999). But in the mid-1970s, their pathways parted. The United States developed its fragmented health care funding, based on a complicated mix of public and private insurance schemes with high out-of-pocket payments. Canada followed the European example of broadening access to health care (Taylor 1987). It expanded the scope and coverage of existing provincial schemes to universal health insurance over the entire country. The 1984 Canada Health Act (CHA) offers Canadian provinces considerable financial support by the federal government on the condition that they comply with the five basic principles framed in the CHA: universal coverage, a comprehensive range of health services, public administration, free access at the point of delivery of care, and portability of insurance from one province to another. Over time, the provincial schemes expanded the range of services to include hospital care and medical care outside hospitals (Taylor 1987). From the late 1950s on, the funding for (independent) hospitals came largely from the Canadian provinces. That system continued with little change for over three decades.

Like the introduction of America's Medicare (limited to the elderly), Canada's Medicare (for the entire population) created an important and relatively stable income source for hospital care. Other components of hospital funding are direct payments by patients, private insurance for services not covered by CHA, and voluntary contributions (the latter mostly for hospital capital investments). Most hospitals in Canada (with the notable exception of the provincial psychiatric institutions) were set up as nonprofit institutions by charitable and religious organizations (Boychuk 1999). That nonprofit character is still dominant in the early 2000s. In fact, provincial health insurance schemes do not allow for-profit hospitals to apply for public reimbursement. Smaller private clinics offer specialized services on a fee-for-service basis, but they operate outside the public system. However, the well-publicized outcome of the 2005 *Chaoulli* case in Quebec (see discussion later in this chapter) has created pressure to allow for private for-profit health care (Flood, Roach, and Sossin 2005; Flood and Lewis 2005).

Geography matters. Surface-wise (like the United States), Canada is a very large country. Most of its thirty million or so inhabitants live in urban centers and regions bordering the United States. The allocation of hospital capacity but also the change in hospital use over time reflects this geographic pattern. Apart from the large city hospitals that serve the vast majority of Canada's population, there are many very small hospitals in remote areas with less than twenty beds. Those small facilities, usually staffed and led by nurses, serve a variety of functions for the local population: place of first contact with the medical system, emergency care, sometimes shelter for the homeless, local clinic, and maternity ward. They do not provide advance medical treatment and doctors have to fly in to see patients or patients fly to the cities to receive specialized medical care. While the urban medical centers are merging and increasing their scale of operations, many smaller ones have closed down or restrict their range of services.

Like other OECD countries, Canada's hospital capacity has decreased rapidly in the last few decades. Between the early 1990s and 2000, the number of hospitals fell from 900 to 774 (Canadian Institute for Health Information [CIHI] 2000). In 2000, they employed 1.1 million people (including over 200,000 nurses), or about 10 percent of the country's workforce (CIHI 2000). The number of acute beds per 1,000 inhabitants went down from 4.6 in 1980 to 4.0 in 1990 and to 3.2 in 2002 (OECD 2005). After a decline in the 1980s and early 1990s, the average length of hospital stay went slightly up again, from 7.2 days in 1995 to 7.4 in 2002. On balance, the occupancy rate declined between 1980 and 1990 from 80.4 percent to 78.6 percent but then went up again to 86.6 percent in 2002, one of the highest in the OECD (OECD 2005). While the number of beds went down, treatment intensity increased. For example, the number of Magnetic Resonance Imaging (MRI) machines went up from twenty-two in 1991 to 176 in 2005, and Computed Tomography (CT) scanners from 205 to 328. The costs of hospital care continued to increase, from about C$25 billion to over C$31 billion in 2002 (CIHI 2005).

The last two decades have witnessed fierce debate over the future of Canada's Medicare. Media coverage highlighted the problems of—perceived and real—wait lists, lack of patient-friendly service, acute shortage of staff, and other shortcomings such as the lack of comparable data about the results of hospital care (CIHI 2005). In the 1980s and 1990s, both federal and provincial governments established expert commissions to study solutions for those problems (National Forum on Health 1997; Canada Senate 2001; Clair Commission 2001; Fyke Commission 2001; Mazankowski Commission 2001; Commission on the Future 2002; Okma 2002). The commissions' proposals ranged from substantial increases in federal funding for the provincial health insurance and the development of quality assurance systems to suggestions to relax the prohibition of private health insurance for services covered by the Canada Health Act. Most commissions found that none of the problems justified a major overhaul of the public funding model. A minority of the reports, for example, the 2001 Mazankowski report in Alberta, advocated opening up the system to private health insurance and for-profit providers to improve the efficiency and quality of the public system. Independent research groups published similar reports as well (Decter et al. 2000; Rachlis et al. 2001).

In the 1990s, Canadian provinces started to regionalize health governance structures and consolidate hospitals. British Columbia had already experimented in the 1970s and 1980s with models of regional governance that brought several hospitals under one larger board. Saskatchewan closed down several of its smallest hospitals, and Quebec forced hospitals to amalgamate into larger groupings. The province of Ontario was one of the last to embrace this model. After the recommendations of an advisory commission headed by Duncan Sinclair, Ontario closed down several smaller hospitals (Ontario Health Services Restructuring Commission 2000). Thus the speed of consolidation varied across the provinces, but the directions were the same: fewer hospital boards and larger, more geographically based delivery organizations, ranging from multisite hospitals to broader health services organizations (Decter 1998). Stand-alone hospitals consolidated into larger groupings and agglomerations. In some cases, the new bodies shifted the emphasis from the treatment of illness to health promotion and population health. A leading example of this evolution is Capital Health in Edmonton, Alberta. A little over a decade ago, fourteen hospitals, myriad nursing homes, several home care services, and other health organizations provided fragmented health services under a plethora of governances in the area. Public health was a complete separate organization, and there was little integration of services. Since the late 1990s, Edmonton's one million residents plus 600,000 from surrounding regions receive their care from Capital Health. One management team under one governance board directs 29,000 health staff and manages a C$2.4 billion budget. Public health, home care, and long-term care are fully integrated with the acute care system. So are 2,700 hospital beds and 6,000 continuing care beds. An electronic health record and a 1–800 nurse call line add to the integrated nature of the services. Nurse call lines are replacing visits to hospital emergency rooms (ERs). Increasingly, Capital Health seeks to target its health promotion and wellness efforts to the population with the highest needs within the region. Patients can access the system via Internet to find their way in the network of health providers. There is a strong link to the research and teaching of University of Alberta. The results are encouraging, judged by both outcomes and efficiencies achieved. The model has not spread over the entire country.

In 2005, in a striking ruling on the *Chaoulli* case, the Supreme Court of Canada decided that if the provincial government failed to take sufficient action to alleviate the problem of waiting lists, it no longer could justify banning private health insurance (Flood and Lewis 2005). At the beginning of 2006, there was much debate about the potential impact of that court decision. Critics fear that it heralds the unraveling of the public (and popular) system of publicly funded and privately provided health care; others are less worried and hope that an infusion of private activities will help to make health care more efficient and patient friendly.

Hospitals are still there, but as we have seen before the nature of their daily activities has shifted dramatically. The trend from inpatient care to day surgery that started in the 1990s had not yet ended by the mid 2000s. One development not foreseen is the rapid increase in elective hospital services that are more cosmetic than medical in nature, for example gastric bypass surgery. That trend can be seen as evidence of the failure of health promotion efforts to reach broader population segments. A recent study of hospital emergency room use in different countries revealed that over 50 percent of the ER visits in Canada and 35 percent in the United States were not urgent. Patients could have seen a regular doctor, had one been available (Schoen et al. 2004). In both countries, but to a greater extent in Canada, ERs still serve as a location for nonurgent care. It is clear that 24/7 primary care is not fully in place to deal with minor ailments and to prevent unnecessary hospital visits.

Changes in hospital care in Canada thus reflect—similar to other OECD countries—a confusing mix of technological and organizational innovation, as well as innovation in governance structures fueled by fiscal pressure and ideological debate. But at the same time, there has been much continuity in the basic features of hospital care: Most Canadian hospitals still are independent, not-for-profit institutions, with budgets paid out of public sources and services free of charge for patients. Much consolidation has occurred, yet Canadian hospitals remain oddly at the center of the health care delivery paradigm. Despite a decade of rhetoric on patient-centered care, primary care reform, and disease state management, the Ptolemaic solar system has remained firmly in place.

One particular change in health policy making that affected the governance of hospitals has been the growing emphasis on regionalization. All Canadian provinces have experimented with different models of regional governance of health services, with different degrees of budgetary autonomy of the regionalized services. The stated purpose of regionalization is the need for better coordination between different services and the creation of a "continuum of care" (though this term is rarely explained in operational detail). Another, less explicitly framed goal is the restructuring of hospitals: It seems to be somewhat easier to scale down, to concentrate services in certain locations, or to close hospitals altogether when they are part of a broader conglomerate of health facilities than to take the highly visible political decision about closure of one particular hospital in the community.

With a few exceptions, efforts to translate publicly framed policy goals of improving population health into actual policy have been less than successful. Changing the focus of health services and changing actual behavior of the population are very hard challenges indeed.

Hospital Care in Germany

The introduction of social health insurance in 1883 created a split in the German population that still exists today (Pfaff and Kern 2005). Low-income and middle-income wage earners and their dependents (as well as some other population groups such as students, elderly, and self-employed with low incomes) are mandatorily insured with a sick fund. In 2003, there were about 300 sick funds, down from 1,200 in the early 1990s (and down from over 22,000 at the beginning of the twentieth century) (Rau 2005). Together, they cover 88 percent of Germany's population. Higher-income families can opt to leave the social health insurance and take out private insurance. About 10 percent of the German population has actually done so. In practice almost 100 percent of the German population has health insurance (see Chapter 4).

The introduction of social health insurance did not change the legal status of providers of care. Traditionally, hospitals have been under the ownership and management of nonprofit charitable or religious organizations, and that tradition was still visible in 2008. In 2003, German hospitals employed 4.2 million people, including over 300,000 physicians and 940,000 nurses

(Statistisches Bundesamt Deutschland [National Bureau of Statistics] www .destatis.de). Chiefs of clinics have a special status, one that allows them to treat patients privately as an additional source of income and status. Most other medical specialists are employed by their hospital. Another group of medical specialists, much smaller in number, is that of the *Belegaerzte*. They work in private practice but also have hospital privileges to treat their patients. Finally, there are the *ermaechtige Aertzte,* who offer outpatient care in academic or other clinics. Medical specialists can set up their own independent practice, and many German specialists do so after gaining experience in a hospital. The last category includes the *Hausärtzte,* or family physicians or general practitioners. In 1998, there were about 77,100 medical specialists with a license for ambulatory care and 44,700 general practitioners (Knieps 1998). The borderline between "primary care" and "secondary care" in Germany is far from clear. Self-employed physicians often have practices that are extensively equipped with MRIs, CT-scanning machines, X-ray machines, laboratory testing equipment, and other medical technology.

Until the 1990s, patients did not need a referral by their general practitioner to seek treatment by a specialist in or outside the hospital. In the late 1990s, the German Ministry of Health announced experiments with "gatekeeping" general practitioners on a voluntary basis. In that model, patients sign up with a GP of their choice, and they cannot see a medical specialist without referral (unless they are willing to pay a higher co-payment). Both patients and physicians opposed the model, and it never became popular. In 2004, one of the series of restructuring laws (the 2004 GKV Modernisierungsgesezt, or Social Health Insurance Modernizing Act) added a financial incentive to this model by charging patients an additional €10 co-payment for direct access to their medical specialist (Pfaff and Kern 2005).

Since the early 1970s, German hospitals have had a dual funding system. The federal states, or Länder, provide the funds for major capital investment whereas the public and private health insurance schemes (as well as modest amounts of co-payments by patients) cover the running costs. The dual funding model has created strong regional constituencies for hospitals. Many hospitals have local notables on their board, and local communities attach great importance to the presence of their hospital. As in other countries, efforts to close down a local hospital often face strong resistance.

Nonetheless, similar to other countries, there has been a gradual decline in hospital capacity because of bed reductions, mergers, and (more rarely) closing down of hospital facilities. Between 1960 and 1989, the number of independent hospitals in Western Germany went down from 2,625 to 1,735 (a decline of 35 percent), in Eastern Germany from 822 to 539 (a decline of 34 percent). In that period, the total number of hospital beds went up in the West by 13 percent, but declined in the East by 34 percent. After the German Reunification in 1989, the total number of hospitals decreased further between 1990 and 2003 from 2,207 to 1,868 (a decline of 10 percent); bed numbers shrunk by about 16 percent. Illustrating the general trend toward "quicker and sicker" patients, the number of patient days in hospitals decreased by 27 percent while the number of admissions increased by 20 percent during the same period (www.destatis.de).

The change in capacity was not distributed evenly across the different categories of hospitals. Between 1960 and 1989, the number of public (government-owned) hospitals declined from 1,043 to 689 (minus 35 percent) and private not-for-profit hospitals from 843 to 737 (minus 13 percent). In striking contrast, the number of for-profit hospitals went up from 321 to 442 (plus 37 percent), with an increase in beds of over 100 percent (but their average size is smaller than the public hospitals). The latter category grew fastest, partly because states and local communities decided to end public ownership and to sell their local hospital to private investors. This also led to the growth of new for-profit hospital chains, a relatively new phenomenon in German health care. The average size of all three categories of hospitals went up, due to mergers and closures of small hospitals (Rau 2005).

Germany's hospitals have traditionally had high average lengths of stay. In fact, until the late 1990s, because of lack of alternatives for elderly and chronically ill patients, hospitals routinely served as nursing homes for long-term care (similar to Japan). The average LOS in German hospitals went down between 1992 and 2002 from 13.2 days to 9.2 days, still the second highest of the OECD after Japan (OECD 2005). The introduction of the Pflegeversicherung, the long-term care insurance of 1995, has prompted a further decline as it offers financial support for nursing home care.

Since the 1970s, there have been continuous efforts to restrain hospital expenditure by a succession of legislative change (see Chapter 4). Those efforts illustrate the incremental nature of the German reform process: a typical case where many small steps may lead to major change (Klein 1995). It also illustrates that the term "reform" includes both major change in the allocation of decision-making power and financial risk, as well as minor adjustments in current policies such as existing payment methods.

The 1972 Hospital Finance Act introduced the dual funding model. At that time, the planning and funding of hospital facilities was seen as a public responsibility. In the 1980s, several expert commissions looked at options to replace that funding model and to develop payment alternatives and mechanisms to contain the growth of health expenditures that in spite of earlier policy measures did not show a decline. Cost-control efforts included new budget models and spending caps, restrictive rules for hospital planning, planning of capital investment, and changes in payment modes. In 1985, global prospective hospital budgets replaced—in principle—per-diem payment, but in practice, hospitals continued to receive full reimbursement for almost all their costs and budget overruns. The hospital budgets also created problems. It "punished" efficient hospitals and rewarded inefficient ones (Wiley et al. 1995, 102). The 1994 Health Restructuring Act announced that the federal states would set budgets for each hospital, with separate payments for capital investments and medical treatment. Next, in 1996, the payment model shifted from global hospital budgets to case-based payments and spending caps, but only for a modest share of total hospital expenditure. In 2004, hospitals still received about 80 percent of their budgets on a per-diem base, and 20 percent as lump-sum payment. From 1970 to 2005, there was a sharp decline in the role of the states as capital funding shifted back to the financial responsibility of hospitals themselves (Rau 2005).

In the early 2000s, Germany decided to introduce case-based payment for hospital care. It imported Australia's DRG model, but—similar to the Dutch experience—the actual implementation took (much) more time than expected (Rau 2005). First, the Australian model had to be slightly adjusted to the German circumstances, and next, it appeared that hospitals needed (much) more time than foreseen to adjust their internal administration to work with DRGs. The government therefore slated that the 900 or so DRGs will serve as the payment base for the largest share of hospital care by the year 2010. The first steps occurred in 2006. The aims of the new payment model are threefold: more transparency of hospital activities, better comparability of results, and more effective cost control. One issue still under debate is whether there will be countrywide tariffs or health insurers will be able to negotiate tariffs with the hospitals on the regional or local level.

Other policy steps included efforts to develop information systems to compare hospital results, as well as experiments with disease management programs (Rau 2005), efforts to improve "integrated delivery" with increased emphasis on primary care (mostly seen as ambulatory medical care), and further experiments with gatekeeping and *fundholding* GPs (that never became popular with German patients used to unlimited access to specialist medical care). Efforts to set up integrated networks of providers, however, were somewhat less than successful. In the second half of the 1990s, almost 400 integrated delivery networks started but very few of those are still operating today (Salfeld and Vaagen 2004). Patient resistance to restricted access to providers and high administrative costs were the core problems.

In summary, similar to other countries, there was a substantial decline in numbers of beds and numbers of hospitals in Germany while the numbers of patients went up. Hospitals are facing the challenge of budgetary restraints and demand pressure aggravated by technological innovation. There has also been some change in the governance, with for-profit organizations taking over public hospitals (still, the not-for-profit ones are dominant). Another important change occurred in hospital funding, where integrated funding for capital costs and running hospital expenditure via health insurance replaced the dual funding system where the states paid for the major capital investments. This also reduced the role of the (regional) states.

However, in spite of several efforts to expand hospital activity beyond inpatient care and to integrate hospital and ambulatory services, the degree of vertical integration between hospitals and other health services has remained modest indeed. Policy efforts to develop transparent information systems that allow patients to compare and choose a hospital of their own preference have not been successful. German physicians still have a strong position. There is little interference in their medical practice and their associations have kept a central role in collective bargaining over their payment mode and level, as well as a strong position in general policy making.

Hospital Care in the Netherlands

With a delay of over half a century, the Netherlands followed the German example of social health insurance and introduced mandatory insurance for low-income workers by the Ziekenfondsenbesluit, or Sick Fund Decree, of 1941. Interestingly, the decree was imposed by the German occupational forces, but the idea itself was not new: Ever since the introduction of social insurance in Germany in 1883, Dutch politicians and policy makers had been looking at their neighbor. The main reason why many successive coalition governments failed to pass similar legislation was that there was a deep division over the governance of sick funds: Right-wing Christian Democrats favored the model of "subsidiarity" and self-governance by employers and employees, while the more liberal politicians favored a stronger role of the state (Lijphart 1968). After the Second World War, the Ziekenfondswet, or Sick Fund Act, enacted in 1962, became the mandatory health insurance for families of low-income employees. Since the 1970s, it covered about 60 percent of the Dutch population. Until January 2006, the remaining 40 percent of the population, mostly higher income groups, the self-employed and civil servants, did not have access to the social health insurance and could opt to take out private health insurance to cover their medical bills and costs of hospitalization. While taking out private health insurance was not mandatory, in practice almost all Dutch had done so: In the late 1990s, less than 1 percent of the population did not have health insurance. Thus public and private insurance became the major sources for hospital funding, with low levels of co-payments by patients. In 2006, a new population-wide health insurance (or rather, a mandate to take out private insurance) replaced this dual model (see Chapter 5).

During the first decades of this dual insurance model, there were systemic differences between the public and private schemes in tariffs (higher tariffs for private patients), in payment methods (capitation for sick fund patients, fee-for-services for privately insured), in payment modes (payment for sick fund patients by their fund, by the privately insured patients themselves, with later reimbursement), and to some extent in the quality of treatment (front-door entrance for private patients, back-door entrance for sick fund patients, with longer wait times as well; first class rooms for private patients). But over time, most if not all of those differences gradually faded away as the egalitarian culture of the Netherlands does not really allow for much class differentiation. At the beginning of the twenty-first century, hospitals no longer had first, second, and third class rooms (in Germany, such distinctions still existed), GPs no longer had a separate entrance for sick fund patients, and the tariffs for both categories of insurance became uniform. The last remaining difference, the payment mode for general practitioners, disappeared with the introduction of the population-wide health insurance as of January 1, 2006 (see Chapter 5). GPs now receive a mix of capitation, fee-for-services, and special payment for particular activities (Ministry of Health, www.minvws.nl). Their income ranks amongst the highest in Europe (MoH 2004). In the early 2000s, the Dutch government announced a shift from the prospective hospital budgets (introduced in the early 1980s) to payment based on "diagnosis-treatment combinations" (*diagnosebehandelcombinaties,* or DBCs), a sort of homegrown adjusted DRG model. But in 2003 and 2004, it admitted delays in the introduction of the DBCs (Raad voor de Volksgezondheid & Zorg, www.rvz.net). In 2006, only about 10 percent of all payments for hospital services were based on the DBC model. Reflecting the decentralized decision making in Dutch health care (every specialty can develop its own DBC), the number of DBCs had risen to over 40,000 in the early 2000s. In early 2007, the health minister announced a drastic simplification of the DBC system before expanding its application (www.minvws.nl).

As in Germany, the introduction of social health insurance in the Netherlands did not affect the independent status of hospitals and other institutions.

Table 8.1 Hospital concentration in the Netherlands, 1950–2002

Number of hospital beds	1950	1980	2002
More than 750	1	8	15
500-749	4	20	23
250-499	30	87	47
125-249	60	45	10
Less than 125	110	15	0
Total	205	175	95

Source: Estimates are based on RVZ 2003, fig. 3.1.

Until the early 1980s, reflecting their historical roots, most hospital facilities were not-for-profit, and most had kept their religious or charitable character. Only the wave of mergers and other collaboration of health services in the late 1990s all but eroded the signs of such backgrounds (Boot 1998; see also Chapter 5). Under budgetary pressure of the 1970s and 1980s, Dutch hospital care underwent extensive change. Innovation in medical technology as well as new managerial thinking fueled a process of reorganization. Prompted by government policy (and enabled by modern medicine), the numbers of hospitals went down rapidly, from 205 in 1950 to 180 in 1980 and to 95 in 2002 (Raad voor de Volksgezondheid & Zorg [RVZ] 2003). The scale of hospitals increased, and the smaller ones all but disappeared (see Table 8.1).

Between 1990 and 2002, the number of acute care hospital beds declined from 4.3 to 3.4 beds per 1,000 habitants. The average LOS declined in that decade from 11.2 to 8.6 days. Still, in spite of shrinking capacity, average occupancy rates dropped faster, from 73 percent to 66 percent, one of the lowest in Europe (OECD 2005). It is important to note that this concentration trend in itself does not mean that over half of all hospital buildings in the Netherlands have closed down. Mergers and takeovers often allowed many smaller hospitals to continue operating, sometimes with a more limited range of medical services, at their location under the umbrella of a larger governance organization. It is also important to note that the number of hospitals or hospital beds is no longer the only defining element of hospital capacity as services are shifting from inpatient care to day care, same-day surgery, and outpatient care.

The Dutch experience shows that there is tension between competing and sometimes conflicting policy goals of increased transparency versus increased competition; and between competition versus the demand for better regional collaboration and the trend of market concentration. Prompted by fashionable ideas about the best model for hospital care, hospital managers

and boards embraced a rapid succession of management models and administrative innovations (see also Chapter 5). To secure a solid market position,
many hospitals and other health facilities engaged in horizontal and vertical
integration. Prompted by external criticism about the lack of transparency
(and by new quality legislation), hospitals joined their association's efforts to
develop quality systems for hospital care based on systematic collection of
data on the results of their activities. At several occasions, the Dutch government announced that it would sponsor efforts to set up benchmarking systems
that allow for a systematic comparison between hospitals (though the actual
realization of such systems turned out to be more difficult than expected). And
finally, prompted by patients' criticism about the lack of collaboration between hospitals and other health services, hospitals reached out to develop
formal and informal regional networks that link up with other providers in
processes of horizontal and vertical integration.

Other developments in Dutch hospital care reflect changing ideological
views and the emergence of new actors in the health policy arena. The 1990s
saw the rise of *zelfstandige behandelcentra,* or ZBCs, independent for-profit
clinics that offered specialized elective services such as eye operations, hip surgery, or cosmetic surgery. They not only drew patients who pay out of their
own pockets but also contracted with public and private health insurance.
Not all of those fared well and within a decade, some had to close their doors
again (*Algemeen Dagblad* 2003; www.rvz.net). There has been some discussion about the quality of their services, but there is little or no evidence that
they do better or worse than the not-for-profit providers. At first, facing concerns about the potential inequitable consequences of the rise of for-profit
care, the government announced measures to rein in that development. Next,
the Minister of Health decided to tolerate for-profit clinics on condition that
they establish formal ties with regular hospitals. After a few years, the opposition waned, and private clinics became an accepted feature in the Dutch
health care system. One particular unanswered question is whether, on balance, they have added to the capacity and thus helped to reduce waiting lists
or just shifted services out of hospitals to another location.

Dutch health policy makers put much emphasis on the importance of close
collaboration between hospitals and other health services (sometimes labeled
as "transmural care"). Changes in payment methods have added to the blur-
ring of the borderlines between the organization of inpatient and outpatient
care. Many hospitals collaborate closely with nursing homes and home care
services, sometimes under the formal umbrella of one governance structure. In
some cases, such networks focus on specific categories of disease, like cardio-

vascular disease or diabetes. The common feature is the fading of the formal distinction between inpatient care and ambulatory treatment, and between *eerstelijnszorg* (primary care defined as services outside the hospital, with some emphasis on nonmedical services) and *tweedelijnszorg* (secondary care defined as specialized medical care in general hospitals).

There are concerns about the high degree of market concentration in hospital care (RVZ 2003). Hospitals have to submit their plans for mergers and takeovers to the National Health Authority (Nederlandse Zorgauthoriteit, or NZa) for approval. The NZa rejects plans if they threaten to lead to regional monopolies. In several cases, NZa has actually done so. In 1992, in a sharp turnaround of previous policy, after two decades of active support for hospital mergers in order to increase the scale of operations, the Dutch government discontinued that support because of lack of evidence of the increased efficiency of larger hospitals (MoH 1992).

International evidence shows that in order to safeguard patient safety, there is need for a critical minimum volume of some core activities and thus for a minimum scale of hospitals (Canadian Health Services Research 2004). Once hospitals have reached that scale, however, with an optimal size of perhaps 200–300 beds, there are also diseconomies of scale (RVZ 2003; Canadian Health Services Research Foundation 2004). In fact, the RVZ concludes, it is more important to look at the different *functions* of hospital care rather than at entire hospitals. Modern technology allows for a wider scope of inpatient and ambulatory treatment settings. Other considerations in the planning of hospital capacity are access, travel time of patients, and the need to centralize certain skill- and capital-intensive services such as heart or skin transplants.

The RVZ 2003 report mentioned above raised a broader issue that is not yet solved in Dutch health care: Who determines the market structure and who allocates capacities in terms of functions rather than in terms of hospitals (RVZ 2003)? Recent policy changes have shifted the role of the government from direct regulator to "market master," or market regulator (MoH 2001). But it is not yet clear what that means, or to what extent government will keep its power to intervene when it does not like the outcome of the market. In a broader sense, this question also reflects the tension caused by the partial transformation of the traditional neocorporatist policy arena with consensual decision making to a model of market allocation in health care. The former model assumes that governments share the responsibility for the shaping and outcome of social policy with organized interests on the national and regional levels, with collective bargaining over the volume, quality and prices of health care (Lijphart 1968; Okma 1997; Visser and Hemereyk 1997). The market model assumes that individual, risk-bearing non-state actors are making decisions over the allocation of resources in health care. The current Dutch health politics reflect the tensions created by the overlay of different and sometimes competing notions of governance in health care (Helderman 2007). In spite of the current government-stated policy of strengthening market competition and lessening the role of government, its actual policies show a strong degree of "hands-on" interference (Chapter 5).

Some of the changes in Dutch hospital care clearly followed the pattern of other countries. There has been a gradual decline in numbers of beds, numbers of hospitals, average lengths of stay, and occupancy rates. The rise of for-profit medicine has not pushed out the dominant position of the traditional not-for-profit hospitals. The last decade has seen a rapid process of horizontal and vertical integration of hospital services with other health care—to a far greater degree than neighboring Germany. Efforts to implement quality systems based on systematic and transparent outcome measurement of hospital care to allow for patient choice, however, have been slow to materialize. Finally, the reorganization process does not seem to pay much attention to issues of population health. Some of the changes are unique to the Netherlands: the long tradition with independent not-for-profit hospitals, the homegrown DBC-based payment model, and the parallel processes of increased competition and increased market concentration. And the process of market concentration of hospitals has masked the fact that there have been fewer actual hospital closures than in other countries.

Hospital Care in the United Kingdom

The introduction of the tax-based National Health Service (NHS) brought the entire U.K. population under one health insurance in 1948 (Klein 1995; Timmins 1995). It also nationalized hospitals and changed the status of physicians to employed consultants. General practitioners (GPs), however, continued to practice as self-employed professionals. That model was still dominant in the early 2000s. But within that model—as seen in Chapter 6—there has been a continuous and seemingly never-ending process of organizational change in the last twenty years (Klein 2007; Oliver 2005). At the funding side, general taxation is still the dominant source of finance, but since the 1970s there is a rising share of (parallel) private health insurance and out-of-pocket payment by patients. Most medical specialists became hospital employees who negotiate over their contracts each year. There is a special reward system under which specialists receive additional payment based on the annual performance review.

In the first decades after the Second World War, GPs continued to work independently, mostly in solo practice. The 1980s saw the rise of group practices of two or more GPs working with other health professionals such as practice nurses, dieticians, and others. In the 1990s, there was a further grouping of GPs into Primary Care Groups (PCGs), and next, in the early 2000s, into Primary Care Trusts (PCTs). In 2005 there were about 300 PCTs (www.nhs.uk), but that number is decreasing following a process of mergers and consolidations (Royal College of General Practitioners 2005). In fact, PCTs have taken over many of the functions of the former district health authorities. They serve as administrative bodies that are responsible for the provision of health care to the patients in their region and the contracting of health care from other providers. In 2006, PCTs managed about 75 percent of the total NHS budget (www.nhs.uk). The remaining 25 percent of the money flows mostly via the twenty-eight Strategic Health Authorities (SHAs), the organizations that replaced the former ninety-nine Health Authorities. The SHAs are responsible for developing plans to improve the health services in the region. The process of mergers of the PCTs and the SHAs means that there is, in fact, a return to the regionalized governance models of the early 1980s (Maynard 2005; Klein 2007). Hospitals (or Hospital Trusts) have to negotiate contracts over their budgets with the Strategic Health Authorities and with PCTs. Interestingly, in spite of such organizational aggregation, general practitioners kept their self-employed status within the PCTs. However, they are facing pressure to change their practice patterns and range of activities (Manyon 2005). For example, practice nurses are taking over some of GP activity, including preliminary diagnosis and the prescription of drugs. But there is no clear division of roles, functions, or levels of expertise of specialist and advanced practitioners, and a lack of evidence of benefits of shifting activities from one professional to another (with the notable exception of midwives replacing doctors in low- or average-risk pregnancies).

Hospital care followed a different organization pathway from that of general practice. In the last two decades of the twentieth century, hospitals regained some of their prewar independence by opting for the status and governance model of NHS Trust (Klein 2007). The Thatcher administration introduced the so-called internal markets in the NHS, with competing and risk-bearing health care providers. This also fueled a process of consolidation in the governance of hospitals. In 1996, there were 350 NHS Trusts, but in 2005, there were 176 Acute Trusts (www.nhs.uk). They manage one or more hospitals under one board and offer services at one or more locations. As a further step toward independence, Acute Trusts can "earn" the status of Foundation Trust. Foundation Trusts have more operational and financial freedom—though within the limits of NHS rules. In late 2005, there were thirty-one Foundation Trusts for acute medical care, ninety-nine Mental Trusts that offer inpatient and ambulatory mental health services, and thirty-three Ambulance Trusts (www.nhs.uk). There were also plans to start separate Trusts for nursing care and for child services. The process of reorganization has not yet ended. For GPs, in 2005, the model of fundholding resurfaced by the introduction of indicative commissioning budgets for PCTs under the label of "practice based commissioning" (Maynard and Bloor 2003). In the last decades, the number of acute care beds went down between 1995 and 2002 from 4.0 to 3.7 beds per 100,000 inhabitants, a lower number than in most other European countries. In that period, the average LOS went down from 9.2 to 6.9 days. The occupancy rate declined a bit from 1980 to 1990 from 74.8 to 74.0 percent, but then it rose again to 84.3 percent in 2002, a much higher rate than other countries in Western Europe (OECD 2005).

While the new Labour government of 1997 kept the Trust model in place, it also emphasized the importance of long-term contracts and regional collaboration with other health providers in offering "continuous and seamless care." At the same time, it kept some of the core features of the "internal market" model of the Thatcher administration intact and even advocated increased competition between the public and the private sector (Maynard 2005). For example, GPs must offer patients who have to wait for care a choice of five alternative providers including at least one for-profit provider. Providers can be in the NHS or in the private sector. The government has also encouraged investment in private sector "diagnosis and treatment centres" (DTCs). DTCs are small-scale facilities that offer specialized elective procedures, similar to the private independent clinics in the Netherlands. Government support for the growing private sector is based on the expectation that it will help alleviate the problem of wait lists and also will serve as a catalyst to induce more flexibility in the public sector (Maynard 2005).

A particular event that shook the world of health care in Britain was the scandal in the Bristol Royal Infirmary, where surgeons continued to operate even after it was clear that the survival rates of their patients were way below those of comparable groups of patients in other hospitals (Bristol Royal Infirmary Inquiry 2001). The 2002 Wanless Review pointed to major shortcomings in the NHS, like excessive waiting times for elective surgery and poor quality of services (Wanless 2002). It also advocated a major expansion of health care funding. In reaction, the New Labour government announced a substantial increase in funding for the NHS to modernize hospital facilities and reduce waiting times (Maynard and Street 2006). The government also set up new institutions that in one way or another expanded the public domain: for the development of protocols and practice guidelines, the National Institute for Clinical Excellence (NICE, www.nice.org.uk), and for monitoring and benchmarking, the Commission for Health Improvement (CHI). CHI was renamed CHAI and next Healthcare Commission (HCC) (www.hcc.org.uk). The government also initiated systems to rate hospital performance with "star ratings," a short-lived system that disappeared again after a few years, and sponsored the development of guidelines for the contracting by the Trusts. The payment for hospital services shifted from per-diem payment and block contracts to case-based payment. Adjusting the DRG-model of other countries, the NHS introduced its own payment model based on "health care resource groups" (HRGs).

Notwithstanding the nominally independent status of Trusts, the government is quick to act when it perceives undesired developments. For example, in 2005 it appeared that over fifty Acute Hospital Trusts had run substantial deficits (estimated to surpass £948 million). Immediately, health secretary Patricia Hewitt ordered "budgetary hit squads" also known as "turnaround teams" to take action in order to reduce the deficits (Carvel 2005).

Thus, the NHS development reveals a somewhat contradictory mix of policy instruments. Like that of the Netherlands, the United Kingdom's government health policy both seeks to strengthen competition and regional collaboration. Competition is based on the assumption that consumers, that is, patients, are interested in shopping around. In practice there is little evidence that they are doing so (Pickard, Sheaff, and Dowlong 2006). Policy steps to decentralize decision-making power are counteracted by (perhaps much stronger) steps that strengthen centralized control. The shift from inpatient to outpatient care and medical treatment at home requires substantial investments in alternative health services and home care—but those are outside the scope of the NHS. The efforts to replace higher-skilled and higher-qualified medical personnel with lower-skilled and lower-qualified staff (for example, practice nurses for physicians, midwives for doctors, shifts from hospital care to GP practices) do not confirm expectations that the modern hospital will drive out less-skilled labor. The continuous process of reorganization of both hospital care and GP practices illustrates the power of a unified one-party government that can overrule objections of stakeholders to a far greater degree than some other countries discussed in this book. Finally, the NHS experience also illustrates that the meaning of "hospital" has become hard to apply as a unit of comparison, as statistical data may refer to different levels of governance (for example, individual Trusts, hospitals, facilities, locations, or numbers of specialties in one region).

Conclusions: Common Pressures, Common Future of Hospital Care?

This concluding section takes up the questions raised in the beginning of the chapter by confronting the general claims and expectations about the future of hospitals in industrialized countries with the evidence presented in the brief country sections.

At first sight, there are good reasons for such generalized claims about expected change in hospital systems. Ever since the oil crises and economic stagnation in the 1970s, policy makers and health care managers in many countries have engaged in extensive debate about the need to adjust, to modernize, and to reorganize hospitals and other health services. Everywhere, fiscal and budgetary pressures fueled organizational change in hospital care: downsizing, integration and specialization. In all countries, new medical technology and changes in payment methods pushed down average lengths of stay. Governments and other third-payers replaced open-ended reimbursement by new case-based payment methods. In all five countries, in varying degrees, for-profit providers of medical care took away business from traditional hospitals (a trend least visible in Canada). Hospital managers and hospital boards embraced new governance models, with chief executive officers (CEOs) replacing medical (or nursing) directors, and hospital divisions as quasi-independent profit centers replacing the old department model. The main focus of management became the rationalization of internal processes. The debate was inspired as much by fiscal realities as by ideas floating around in national and international publications, management journals, expert commissions, management consultancy firms, and international organizations. Nationally and internationally, there was a crossover of ideas from the business world to the world of health care, exposing hospital to modern management jargon and methods.

All five countries have embraced the notion of "healthy policy" by signing the Alma-Ata declaration of 1978 (WHO 1978). The expected shift toward population-health-oriented policies, however, has not gained much ground. Three decades later, with few exceptions, government support for that idea has hardly translated into reality. Only in situations where one large (regional) body has "captured" the (regional) provision of health services, has such a body been able to frame "population health" policy and, to a modest extent, actually implement measures.

The evidence of success of "consumer-driven" change is somewhat mixed. In the last decades, governments and health care providers alike sought to improve the quality, efficiency, and (cost-)effectiveness of hospital care. Following the U.S. example (or perhaps more accurately, following perceptions of that example), several countries have sought to expand consumer choice in health based on competing health insurers and providers. In reality, fiscal and budgetary pressure often trumped such considerations and forced governments to go back to the good old cost-controlling devices such as imposing global budgets on providers, delisting services from social insurance or increasing patient co-payment. The efforts also included the development of quality systems, quality legislation, practice protocols, and disease management. There is not much evidence that change in this area is attributable to the actions of dissatisfied patients. Popular media like television, daily newspapers, and glossy journals have fueled public debate and prompted political action. In that sense there has been less of a direct consumer revolution than a media revolution, one that has brought news over financial scandals, unduly long wait lists or lack of collaboration between services in the open in much more detail than ever before.

In most countries, neither the market-driven concentration in hospital ownership nor state-sponsored collaboration between hospital care and other services has done away with the independent management of hospitals. The vertical integration of services still faces the hurdle of separate funding streams.

Another common force of change is medical technology. In all countries, medical innovation has enabled the shift of treatment from inpatient settings to ambulatory care or treatment at home, thus adding to the decline of average LOS in hospitals. That innovation has also aggravated cost pressure everywhere, because of increased intensity of treatment, new technologies and expanding application of existing ones. For example, the number of MRI and CT-scan machines in hospitals greatly varies across countries, but has risen everywhere (OECD 2005). Efforts to develop information systems that help patients to select hospitals or other health care providers are still embryonic.

Policy documents in all countries refer to financial and budgetary pressure— regardless the actual fiscal and budgetary situation. Perhaps this force of change should be labeled "perceptions of fiscal and budgetary crises."

But in spite of the above common pressure for change there are marked differences in the development of hospitals since the 1980s. A brief summary of country-specific changes includes the following:

American citizens have the lowest (and declining) degree of health insurance coverage of all countries. There is less public funding for hospitals in the United States than elsewhere. Most physicians are self-employed (except residents and physicians who work in academic hospitals), and there is no general system of gatekeeping by family physicians or GPs in place. The rise of "managed care" in the 1970s imposed new restraints on hospitals and accelerated the shift from inpatient to outpatient care. In the 1990s, chafed by direct interference in the medical practice, physicians took the managed care organizations to court. Several states passed laws that restrained the restraining practices of HMOs. Still, there is widespread dissatisfaction among patients (who see their access to care limited because of the selective contracting of their insurer), physicians (facing enormous administrative burdens of dealing with a large number of third-payers and the mounting threat of litigation), and hospital managers (pressured by investors to push up profits).

In many ways, American medical care has been the most innovative of all systems. The Medicare administration sponsored the studies that led to the development of benchmarking, quality measuring, and new payment methods; most of the innovation in medical technology, pharmaceutical care, and health information technology still originates from the United States. Many new management ideas and organizational models of hospitals trace their roots to American institutions. Many policy ideas, good and bad ones, seem to be inspired by change in the United States. The United States was the first to introduce case-based (DRG-based) payment. As in other countries, not-for-profit hospitals are still in the majority, but there are more independent specialty clinics than elsewhere. In some cases, investor-owned for-profit medicine has fraud and abuse of managers whose incomes depended on financial results to an extent rarely seen in any other country.

Canada's health care system was very similar to that of the United States until the 1970s when the countries split their ways. In 1984, the Canada Health Act provided the base for the population-wide health insurance administered by the provinces. Since the 1980s, those provincial schemes provide a reliable and stable source of income for hospitals. By law, health providers have to be not-for-profit if they want to receive public funding, and private health insurers cannot offer coverage of services under the CHA. However, the 2005 *Chaoulli* case in Quebec opened to the door for private health insurance. Apart from the urban centers, Canada's hospitals are smaller than elsewhere. In remote rural areas they offer a limited range of medical care but also serve other functions in the local community. In the last three decades, the Canadian provinces initiated a variety of regionalization models of health governance. In most cases, this effort led to larger bodies under common governance; in some cases, it led to increased focus on population health issues. In the 1980s and 1990s, federal and provincial expert commissions proposed a wide range of reform measures to address the short-comings of the public system. The vast majority of those committees concluded that solving the problems does not require abandoning the CHA but adjustment within that public funding model.

Germany was the first country to introduce social health insurance for industrial workers in 1883. This created a split in the populations served by public and private insurance. The social health insurance is based on mandatory participation of all eligible families and decentralized administration by independent sick funds (the not-for-profit health insurers) under strong government controls. The long tradition of nongovernment provision and funding of health care has created the typical neocorporatist style of governance where government shares the responsibility for social policy with the sick funds, the associations of physicians, and other organized stakeholders. As in the Netherlands (see Chapter 5), this permanent involvement of other actors on the federal and state levels has created strong popular support and stability but also veto positions of the key players, and it does not allow for rapid change. In fact, it has been hard if not impossible for German policy makers to frame and implement structural health reforms or even to pass more modest change, as illustrated by the slow speed of introducing case-based payments or the unwillingness to adopt gatekeeping. For over twenty years, German hospitals had a dual funding system: The states provided the capital investment funds, the public and private health insurance provided the budgets for running costs. The abandoning of that dual model in fact depoliticized decisions on hospital closure by eliminating the role of states in hospital planning. It also weakened the ties with local constituencies and opened the door for new governance models and for-profit hospital chains. Traditionally, German hospital capacity ranked amongst the highest in the world (as in Japan, partly explained by the lack of an alternative setting for long-term nursing care). In the late twentieth century, similar to other countries, financial pressure and technological change forced hospitals to reduce beds. The 1990s saw the rise of for-profit hospital chains that in some cases took over public hospitals. However, there is less concentration than other countries, and the charitable and religious roots of hospitals are still visible today. There has not been much success in developing health care networks, as the separate funding streams for acute medical care in hospitals, ambulatory care, and long-term care hinder the development of vertically integrated conglomerates of health care providers. Even while Germany has been one of the first countries to emphasize prevention and healthy lifestyles in the beginning of the twentieth century, there is no evidence of substantial shifts toward "healthy policies," or an increased focus on population health.

The Netherlands has copied much of the core institutions of Germany during and after the Second World War. In 2006, a new model of mandatory health insurance for all residents replaced the former mix of public and private health insurance (in Germany, the 2006 Christian Democrat and Social Democrat coalition discussed a similar shift, but could not reach agreement). Similar to other West European countries, hospitals have a long tradition of charitable and religious ownership and management. After a wave of mergers and takeovers that accelerated the concentration of Dutch hospitals in the 1980s and 1990s—and parallel to a general process of rapid secularization of Dutch society—those religious and charitable roots are hardly visible today. At the beginning of the twenty-first century, Dutch social policy reflects intricate layering of overlapping, competing, and sometimes conflicting ideologies and governance notions. There is emphasis on both regional collaboration and (some degree of) market competition. There is striking continuity in the willingness of health care providers and insurers to participate in collective action even after the government dismantled traditional neocorporatist structures (Okma 1997, Chapter 5). The system saw a hesitant and not always successful start of for-profit clinics. Like patients in other countries, Dutch patients are generally happy with their own physician and hospital and are not keen to shop around.

The United Kingdom was the first country in Western Europe to introduce the National Health Service. The NHS combines tax-based funding with nationalized hospitals but independent general practitioners (GPs). Long-term nursing is mostly part of local social services. In the 1980s and 1990s, the NHS has seen a never-ending process of change. The Thatcher administration first tried to replace the tax funding with (private) health insurance, but faced too much opposition and thus shifted to the internal market model (a model copied from the United States, but copied by other countries too). Successive governments encouraged GPs to collaborate in group practices or "primary care groups" and then in the larger grouping of the "primary care trusts" (PCTs). Hospitals regained some of their former independence as "hospital trusts" under independent boards. The Labour administration formally abandoned the internal market, but kept the core features; it also encouraged regional collaboration and long-term contracts between independent providers. The Labour administration declared more independence of hospitals and other health care providers and set up all sorts of new monitoring and control mechanisms that in fact greatly expanded the public domain. In striking contrast with other countries, the government announced an enormous expansion of public funding for the NHS (Klein 2007). It wanted to bring up health spending to the average of OECD countries.

The wide variety in national experiences with hospital change supports the need for competing, alternative factors explaining change and nonchange in hospital care. It also leads to a reframing of the issue, based on a less universalistic approach that takes into account country-specific features that are crucial in the shaping and outcome of social policy.

The country evidence illustrates that there are common forces that fuel and enable change or counterforces that block, thwart, or slow down efforts to change hospitals. One clear example of such counterforce is the almost universal resistance in the local community against the closure of a hospital. Hospitals do not only provide specialized medical care, but they serve multiple functions: center for research and teaching, major employer, shelter for homeless or elderly, or long-term care facility. Such multiple purpose character has also created multiple constituencies. It is interesting to see that the recent changes in governance structures—the regionalized models of Canada, the Acute Hospital Trusts in the United Kingdom, and the commercial hospital chains in Germany—have created a new organizational environment that allows for closing down hospitals in a less disputed way than direct government decisions. Those broader governance structures have taken over decision-making power from the government over hospital closure and also serve as a buffer to absorb the blame for such unpopular decisions. Perhaps the closing down of hospitals by private actors is somewhat more acceptable than such action by public authorities.

The country examples show new developments that were not on the radar screen in the mid-twentieth century. For example, the breakaway sections of elective specialist services in independent for-profit clinics and the rise of independent clinics for cosmetic and other surgery in Germany and in the Netherlands seem to be less inspired by the population health needs rather than returns on private investment and elite beauty concerns. But there are marked differences between countries in the degree to which they are able to block or slow down such developments of for-profit health care.

Country-specific politics matter more than general pressure for change. For example, the centralized nature of decision making in the United Kingdom allows the NHS to impose strict rules on independent Hospital Trusts. The federal structure of Canada leaves the provinces almost fully autonomous in the way they organize their health care systems; in turn, provinces can opt to shift decision-making powers and financial risks further down to regionalized governance models. There is no way the Canadian federal government can impose centralized rules on the administration of hospitals. Another explanation of the diverging directions and pace of change is the difference in the style of policy making across countries explained by institutional legacies. For example, in the German and Dutch neocorporatist model, policy makers consider measures such as the introduction of case-based DRGs as a consultative process with the main stakeholders. The Dutch government originally left the development of DRGs (in its own model of DBCs) largely in the hands of medical specialists and hospitals (a decentralized process that originally resulted in over 40,000 DBCs, later to be scaled down to a smaller number). Such consultative and decentralized approaches offer organized stakeholders strong veto positions and require (much) time for implementing change. In the much more centralized NHS, the government has more power to impose its decisions and adjust the system, sometimes in a breathtaking speed of change.

In all countries of this study, the rhetoric about population health did not translate into substantial action. Nor did the rhetoric about the promises of health information technology translate into major efficiency gains. In those two fields, policy change has been modest and fragmented everywhere.

Thus, generalized claims do not settle matters. Health systems are as much about values, history, and cultural context as about change in funding sources, payment models, or governance structures of health care. The same apparent reform may evolve at quite different speeds and in quite different directions in one nation than in another.

References

Algemeen Dagblad. 2003. Privé-klinieken geen vetpot [For Profit Clinics Barely Successful]. October.

Altenstetter, C., and S. C. Haywood. 1991. *Comparative health policy and the new right: From rhetoric to reality.* Hong Kong: Macmillan.

Bloomberg News. 2005. Doctors to pay to settle probe of company. *Washington Post,* November 18.

Boot, J. M. 1998. Schaalvergroting en concentratie in het Nederlands ziekenhuiswezen [Increased scale of operation and market concentration in Dutch hospitals]. *Bestuurskunde* 7 (1): 29–37.

Boychuk, T. 1999. *The making and meaning of hospital policy in the United States and Canada.* Ann Arbor: University of Michigan Press.

Bristol Royal Infirmary Inquiry. 2001. *Learning from Bristol: The report of the public inquiry into children's heart surgery at the Bristol Royal Infirmary 1984–1995.* Norwich, UK: Stationery Office.

Canada Senate Committee on Social Affairs, Science and Technology. 2001. *The health of Canadians: The federal role.* Vol. 4. 37th Parliament, 1st sess. http://www.parl.gc.ca/37/1/parlbus/commbus/senate/com-e/SOCI-E/rep-e/repintsepo1-e.htm.

Canadian Health Services Research Foundation. 2004. Bigger is always better when it comes to hospital mergers. *Journal of Health Services Research and Policy* 9 (1): 59–60.

Canadian Institute for Health Information. 2000. *Health care in Canada, 2000: A first annual report.* Ottawa: CIHI.

Canadian Institute for Health Information. 2005. *Understanding emergency depart-ment wait times: Who is using emergency departments and how long are they wait-ing?* Ottawa: CIHI.

Carvel, J. 2005. NHS crisis as trust deficits top £900m: Hewitt sends in budget hit squads. *Guardian,* December 2.

CIHI. *See* Canadian Institute for Health Information.

Clair Commission. 2001. *Les solutions émergentes.* Commission d'étude sur les services de santé et les services sociaux [Emerging solutions. Commission on health and social services]. http://www.cessss.gouv.qc.

Commission on the Future of Health Care in Canada. 2002. *Shape the future of health care: Interim report.* Ottawa: Government of Canada.

Decter, M. B. 1998. Winds of change shaping the future of hospitals. In *Four Country Conference: The future of the hospital,* 15–18. Conference Report. New Haven, CT, June 9–11.

Decter, M. B. 2000. *Four strong winds: Understanding the growing challenges to health care.* Toronto: Stoddard Publishing.

Decter, M. B., C. Flood, C. Forget. H. Friesen, M. Quigley, D. Sinclair, and C. Tuohy. 2000. *IRPP task force on health policy: Recommendations to first ministers.* Mon-treal: Institute for Research on Public Policy.

DesRoches, C. M., E. Raleigh, and R. Osborn. 2004. *A cross-national look at hospitals and their health care systems: Views of US hospital executives in comparison to four other countries.* New York: Commonwealth Fund.

De Swaan, A. 1988. *In care of the state: Health care, education and welfare in Europe and the USA in the modern era.* Oxford, UK: Polity Press.

Flood, C., and S. Lewis. 2005. Courting trouble: The Supreme Court's embrace of pri-vate health insurance. *Healthcare Policy* 1 (1): 26–35.

Flood, C., K. Roach, and L. Sossin, eds. 2005. *Access to care, access to justice: The legal debate over private health insurance in Canada.* Toronto: University of Toronto Press.

Four Country Conference: The future of the hospital. 1998. Conference Report. New Haven, CT, June 9–11.

Fyke Commission. 2001. *Caring for Medicare: Sustaining a quality system.* Regina, Saskatchewan: Government of Saskatchewan.

Healy, J., and M. McKee. 2002. The evolution of hospital systems. In *Hospitals in a changing Europe,* ed. M. McKee and J. Healy, 14–34. Philadelphia: Open University Press.

Helderman, J. K. 2007. Institutional complementarity in Dutch health care reforms: Going beyond the pre-occupation with choice. Paper presented at meeting of the Eu-ropean Health Policy Group, Berlin.

Illich, I. 1973. *Medical nemesis: The expropriation of health.* Boston: Beacon Press.

Kingdon, J. 1984. *Agendas, alternatives and public policies.* Boston: Little, Brown.

Klein, R. 1995. Learning from others: Shall the last be the first markets? In *Four Coun-try Conference on Health Care Reforms and Health Care Policies in the United States, Canada, Germany and the Netherlands,* 95–102. Conference Report. Amster-dam, February 23–25.

Klein, R. 2001. *The new politics of the National Health Service.* 4th ed. Harlow, Essex, UK: Longman.

Klein, R. 2007. The new model NHS: Performance, perceptions and expectations. *British Medical Bulletin* 81–82 (1): 39–50.

Kleinfield, N. R. 2006. Costs of a crisis: Diabetics confront a tangle of workplace laws. *New York Times,* December 26.

Knieps, F. 1998. The present situation of non-primary care, especially hospital care, in Germany. In *Four Country Conference: The future of the hospital,* 30–32. Conference Report. New Haven, CT, June 9–11.

Kohn, L. T., J. M. Corrigan, and M.S. Donaldson, eds. 2000. *To err is human.* Washington, DC: Institute of Medicine.

Lalonde, M. 1974. *A new perspective on the health of Canadians.* Ottawa: Government of Canada.

Leape, L. L., and D. M. Berwick. 2005. Five years after "To Err is Human": What have we learned? *Journal of the American Medical Association* 293: 2384–2390.

Lijphart, A. 1968. *Verzuiling, pacificatie en kentering in de Nederlandse politiek* [Pillarization, pacification, and change in Dutch politics]. Amsterdam: J. H. de Bussy.

Manyon, R. 2005. Practice based commissioning: A summary of the evidence. *Health Policy Matters,* no. 11.

Marmor, T. R. 1998. Hype and hyperbole: The rhetoric and realities of managerial reform in health care. *Journal of Health Services Research and Policy* 3 (1): 62–64.

Marmor, T. R., J. Mashaw, and P. L. Harvey. 1990. *America's misunderstood welfare state: Persistent myths, enduring realities.* New York: Basic Books.

Maynard, A. 2005. UK healthcare reform: Continuity and change. In *The public-private mix for health,* ed. A. Maynard, 63–82. London: Nuffield Trust.

Maynard, A., and K. Bloor. 2003. Do those who pay the piper call the tune? *Health Policy Matters,* no. 8.

Maynard, A., and A. Street. 2006. Seven years of feast, seven years of famine: Boom to bust in the NHS? *BMJ* 332 (7546): 906–8.

Mazankowski Commission. 2001. A framework for reform. *Report of the Premier's Advisory Council on Health.* Edmonton.

Ministry of Health. 1992. *Positioning Hospital Care.* The Hague: Ministry of Health.

Ministry of Health. 2001. *Demand at the Centre.* The Hague: Ministry of Health.

Ministry of Health. 2004. *Renumeration of Medical Specialists and GPs in Europe.* (White Paper.) The Hague: Ministry of Health.

National Forum on Health. 1997. *Canada health action: Building on the legacy.* Ottawa: Health Canada Communications.

OECD. *See* Organization for Economic Co-Operation and Development.

Okma, K. G. H. 1997. *Studies of Dutch health politics, policy and law.* Utrecht: University Utrecht.

Okma, K. G. H. 2001. Over wortels en stokken [About carrots and sticks]. *ESB* 86: D26–28.

Okma, K. G. H. 2002. What is the best public-private model for Canadian health care? *Policy Matters* 3 (6).

Oliver, A. 2005. The English National Health Service 1979–2005. *Health Economics* 14: S75–99.

Ontario Health Services Restructuring Commission. 2000. *1996–2000: Looking back, looking forward; A legacy report.* Ottawa: Health Services Research Foundation.

Organisation for Economic Co-operation and Development. 1992. *The reform of health care: A comparative analysis of seven OECD countries.* Health Reform Studies no. 2. Paris: OECD.

Organisation for Economic Co-operation and Development. 1994. *The reform of health care: A review of seventeen OECD countries.* Health Reform Studies no. 5. Paris: OECD.

Organisation for Economic Co-operation and Development. 2005. *Health at a Glance: OECD Indicators 2005.* Paris: OECD.

Pérez-Peña, R. 2006. Dialysis in NY lags as diabetes ruins kidneys. *New York Times,* December 28.

Peterson, M. A., ed. 1999. Healthy markets? The new competition in medical care and the managed care backlash. Special issue, *JHPPL* 24 (1).

Pfaff, M., and A. O. Kern. 2005. Public-private mix of healthcare in Germany. In *The public-private mix for health,* ed. A. Maynard, 191–218. London: Nuffield Trust.

Pickard, S., R. Sheaff, and B. Dowlong. 2006. Exit, voice and user-responsiveness: The case of English primary care trusts. *Social Science Medicine* 63 (2): 373–83.

Preker, A. S., A. Harding, and P. Travis. 2000. "Make or buy" decisions in the production of health care goods and services: New insights from institutional economics and organizational theory. *Bulletin of the World Health Organization* 78 (6): 830–44.

Raad voor de Volksgezondheid & Zorg. 2003. *Marktconcentratie in de Ziekenhuiszorg* [Market concentration in Dutch hospital care]. Zoetermeer, the Netherlands: RVZ.

Rachlis, M., et al. 2001. *Revitalizing Medicare: Shared problem, public solutions.* Vancouver: Tommy Douglas Research Institute.

Ranade, W. ed. 1998. *Markets and health care: A comparative analysis.* New York: Addison Wesley Longman.

Rau, F. 2005. Changes in the hospital care sector in Germany. Seminar on German Health Reforms in the Last Decades, Bremen.

Relman, A. S. 1988. Assessment and accountability: The third revolution in medical care. *New England Journal of Medicine* 319 (18): 1220–22.

Royal College of General Practitioners. 2005. *General practice in the UK: A basic overview.* http://www.rcgp.org.uk/pdf/ISS_INFO_04_MAY05.pdf.

RVZ. *See* Raad voor de Volksgezondheid & Zorg.

Salfeld, R., and M. Vaagen. 2004. The road to reform in Europe. *Health Europe,* 3 (March): 14–29.

Schoen, C., R. Osborn, P. T. Huynh, M. Doty, J. Peugh, and K. Zapert. 2004. Primary care and health system performance: Adult's experience in five countries. *Health Affairs,* Web Exclusive: www.cmwf.org, W4–487–503.

Sekhri, N. K. 2000. Managed care: The US experience. *Bulletin of the World Health Organization* 78 (6): 830–44.

Skrabanek, P. 1994. *The death of humane medicine: And the rise of coercive healthism.* London: Social Affairs Unit.

Starr, P. 1982. *The social transformation of American medicine.* New York: Basic Books.

Stevens, R. 1971. *American medicine and the public interest.* New Haven, CT: Yale University Press.

Taylor, M. G. 1987. *Health insurance and Canadian public policy: The seven decisions that created Canadian health insurance and their outcomes.* Montreal: McGill-Queen's University Press.

Timmins, N. 1995. *The five giants: A biography of the welfare state.* London: Fontana Press.

Visser, J., and A. Hemereyk. 1997. *A Dutch miracle: Job growth, welfare reform and corporatism in the Netherlands.* Amsterdam: Amsterdam University Press.

Wanless, D. 2002. *Securing our future health: Taking a long-term view.* London: HM Treaury.

Wennberg, D. E., and J. E. Wennberg. 2003. Addressing variations: Is there hope for the future? *Health Affairs,* Web Exclusive: W3–614–17.

Wennberg, J. E. 1973. Small area variations in health care delivery. *Science* 182: 1102–8.

Wennberg, J. E. 2005. *Variations in use of medical care services among regions and selected academic medical centers: Is more better?* New York: Commonwealth Fund.

WHO. *See* World Health Organization.

Wiley, M., M. A. Laschober, and H. Gelband, eds. 1995. *Hospital financing in seven countries.* U.S. Congress. Office of Technology Assessment. Washington, DC: U.S. Government Printing Office.

World Health Organization. 1978. Declaration of Alma-Ata. *Primary health care: Report of the International Conference on Primary Health Care,* Alma-Ata, USSR, September 6–12, 1978. Geneva: World Health Organization.

Websites

Bundesministerium für Gesundheit [Ministry of Health, Germany]. www.bmg.org.de

Canadian Institute of Health Information. www.cihi.ca

Commonwealth Fund. www.cmwf.org

Department of Health, UK. www.dh.gov.uk

Health Canada. www.hc-sc.gc.ca

Healthcare Commission, UK. www.hcc.org.uk

Ministry of Health, the Netherlands. www.minvws.nl

National Health Services, UK. www.nhs.uk

National Institute for Clinical Excellence. www.nice.org.uk

Royal College of General Practitioners, UK. www.rcgp.org.uk

Raad voor de Volkgezondheid & Zorg [Council of Health and Care, the Netherlands].www.rvz.net

Statistisches Bundesamt Deutschland [Federal Statistic Office, Germany]. www.destatis.de

University of York, Health Sciences. www.york.ac.uk/dept/healthsxciences/hpmindex.htm

Pharmaceutical Policy and Politics in OECD Countries

RICHARD FREEMAN

Perhaps the key difference in the practice of medicine at the beginning of the twenty-first century compared to a hundred or even fifty years ago is the prescription and use of therapeutic drugs. With this change, health politics has changed, too.

For health care is a problem of political economy. When health care states were established, the problem became the distribution of its costs, between capital and labour, employers and employees, tax payers and patients. And in most countries and systems, the question of who bears the health financing is still contentious. As far as pharmaceuticals are concerned, however, what is consumed in one part of the economy is produced in another. There is therefore a trade-off to be made between benefits to doctors and patients in the health care state, and those that accrue to firms and shareholders private sectors within the health care industry.

The health care state, as Michael Moran famously explained, is not only a welfare state but also an industrial capitalist state, as well as a liberal democratic state (Moran 1995, 1999). As such, it faces dilemma and compromise at every turn. To guarantee access to health care means ensuring the availability of medicines, and doing so means addressing familiar distributional issues of who gets what, when, how. Governments are concerned with promoting therapeutic innovation but also with protecting patients from risks. Meanwhile, major pharmaceutical firms are emblematic of national economic success: They often provide high quality and high volume employment, their production generates considerable added value, and they are a principal source of foreign export earnings. Thus governments face the dual task of sponsoring and disciplining industry, to maximize its possible earnings and contribution to health but to minimize its potential cost. This dilemma—a "quadrilemma," in Weisbrod's (1991) phrase—is the more difficult in democratic states, where decision making is subject to powerful lobbying by producer interests and subject to electoral approval (or otherwise) by consumers. Furthermore, as Weisbrod suggests, it has an accelerating, dynamic quality. The market for new drugs depends in large part on public coverage of much of their costs, which in turn feeds new and increased demand (Weisbrod 1991).

Yet things are more complicated still. More than other elements of health care systems, pharmaceutical research, production, and marketing are unusually internationalized. This global aspect has been a feature of the industry since its development in the later decades of the nineteenth century. It contrasts markedly with the predominantly national organization and regulation of the medical profession, for example. National economies and health systems are exposed to the global market in pharmaceuticals to different degrees and in different ways, though all are subject to changes in an environment essentially beyond their control. While attempts at the international regulation of that market began in the 1990s, it remains dominated by global networks of global producers.

Across Organisation for Economic Cooperation and Development (OECD) countries, total expenditure on pharmaceuticals amounts, on average, to slightly more than 1.3 percent of GDP (Table 9.1) and to around 17.5 percent of all health spending (OECD 2006).[1] In most countries, more than half of pharmaceutical expenditure is reimbursed by public funds. Pharmaceuticals represent about 13.8 percent of total public health spending (Table 9.2). Between 1970 and 2000, the average share of GDP devoted to pharmaceuticals increased in OECD countries by around 50 percent. Even in countries with relatively moderate health expenditure growth, such as the United Kingdom or the Netherlands, the growth of the share of pharmaceuticals in GDP has been significant.

Public expenditure on pharmaceuticals (Table 9.2) tends to be highest in countries that combine extensive coverage with high levels of consumption, such as Japan, Germany, and France. In the United States, where public coverage is limited, public expenditure on drugs is low although total pharmaceutical spending is at the OECD mean. Pharmaceutical expenditure levels per capita are highest in Japan, the United States, France, Belgium and Germany. They

Table 9.1 Total spending on pharmaceuticals in selected OECD countries, 1970–2000 (% GDP)

	1970	1980	1990	2000
Canada	0.6	0.6	1.0	1.4
Germany	1.0	1.2	1.2	1.4
The Netherlands	–	0.6	0.7	0.9
United Kingdom	0.7	0.7	0.8	1.1
United States	0.9	0.8	1.1	1.5
OECD 17 mean	0.81	0.84	0.95	1.25
OECD 30 mean	–	–	–	1.34

Source: OECD (2006). The Netherlands 1970 figures are in fact taken from 1972, and the United Kingdom's 2000 figures from 1997. OECD 17 countries are Australia (1970 = 1971), Belgium (2000 = 1997), Canada, Finland, France, Germany, Greece, Iceland, Ireland, Luxembourg, the Netherlands (1970 = 1972), New Zealand (1970 = 1971), Norway, Portugal, Sweden, United Kingdom (2000 = 1997), and the United States.

Table 9.2 Public spending on pharmaceuticals in selected OECD countries, 1970–2000 (% public spending on health)

	1970	1980	1990	2000
Canada	0.3	2.8	5.1	8
Germany	14.1	12.5	13.7	12.3
The Netherlands	10.2	7.7	9.5	10.8
United Kingdom	10	9.7	10.8	12.6
United States	1.9	1.9	2.9	5.1
OECD 17 mean	13.1	9.9	10.9	12.4
OECD 30 mean	–	–	–	13.8

Source: OECD (2006). The Netherlands 1970 figures are in fact taken from 1972, and the United Kingdom's 2000 figures from 1997. OECD 17 countries are Australia (1970 = 1971), Belgium (2000 = 1997), Canada, Finland, France, Germany, Greece, Iceland, Ireland, Luxembourg, the Netherlands (1970 = 1972), New Zealand (1970 = 1971), Norway, Portugal, Sweden, United Kingdom (2000 = 1997), and the United States.

tend to be lower in northern European countries, where doctors are paid mainly by salary and capitation (and thus have no direct incentive to prescribe more).

Pharmaceutical production is disproportionately concentrated in five to ten countries. The United States remains the major producer. Its market share declined between 1970 and 1980, but it has remained stable since then. The U.S. position has been sustained by strict requirements for market entry as well as by high levels of domestic consumption. Pharmaceuticals are manufactured goods. Most originate from countries such as the United States, Sweden, Switzerland, Germany and the United Kingdom that have high living standards and high labor costs. This origin means that the cost of drugs tends to be a relatively heavier burden for health care systems in poorer countries. Hence, pharmaceutical spending as a proportion of GDP is highest in countries such as Portugal, Greece, Hungary, and the Czech Republic, and much lower in countries such as Denmark, Norway, Luxembourg, Switzerland, and the Netherlands.

A ranking of trade balances underlines the strong position of countries with a research-based pharmaceutical industry, such as Switzerland, Germany, and the United Kingdom. Belgium, Sweden, Denmark, and Ireland also have a significant surplus, while the French surplus is relatively small in comparison to its overall domestic production. It is notable that, in relative terms, the United States is not a big exporter of pharmaceutical goods. Japan is the biggest importer of drugs, which reflects the limitations of its own industry (Balance, Pogany, and Forstner 1992; Thomas 1995). Adjusting trade performance to the size of the domestic market underlines the success of the industry in Denmark, Sweden, the United Kingdom, and Germany. By contrast, other European countries such as Greece, Finland, Portugal, and Norway have large deficits. Australia, Canada, and Austria import a significant share of their drugs.

Not surprisingly, countries with a strong trade position are also the home countries of large multinational exporting companies. This pattern is particularly true for Switzerland (Roche, Novartis), the United Kingdom (GlaxoSmithKline), Sweden (AstraZeneca), and Germany (Bayer). The United States (Merck, Pfizer, Johnson & Johnson, Bristol Myers Squibb, Eli Lilly) ranks highly in international terms simply due to the size of the U.S. market (around a third of the total OECD markets). That also means that U.S.-based firms control roughly half of all pharmaceutical production in the OECD area.

In sum, pharmaceuticals absorb a significant share of health expenditure and, critically, an increasing share of public spending on health in most OECD countries. Pharmaceutical spending, like health spending in general, is closely associated with national wealth. It is also subject to specific institutional effects. The next section of this chapter discusses the range of regulatory instruments used by the governments of OECD countries to steer the production, trade, and use of medicines.

Policy Instruments

Given the wide range of objectives governments have in formulating pharmaceutical policy, it is unlikely that they will find a single measure or "magic bullet" to meet their needs or cure all ills. Instead, they deploy a range of instruments, targeted at various aspects of demand and supply, in something like a policy variant of combination therapy.

DEFINING THE MARKET

Pharmaceutical policy starts with defining the scope and extent of the market itself. Next, governments have to set rules for market entry, such as establishing the efficacy and safety criteria the industry must meet before it can sell or distribute a given drug. The Food and Drug Administration (FDA) in the United States and its equivalents in other countries administer such tests and monitor the market.

Where medicines are covered by public schemes, as for example by social insurance in Germany and the Netherlands or the National Health Service (NHS) in the United Kingdom, a second task is to define the entitlements. Adjusting and updating this list is the most immediate way governments influence demand. Most OECD countries revise their lists several times a year, either through the relevant Ministry (usually Health) or a specific body in charge of pharmaceuticals, such as PHARMAC in New Zealand. Sometimes lists are subject to more extensive reevaluation. In France, the government conducted an extensive reevaluation in 1999. In Germany, the government excluded over-the-counter drugs from reimbursement in 2004.

However, not all countries provide universal coverage for pharmaceuticals. In the United States, each insurer or health maintenance organization (HMO) has to draw up its own list or formulary. In Canada, while Medicare does not cover pharmaceuticals, the federal government provides drug coverage to specific groups (Vandergrift and Kanavos 1997). For their part, provincial and territorial governments subsidize the cost of prescription drugs for at least some sectors of the population, notably seniors, social assistance recipients, individuals with specific disease conditions, and in some cases, home and community care recipients.

PATIENT CO-PAYMENTS

The very function of insurance is to separate immediate financial considerations from access to services. But where demand does not face price, as is the case with pharmaceuticals fully covered by a public scheme, there is a risk of over-consumption. In general, this risk is much greater for pharmaceuticals than other elements of health care such as hospital stays. Almost all insurance schemes, both public and private, therefore include some level or type of co-payment (or deductible) for pharmaceuticals to restrain consumption. Even the tax-funded NHS in the United Kingdom introduced co-payments soon after it was established, extending them significantly in the early 1980s.

Co-payments certainly have an effect on drug consumption. They seem to have more effect when related to the price of the drug than when set at a fixed rate per prescription. Maximum efficacy in terms of reducing consumption seems to be reached at rates of about 25 percent (Newhouse 1993), though this figure may be country and context specific. Cross-national evidence suggests that limiting the level and scope of patient reimbursement inhibits the use of essential drugs as much as nonessential drugs. This finding means that while such measures may reduce overall (public) spending, they may also reduce the cost-effectiveness of drug use (Freemantle and Bloor 1996).

The distributional effects of direct payments by patients are regressive. They tend to disproportionately affect lower-income groups and those with chronic and serious illness. Many OECD countries counter this problem by extensive exemption schemes and safety nets. In the United Kingdom, for example, almost 50 percent of the population (namely, the elderly and chronically ill who consume most of the drugs) is virtually exempt from co-payments on prescription drugs. The United Kingdom also has a more restricted list of such drugs than does Germany or France. On the other hand, some countries have co-payment schemes that appear more illusory than real. In France, for example, the vast majority of insured have supplementary insurance that reimburses most or all of the co-payments set by the principal public schemes. Germany and the Netherlands, meanwhile, like Japan and some other countries, have banned this kind of cost shifting by reinsurance, precisely because it erodes the incentives put in place elsewhere in the system.

PHYSICIAN PRESCRIBING

Often, governments first try to contain public drug spending by introducing or extending co-payments, a step aimed to increase the "financial responsibility" of patients. Targeting providers comes second. Most Western European countries, as well as managed care schemes in the United States, monitor physician prescription and use other tools to influence prescribing, including auditing, the use of guidelines, and fixed drug budgets.

The United Kingdom has long made considerable efforts to influence doctors' prescribing (Rochaix 1993; GAO 1994b). Physicians have been able to compare their patterns of prescription to those of their colleagues. The Prescription Pricing Authority has provided Prescribing Analysis and Cost (PACT) data that serve as benchmarking information. France, too, periodically reviews physicians' individual prescribing activity and publishes the *Tableaux Synthétiques d'Activité des Praticiens (TSAP)*. The NHS in the United Kingdom has used targets and budgets to constrain general practitioner (GP) prescribing. Doctors' willingness to prescribe generic rather than brand-name drugs and to use computerized prescription management systems has generated savings. Although direct evidence of the impact of these initiatives is scarce, U.K. prescription patterns appear more cost-efficient than those of other countries. U.K. physicians have lower rates of unnecessary prescribing and relatively expensive drugs.

Most OECD countries have applied prescription guidelines since the mid-1990s (Mitchell 1996). They can be either positive, listing appropriate prescribing, or negative, as in France, where they state what physicians should not do (with possible sanctions). Meanwhile, reform legislation of 1993 set global pharmaceutical budgets for the physicians in Germany (see Chapter 4). The Juppé Plan of 1996 introduced budgets in a similar fashion in France. In both countries, pharmaceutical companies may also receive financial penalties for oversupply. Finally, where physicians hold both prescribing and dispensing functions, as in Japan and to a limited extent in the Netherlands, they have clear incentives to overprescribe. In both countries, in consequence, governments have been concerned with separating these essentially different tasks (Seo 1994).

One problem underlying all attempts to modify prescription patterns is that evidence of what determines doctors' behavior in the first place remains scant. Budgetary and other incentives appear to have more effect than the simple provision of information. Few of these various methods, however, have been subject to rigorous testing (Bloor and Freemantle 1996). Public authorities and associations of providers have collected information and framed guidelines. Such efforts compete with information disseminated by manufacturers through advertising, sponsored conferences and other benefits, and personal visits to physicians by sales representatives. In this respect, pharmaceutical policy is a battle between government and industry to influence doctors. Meanwhile, prescribing behavior appears to be strongly based on habit. Studies in France, for example, showed that doctors tend to remain insensitive to economic considerations as long as they do not themselves bear the cost of the decisions they make (Lancry and Paris 1995). This finding reveals the extent to which improving the appropriate and cost-effective use of medicines turns on the regulation of not only markets but also professionals, and is likely to be possible only through extensive collaboration with them.

PRICE FIXING AND REFERENCE PRICING

Pharmaceuticals have long been subject to extensive and wide-ranging price fixing in OECD countries.[2] Today, pharmaceutical prices are free in only a minority of OECD countries, though this minority includes some major players such as the United States and Germany. In Canada, for example, a Patented Medicine Prices Review Board has set maximum prices for patented drugs since 1987. The Netherlands combines reference pricing with other price controls as well as measures to influence physician prescription and patient drug use.

The U.K.'s Pharmaceutical Price Regulation Scheme (PPRS) determines an initial or "benchmark" price for a drug. In the knowledge that this launch price will subsequently be contained, if not fixed, manufacturers seek to set the benchmark as high as possible. This scheme makes the United Kingdom a lead market of some significance in determining how others work.

The difficulty with price fixing of pharmaceuticals is to determine the unit of control. Prices are fixed for what is apparently traded on the market, namely boxes. What is actually bought is a certain set of chemical substances with therapeutic properties. In the case of pricing by the box, the price-fixing mechanism is highly vulnerable to manipulation (Abbott 1995; Schönhöfer 2000). Minor changes in strength, packaging, or some recomposition of the chemical formula all create "new" products. This means manufacturers can push up price by differentiating products with the same therapeutic properties.

The effectiveness and appropriateness of price controls also depend on the level at which the price is fixed. OECD countries use a combination of criteria to fix the prices for drugs under public schemes. These include the therapeutic value of the drug, reference to existing products or to international comparisons, and the contribution of pharmaceuticals to the national economy. In Canada, the guidelines of the Patented Medicine Prices Review Board include several tests. First, it measures a new drug against others with a comparable molecular structure. For breakthrough products (drugs that promise substantial therapeutic innovation), the board makes international price comparisons based on average exchange rates over the previous thirty-six months. Drugs that only promise a modest therapeutic improvement are assessed with comparable medicines of comparable dosage in a therapeutic class.

Reference pricing sets a standard rate of reimbursement for specific drugs. Strictly defined, a reference price compares a name-brand product with its generic equivalents. In a more general sense, however, it may involve similar products of the same therapeutic class though not necessarily the same chemical formula. Reference pricing started in countries with a dominant public reimbursement system and a strong, research-oriented pharmaceutical industry, mainly in northern Europe.[3] The most extensive is that in Germany. Denmark, Sweden, and the Netherlands also have reference pricing, as well as Italy since 1996. Since 1999, reference prices in Germany may not exceed the price at the first tercile of the products within a given reference group. For drugs without reference prices, public health insurance reimburses the price of the drug at a discount. The introduction of this system led initially to significant savings of several billion euros a year. Over time, however, its effect faded.

In the German scheme, patients bear the difference between the name-brand price and the reference price. In theory, this gives the patient a strong incentive to be discriminating in his use of medicines. However, patients' ability to switch to generic products is limited by a lack of appropriate information. This mechanism puts some patients at risk of incurring high out-of-pocket costs. It is often the pharmacist who guides a patient's decision. For this reason, reference pricing is often linked with a pharmacist's right to substitute one product for another, coupled with incentives to sell generics.

PROFIT CONTROLS

Governments use profit controls to a lesser extent than price controls. The Pharmaceutical Price Regulation Scheme in the United Kingdom specifies a permitted rate of return on capital when companies submit new products for approval. Drug companies are free to set their own prices but may not exceed a predetermined profit ceiling. By the same token, prices for existing products cannot be raised. The scheme has been in operation in various forms since 1957 and covers all licensed, name-brand prescription medicines sold to the NHS (80 percent of all NHS pharmaceutical spending). Over time, the government has both lowered the rate of return and adopted a more restrictive approach in its approval of drugs.

The U.K. scheme (U.K. Department of Health 1997) has attracted much attention. It combines a strong performance by U.K.-based pharmaceutical firms with a relatively low level of domestic health spending by the NHS (GAO 1994a, 1994b; Thomas 1995). In practice, however, the scheme is less than transparent (Bloom and van Reenen 1998). Its success is largely due to the ability of public authorities to establish and maintain a flexible and reliable relationship with pharmaceutical manufacturers. Agreements between the two have allowed some leeway for newer products in exchange for reduced prices for existing drugs (U.K. Department of Health 1997). It is notable, too, that the U.K. pharmaceutical industry has become one of the most concentrated in the OECD, as smaller firms have virtually disappeared.

GLOBAL BUDGETS

Faced with both slower economic growth and rising health care spending in the 1980s and 1990s, governments faced pressure to stabilize or reduce public spending. The measures included price freezes and sometimes price cuts on pharmaceuticals. Such measures took place in all public coverage schemes in northern, central, and southern Europe.

France and Germany, two countries with high levels of expenditure, developed global budgets. France essentially followed Germany's example (Schneider 1995) in setting a national target for drug expenditure. Doctors and the pharmaceutical industry faced penalties if pharmaceutical expenditure exceeded a specified target. In France, penalties apply when total prescribing, whether reimbursed or not, exceeds a certain limit; in Germany, when total drug payments made by sickness funds exceed a certain amount. These measures significantly reduced expenditure in the short term, as doctors in both countries have decreased prescribing or (in Germany) substituted cheaper drugs for more expensive ones. However, such unilateral measures have generally come at the price of considerable disaffection among doctors. Germany suspended the measures in 2000.

GENERIC DRUGS

Most OECD countries now have explicit policies to promote the use of generic drugs. Generics are drugs with the same chemical compound and the same International Common Denomination as brand-name drugs. Once products are off-patent, they can be sold as generic drugs at a much lower price. With the time limit on patents expiring for an increasing number of products, as well as the need to control costs, this interest in generic drugs has grown.

The rising number of patent expirations and the declining number of effective years of patent protection prompted the U.S. industry to seek government support to restore protection for future drugs. The industry also wanted to protect its high initial returns on innovation by delaying the shift to generics. In 1984, the Drug Price Competition and Patent Term Restoration Act, also known as the Waxman-Hatch Act, repealed existing laws that prohibited substitution and tried at the same time to ensure the passing on of savings to consumers (Grabowski and Vernon 1992; Congressional Budget Office 1998). Other countries followed suit at the end of the 1980s, mainly

European countries with sophisticated regulation systems and high prices, such as Germany, the Netherlands, and the United Kingdom.

Special rapid-approval processes allow generics to enter the market. Sometimes additional legislation (or some deregulation of antisubstitution provisions) was necessary to effectively promote their use. By 1989, all U.S. states had passed drug product substitution laws to allow pharmacists to dispense generics instead of brand-name drugs. Meanwhile, buyers effectively sought to speed up the diffusion of generics (see discussion later in this chapter).

They did so by providing either information or economic incentives, or some combination of the two. Information may take the form of advice to patients and guidelines for physicians (discussed in a preceding section). Both forms are widespread in Germany, New Zealand, Sweden, and Switzerland. Countries differ, however, in the extent to which guidelines are backed by financial incentives. Simple budget constraints serve as one way to increase the prescription of generics, as seen in the United Kingdom, France, Germany, and the Netherlands. Economic incentives directed at the consumer, in the form of reference pricing (for example, in Germany and the Netherlands), can also increase the use of generics. On the whole, generic drugs appear to have gained ground only where patients, pharmacists, and physicians faced strong financial incentives.

MANAGED CARE AND CHANGED DISTRIBUTION SYSTEMS

In the United States, managed care organizations have done much to keep pharmaceutical costs down. Instead of specifying standard co-payments for all drugs, for example, HMOs differentiate between generic and nongeneric. They use positive lists and reference pricing for reimbursement purposes. They have also fostered more aggressive buying practices. Pharmaceutical Benefit Management companies (PBMs), for example, aim to restrain high prices and lower the relatively high distribution costs of pharmaceutical retailing. PBMs began by drafting formularies and negotiating rebates from manufacturers. This role put them in a position to offer cheaper, integrated delivery service and payment systems to HMOs and other major purchasers. This changed market dynamic led to a pattern of implicit cross-subsidy among customer categories. Patients in retail pharmacies now pay more in order to compensate producers for those sales for which prices have been bargained down.

A new form of delivery is mail-order pharmacies, partly linked to PBMs. They cover around 10 percent of the U.S. market and are particularly important for chronically ill and older patients (Kane 1997). Mail order is also important in Australia and New Zealand, but it remains relatively uncommon in most European countries. However, its growth may be stimulated by the increasing use of electronic commerce.

In some countries, distribution of drugs remains a full part of the public system. Sweden nationalized all pharmacies in 1970 to form the Apoteksbolaget, a public agency. Elsewhere chain stores selling health-related products have begun to transform over-the-counter (OTC) drug markets. They may be seen as a response to delisting drugs from public insurance on one hand and a rising demand for health care products on the other.

In all of this, pharmaceutical companies themselves have remained far from passive. They adopted two key organizational strategies. They engaged in horizontal integration (merging with or acquiring other companies) to capture a larger share of the market and to build on a wider portfolio of research and development (R&D). In Europe, for example, Novartis is the result of a merger between the Swiss companies Sandoz and Ciba-Geigy; Sweden's AstraZeneca is a merged firm, as is Aventis (between the German firm Hoechst and the French Rhône-Poulenc), while GlaxoSmithKline is the result of a merger between the already merged firms Glaxo Wellcome and SmithKline Beecham. The critical synergetic effect of such alliances lies in acquiring products for a company's own pipeline or in reducing the time-to-market for new drugs (de Wolf 2000). Vertical integration, meanwhile, has meant buying up or contracting with one or more agents operating downstream in order to obtain better conditions of access to the distribution system. In short, pharmaceutical companies have acquired rivals or generics companies in order to gain new market shares for their products, and specific organizations such as PBMs to control their distribution.

RESEARCH AND DEVELOPMENT

In an important sense, the whole pharmaceutical industry is a product of the patent system. In the past, countries without a patent system have been unable to develop a significant, innovative pharmaceutical industry. Developing new drugs is extraordinarily expensive. In order to make innovation worthwhile, innovators must be allowed not only to recover their costs but also to make higher than normal profits, at least in the short term. The patent system works by conferring temporary monopoly power on successful new drugs that pass regulatory tests for safety and efficacy.

The use of scientific methods to develop new drugs is fairly recent and has been greatly influenced by the regulatory process (Scherer 2000). The drug approval process in the United States began with the creation of the Food and Drug Administration in 1938. The Kefauver-Harris Amendments in 1962 further strengthened the process by requiring the FDA to assess the safety and efficacy of new drugs. Firms seeking to test a new drug must obtain an "Investigation of New Drug" authorization, based on tests of its innocuousness on animals, before they may start human testing. Clinical trials comprise three phases, including blind tests and long-term toxicity tests, lasting for a period up to six years. In some cases, the FDA can require a fourth phase. Some countries (for example, Australia) also require a test of cost-effectiveness.

The American example has strongly influenced the regulation of pharmaceutical R&D in Japan and Europe, especially in the United Kingdom and Germany (Thomas 1995). By setting high standards for market entry of new drugs, these countries forced their domestic drug makers to target the development of drugs of superior efficacy. This strong filtering of market entry by regulating product safety and efficacy has affected costs, quality, and the competitiveness of the industry. In France, by contrast, regulation was for a time much less strict, resulting in far shorter admission times. By the time formal market authorization was strengthened at the end of the 1970s, the French pharmaceutical industry had lost much of the comparative advantage of the early 1960s (Thomas 1995).

It is important to distinguish "breakthrough" from "me too" pharmaceutical products. Where research incentives are weak and market entry is relatively easy, the industry may tend to concentrate on what are known as "me too" drugs. For those, innovation at the margin (in packaging, for example) plays a key role. In countries with strict price regulation, the industry uses "me too" innovation as a tool to bypass price controls while contributing only marginally to therapeutic improvements (Jacobzone 1998). All countries face the need to balance "breakthrough" and "me too" innovation. Several countries have set up health technology assessment and clinical evaluation agencies. Well-known examples are the National Institute for Clinical Excellence (NICE) in the United Kingdom, the Institute for Quality and Economy in Healthcare in Germany, and the Transparency Committee in France. Those agencies advise governments on the therapeutic value of health care products, including pharmaceuticals.

OECD countries differ greatly in their interest in pharmaceutical R&D, but policy in one country may affect another. A study for the U.S. Congress, for example, argued that price controls in other OECD countries slowed the rate of innovation in the United States by reducing returns on patented drugs (U.S. Department of Commerce, International Trade Administration 2004). Research-based industry benefits from higher prices. Countries without a research base are not inclined to pay prices that do not support their own scientific and production systems. In Australia, the government allocates funds for R&D. In 1988, it set up the so-called factor F scheme, now called the Pharmaceutical Industry Investment Program (PIIP) (Australia Pharmaceutical Benefits Pricing Authority 1997). The scheme grants support to companies that locate part of their R&D activities in Australia. Although E.U. trade rules prohibit similar government subsidy in Europe, many European countries have tried to attract industry by offering higher prices. The Canadian government made its extension of patent protection contingent on industry commitments to increase R&D spending from 5 to 10 percent of sales. In short, OECD governments are often ready to allow prices to reflect the high investment costs of R&D if doing so benefits their own economies.

Supranational Regulation

In the European Union, trade and industry interests often trump consideration of health and welfare in the regulation of pharmaceuticals. It was the Industry Directorate of the E.U. Commission that convened roundtables with working groups on a single market for pharmaceuticals from 1996 to 1998. It reviewed the principal policy options for pharmaceutical markets, discussing price controls, profit controls, and contractual policies (COM 1998, 588). It supported the increase in the provision of generic drugs and advocated least-cost purchasing strategies. The latter included providing prescribers with more comparative information on drug costs and, where necessary, requiring prescribers to share the cost of expensive practice.

Because Europe represents such a large share of the world market, the European Union has a significant impact on pharmaceutical activity worldwide. In 1989, a European Council (EC) Directive (89/105/EEC) took up the issue of the transparency of national drug prices and entitlements regulations. Moreover, the European Monetary Union (EMU) had some indirect effect on pharmaceutical trading by increasing price transparency. Finally, the Supplementary Protection Certificate (SPC) extended patent protection at the European level (Regulation 1768/92).

European countries first developed drug licensing systems on the national level. Under EC Regulation 2309/93, the European Medicines Evaluation Agency (EMEA) offers a centralized procedure for gaining marketing approval.[4] Since January 1998, firms have the option to apply for drug licenses either country-by-country or on a pan-European basis. The pan-European license saves time and resources in bringing a drug to the market. It also harmonizes the conditions for which the drug is licensed. This legislation covers product classification, advertising, good manufacturing practice, and provisions relating to labeling and wholesale distribution. It does not address the provision of drug safety information either to health professionals or the public (Earl-Slater 1997; Mossialos 1998; Kanavos and Mossialos 1999). An important difference between the EMEA and the FDA is that the former is not subject to freedom-of-information legislation in the way that the latter is.

The organization and financing of health care, however, remain the responsibility of national authorities. In this way, Europe escapes some of the dilemma (see the introductory section of this chapter) that confronts national governments. Though it has been able to develop standard licensing arrangements, its pro-competition industrial policy leaves no basis for common pricing (EC Regulation 2309/93). Only at the national level does monopsony power continue to provide opportunities for price regulation. Thus the enlarged European Union still comprises twenty-five different pharmaceutical pricing and reimbursement systems. This variety of systems makes for a picture of the EC "coordinating divergence" in which a single market in medicines seems unlikely to emerge (Hancher 2004; Permanand and Altenstetter 2004).

One effect of Europeanization has been that disputes between national authorities and providers (and in some cases, patients) over pricing and reimbursement policies have increasingly appealed to European rules (Earl-Slater 1997; Kanavos and Mossialos 1999). The European Court of Justice has ruled in favor of parallel imports, for example, and permitted patients to buy over-the-counter drugs more cheaply in other member states, provided that they are for personal use and the product is authorized in their home country.[5]

Meanwhile, in 1990, the International Federation of Pharmaceutical Manufacturers and Associations invited representatives of both industry and regulatory agencies to meet regularly under the auspices of the International Conference in Harmonisation of Technical Requirements for Registration of Pharmaceuticals for Human Use (ICH). This body constitutes a higher level of regulation and coordination again. ICH includes the regulatory agencies of the European Union, the United States, and Japan, who invariably endorse and adopt its guidelines. The purported logic of harmonization of this kind is to bring drugs more quickly and more efficiently to larger markets. Both industry and regulators employ a discourse of improved safety and enhanced innovation. Compromise between different standards in competing jurisdictions, however, invariably is made down rather than up. This process entails a relaxation of toxicological standards that seems to favor, at least initially, the interests of those developing innovative products over those who might use them (Abraham and Reed 2002).[6]

Few accounts of this increasingly sophisticated and extensive regulation of pharmaceutical supply suggest any decline in the corporate power of producers (Abraham and Lewis 2000, 2002). This begs the key question of what regulation is for. Germany and the United Kingdom effectively implemented regulation after the sedative Thalidomide had been found to cause fetal abnormality in the early 1960s. This regulation served to protect the industry as much as patient safety. Thalidomide had damaged public trust in the pharmaceutical industry. Regulation was needed to restore and protect it (Abraham and Reed 2002). In most countries, drug regulation is essentially corporatist. It reflects the interdependence of government and industry. Consumer or patient interest is in effect absent or marginalized. Meanwhile, through the 1980s and 1990s, the neoliberal position adopted by the "competition state" tends to have made state and industry interests more rather than less congruent.

This pattern is reinforced in supranational regulation, especially in Europe. The Single European Market removes regulation even further from the limited opportunities for participation in national policy making. But it is also due to the way in which national regulators compete to carry out assessments on behalf of the European Union, which they do by speeding up the process and adopting revised criteria that suit producers before patients (Lewis and Abraham 2001).

Discussion: Regulation and Learning

The regulation of pharmaceuticals is a domain in which governments in OECD countries—states with Moran's three faces (Moran 1995 and the introductory section of this chapter)—must pursue multiple goals. Some of these are complementary, some susceptible to reasonable trade-offs, others barely compatible. In choosing and advancing these various goals, governments are playing several multilevel games.

It is difficult for its constituent actors or analysts to make sense of what is going on. Pharmaceutical regulation offers "little new, and much that is unconsciously replicated, with scant recourse to the evidence base" (Maynard and Bloor 2003, 39). Yet it is precisely here, in a domain that is highly internationalized, comprising powerful and autonomous actors (nation-states, transnational corporations, and international agencies), in which competitive advantage is at a premium, that we might expect to find evidence of learning (even if not from "evidence").

Some of this learning is familiar from other chapters in this volume. The development of innovative organizational forms such as PBMs in the United States has often been used as a sort of in vivo social experiment by other countries. Likewise, many of the regulatory instruments in use in the OECD area have been influenced by policies originating in the United States. In Europe, the United Kingdom represents a lead market, which makes U.K. institutions and initiatives of Europe-wide significance.

Simple learning in pharmaceutical regulation is then inherently unlikely. The dilemmas of government do not lend themselves to single or perfect solutions. Though they draw on a common set of instruments, governments select and apply them differently. Each faces a variety of interests, institutions, and ways of thinking about relationships between government, industry, and welfare. The effect of any single regulatory initiative is specific to local or national circumstances and difficult to test comparatively. Governments simply cannot take up the tools used by others, at least not to any equivalent purpose or effect (Mossialos, Walley, and Mrazek 2004; Permanand and Altenstetter 2004; Mossialos and Oliver 2005).

The particular technical complexity of pharmaceuticals and policy issues (principally licensing and pricing) create barriers for learning.[7] They also reduce public participation in debate. The information and research resources of industry often outstrip those of government. Corporations often understand the respective behavior of different national and international markets better than governments do and are consistently able to predict and manipulate the consequences of different regulatory interventions. Indeed, it is their business to do so.

Government appreciation and action is further constrained by divided (and sometimes competing) ministerial competences: between trade and industry on one hand, and health and social affairs on the other. This holds at the European level too: EMEA works for the Directorate-General for Enterprise and Industry, not Health and Consumer Protection. Though the United Kingdom is generally notable for its relative institutional strength, it is worth specific mention again here. It generates the greatest volume of what might be described as state-sponsored information about pharmaceuticals, including the *British National Formulary* and the *Drug and Therapeutics Bulletin* as well as PACT data, the National Prescribing Centre's *Effectiveness Bulletins,* and other material generated by standards and monitoring agencies such as NICE.

Policy learning, then, takes place within and between public and private sectors as much as across countries. Pharmaceutical companies are skilled and resourceful agents in acquiring and using cross-national, comparative knowledge about pharmaceutical markets. As a combination of science and commerce, the industry is uniquely equipped for the diffusion of both hard and soft knowledge about new products. It also has a unique understanding of markets and ways of relating one to the other. This advantage generates an isomorphic response on the part of governments. They must equip themselves with awareness of multilateral business strategies and ways to anticipate and influence them. Regulatory transfer is not the result of a collaborative undertaking among governments to face down industry, but of competition between states for economic and industrial advantage both at home and abroad. In terms of price control, for example, governments' interest may lie in importing effective price-setting instruments. Yet the point is not to achieve common pricing, but to set prices that serve both the interests of domestic pharmaceutical producers and consumers.

The multilevel and multilateral game between states and pharmaceutical companies reflects their reciprocal interdependence. Governments want firms to produce therapeutically effective products but not at levels or prices that put the viability of public health coverage at risk. Firms want governments to provide them with secure markets and income streams (which is what patent licensing and public coverage do) but not on terms that offer them limited return. Innovation and regulation, in both policies and products, are bound up together.

Notes

This chapter is based on S. Jacobzone (2000), http://www.olis.oecd.org/OLIS/2000DOC.NSF/LINKTO/DEELSA-ELSA-WD(2000)1. I am grateful to Peter Schönhöfer for comments on an earlier draft and to Achim Schmid for supplying the data used in Tables 9.1 and 9.2. Mistakes and misconceptions that remain are my own.

1. The expenditure patterns described and analyzed here do not include pharmaceuticals in hospitals. Drugs in hospitals are estimated to represent roughly 10 to 15 percent of the total pharmaceutical market, and in most budgets are included under inpatient care. While innovative patented drugs play a more important role in inpatient settings, trends for hospital drugs are similar to those observed for drugs used in ambulatory care.

2. For a review of price regulation in the European Union, see Mrazek and Mossialos (2004).

3. For a discussion of the possible application of reference pricing in the United States, see Kanavos and Reinhardt (2003).

4. For a description and a discussion of the workings of the EMEA, see Garattini and Bertelè (2004).

5. In Europe, the effect of parallel imports on prices seems minimal since such drugs tend to be priced just below those from original sources. Generics are much more important in price competition (Kanavos and Costa-Font 2005).

6. Although the process of compromise at the ICH might seem to favor those who develop innovative drugs over those who will use them, patient interests are perhaps less than obvious. The key achievement of "treatment activists" in respect to AIDS, especially in the United States, has been to speed up the release of experimental drugs, overcoming established requirements for medical trials (Epstein 1996).

7. For discussion of the fundamental methodological challenges of price measurement, see Jacobzone (2000, 46–48); on measuring policy outcomes, Kanavos et al. (2004).

References

Abbott, T. A. 1995. Price regulation in the pharmaceutical industry: Prescription or placebo? *Journal of Health Economics* 14 (5): 551–67.

Abraham, J., and G. Lewis. 2000. *Regulating medicines in Europe: Competition, expertise and public health.* London: Routledge.

Abraham, J., and G. Lewis. 2002. Citizenship, medical expertise and the capitalist regulatory state in Europe. *Sociology* 36 (1): 67–88.

Abraham, J., and T. Reed. 2002. Progress, innovation and regulatory science in drug development: The politics of international standard-setting. *Social Studies of Science* 32 (3): 337–69.

Australia Pharmaceutical Benefits Pricing Authority. 1997. *Annual Report.* Canberra, AU: Department of Health and Ageing.

Balance, R., J. Pogany, and H. Forstner. 1992. *The world's pharmaceutical industries: An international perspective on innovation, competition and policy.* Cheltenham, UK: Edward Elgar Publishing.

Bloom, N., and J. van Reenen. 1998. Regulating drug prices: Where do we go from here? *Fiscal Studies* 19 (3): 321–42.

Bloor, K., and N. Freemantle. 1996. Lessons from international experience in controlling pharmaceutical expenditure II: Influencing doctors. *British Medical Journal* 312: 1525–27

Congressional Budget Office. 1998. *How increased competition from generic drugs has affected prices and returns in the pharmaceutical industry.* Washington, DC: CBO.

de Wolf, P. 2000. Pharmaceuticals as an international industry. In *Four Country Conference 2000: Pharmaceutical policies in the US, Canada, Germany and the Netherlands.* Conference Report. IJmuiden, Netherlands, July 13–15.

Earl-Slater, A. 1997. A study of pharmaceutical policies in the EU. *Policy Studies,* 18: 251–67.

Epstein, S. 1996. *Impure science: AIDS, activism, and the politics of knowledge.* Berkeley: University of California Press.

Freemantle, N., and K. Bloor. 1996. Lessons from international experience in controlling pharmaceutical expenditure I: Influencing patients. *British Medical Journal,* 312: 1469–71.

GAO. *See* U.S. General Accounting Office.

Garattini, S., and V. Bertelè. 2004. The role of the EMEA in regulating pharmaceutical products. In *Regulating pharmaceuticals in Europe: Striving for efficiency, equity and quality,* ed. E. Mossialos, M. Mrazek, and T. Walley. Maidenhead, UK: Open University Press.

Grabowski, H. G., and J. M. Vernon. 1992. Brand loyalty, entry and price competition in pharmaceuticals after the 1984 Drug Act. *Journal of Law and Economics* 35 (2): 331–50.

Hancher, L. 2004. The European Community dimension: Coordinating divergence. In *Regulating pharmaceuticals in Europe: Striving for efficiency, equity and quality,* ed. E. Mossialos, M. Mrazek, and T. Walley. Maidenhead, UK: Open University Press.

Jacobzone, S. 1998. Le rôle des prix dans la régulation du secteur pharmaceutique [The role of prices in the regulation of pharmaceuticals]. *Economie et Statistique,* 312–313: 35–54.

Jacobzone, S. 2000. *Pharmaceutical policies in OECD countries: Reconciling social and industrial goals.* Labour Market and Social Policy Occasional Papers, no. 40. Paris: OECD.

Kanavos, P., and J. Costa-Font. 2005. Pharmaceutical parallel trade in Europe: Stakeholder and competition effects. *Economic Policy* 20 (44): 751–98.

Kanavos, P., and E. Mossialos. 1999. Outstanding regulatory aspects in the European pharmaceutical market. *Pharmacoeconomics* 15 (6): 519–33.

Kanavos, P., and U. Reinhardt. 2003. Reference pricing for drugs: Is it compatible with US health care? *Health Affairs* 22 (3): 16–30.

Kanavos, P., D. Ross-Degnan, E. Fortess, J. Abelson, and S. Soumerai. 2004. Measuring, monitoring and evaluating policy outcomes in the pharmaceutical sector. In *Regulating pharmaceuticals in Europe: Striving for efficiency, equity and quality,* ed. E. Mossialos, M. Mrazek, and T. Walley. Maidenhead, UK: Open University Press.

Kane, N. 1997. Pharmaceutical cost containment and innovation in the United States. *Health Policy.* Suppl. 41: S71-S89.

Lancry, P. J., and V. Paris. 1995. Age, temps et normes: une analyse de la prescription pharmaceutique (Age, time and norms: an analysis of pharmaceutical prescribing) *Economie et Prévision,* 129–130: 173–88

Lewis, G., and J. Abraham. 2001. The creation of neo-liberal corporate bias in transnational medicines control: The industrial shaping and interest dynamics of the European regulatory state. *European Journal of Political Research,* 39: 53–80.

Maynard, A., and K. Bloor. 2003. Dilemmas in regulation of the market for pharmaceuticals. *Health Affairs* 22 (3): 31–41.

Mitchell, A. 1996. Update and evaluation of Australian guidelines: Government perspective. *Medical Care* 34 (1): DS216–225.

Moran, M. 1995. Three faces of the health care state. *Journal of Health Politics, Policy and Law* 20 (3): 767–81.

Moran, M. 1999. *Governing the Health Care State.* Manchester, UK: Manchester University Press.

Mossialos, E. 1998. Pharmaceutical pricing, financing and cost containment in the European Union member states. In *Health care and its financing in the single European market,* ed. R. Leidl. Amsterdam: IOS Press.

Mossialos, E., and A. Oliver. 2005. An overview of pharmaceutical policy in four countries: France, Germany, the Netherlands and the United Kingdom. *International Journal of Health Planning and Management,* no. 20: 291–306.

Mossialos, E., T. Walley, and M. Mrazek. 2004. Regulating pharmaceuticals in Europe: An overview. In *Regulating pharmaceuticals in Europe: Striving for efficiency, equity and quality,* ed. E. Mossialos, M. Mrazek, and T. Walley. Maidenhead, UK: Open University Press.

Mrazek, M., and E. Mossialos. 2004. Regulating pharmaceutical prices in the European Union. In *Regulating pharmaceuticals in Europe: Striving for efficiency, equity and quality,* ed. E. Mossialos, M. Mrazek, and T. Walley. Maidenhead, UK: Open University Press.

Newhouse, J. 1993. *Free for all? Lessons from the RAND health insurance experiment.* Cambridge, MA: Harvard University Press.

OECD. *See* Organisation for Economic Co-operation and Development.

Organisation for Economic Co-operation and Development. 2006. *OECD Health Data 2006.* Version 2. Paris: OECD.

Permanand, G., and C. Altenstetter. 2004. The politics of pharmaceuticals in the European Union. In *Regulating pharmaceuticals in Europe: Striving for efficiency, equity and quality,* ed. E. Mossialos, M. Mrazek, and T. Walley. Maidenhead, UK: Open University Press.

Rochaix, L. 1993. Le suivi de la prescription pharmaceutique en Grande Bretagne: Développements récents et perspectives pour la France (Monitoring pharmaceutical prescribing in Great Britain: Recent developments and lessons for France). *Journal d'Economie Médicale,* 11: 243–50.

Scherer, F. M. 2000. The pharmaceutical industry. In *Handbook of health economics,* ed. J. P. Newhouse and A. J. Culyer. Amsterdam: Elsevier.

Schneider, M. 1995. Evaluation of cost-containment acts in Germany. In *Health: Quality and choice,* Health Policy Studies, no. 4, 63–81. Paris: OECD.

Schönhöfer, P. 2000. Drugs substituting for hospital care. In *Four Country Conference 2000: Pharmaceutical policies in the US, Canada, Germany and the Netherlands.* Conference Report. IJmuiden, Netherlands, July 13–15.

Seo, T. 1994. Prescribing and dispensing of pharmaceuticals in Japan. *PharmacoEconomics* 6 (2): 95–102.

Thomas, L. G. 1995. Industrial policy and international competitiveness in the pharmaceutical industry. In *Competitive strategies in the pharmaceutical industry,* ed. R. B. Helms. Washington, DC: AEI Press.

U.K. Department of Health. 1997. *Pharmaceutical price regulation scheme.* Second report to Parliament. London, December.

U.S. Department of Commerce, International Trade Administration. 2004. *Pharmaceutical price controls in OECD countries: Implications for US consumers, pricing, research and development, and innovation.* Washington, DC: U.S. Department of Commerce, International Trade Administration.

U.S. General Accounting Office. 1994a. Companies typically charge more in the United States than in the United Kingdom. Pub. No. GAO/HEHS 94–29. Washington, DC: GAO.

U.S. General Accounting Office. 1994b. Spending controls in four European Countries. Pub. No. GAO/HEHS 94–30. Washington, DC: GAO.

Vandergrift, M., and P. Kanavos. 1997. Health policy versus industrial policy in the pharmaceutical sector: The case of Canada. *Health Policy,* 41: 241–60.

Weisbrod, B. 1991. The health care quadrilemma: An essay on technological change, insurance, quality of care, and cost containment. *Journal of Economic Literature* 29 (2): 523–52.

Comprehensive Long-Term Care in Japan and Germany
Policy Learning and Cross-National Comparison

JOHN CREIGHTON CAMPBELL AND
NAOKI IKEGAMI

In an era when retrenchment and constraints seem to dominate welfare-state agendas, long-term care (LTC) stands out as an area of expansion in several countries. As in other areas of social policy, Scandinavia was the first to see the problems of frail elderly people and those who care for them as a proper object of national concern. Sweden (in the 1970s) and Denmark (in the 1980s) substantially expanded LTC. Municipal governments delivered the care, paid from taxes (Sundström and Thorslund 1994). In the 1990s, both Germany and Japan took another tack by creating public, mandatory long-term care insurance (LTCI) programs that cover the entire population.[1] In 1968, The Netherlands had already implemented a similar social insurance scheme.

This chapter has four goals. First, we describe the key elements of "comprehensive LTC policy" and make the case that it is a reasonable policy target for advanced industrial nations. Second, we explain the two "ideal models" for comprehensive LTC: direct public services and social insurance. Third, we analyze the policy process. We examine how Japan first opted for direct services and then switched to an approach similar to Germany. Here, we pay particular attention to the role of cross-national policy learning. Fourth, we turn to comparative analysis to try to explain how and why the Japanese program differs from that in Germany.

Comprehensive Long-Term Care

Why did several industrial nations decide to incorporate a broad or "comprehensive" long-term care program in their social security systems? The answer is that establishing a new, publicly funded LTC system, daunting as the prospect might be, appeared to be the best or only solution to a set of major social problems. That was certainly true of Germany and Japan.

Population aging is at the core. As the number of old (especially very old) people goes up, so does the number of those so frail that they cannot lead a decent life without assistance. Germany and Japan are prominent cases of these developments. Traditional sources of care are declining. Changes in demography and family patterns mean that fewer (and older) spouses and fewer children will be available to help. More women are growing dissatisfied with family responsibilities and would prefer paid employment. German policy makers, given high unemployment in the mid-1990s, aimed to keep women out of the formal labor force by providing payment for informal caregivers; Japan took the opposite tack.

Growing LTC burdens can cause fiscal strains in programs designed for other purposes, such as health insurance, social welfare, and housing. In Germany, nursing home stays imposed a growing burden on municipal public-assistance budgets. In Japan, with hospitals as the main providers of institutional care, it was pressure on health insurance.

Perceptions of unfairness among the public were another factor—whether about poor-quality nursing homes, arbitrary and rigid welfare bureaucrats, family caregivers facing intolerable burdens, even potential heirs resenting "spend-downs" of bank accounts or the family home being sold off to pay for grandpa's or grandma's care. Such dissatisfactions made new proposals politically attractive. In the event, in both Germany and Japan, a leading politician in the conservative governing party, prior to an election, recognized this potential.

Similar pressures in other advanced nations led to programs and policy experiments aimed variously at lessening burdens on families, rationalizing program structures, containing costs, and emphasizing "community-based" services rather than institutional care. Reflecting on these trends, OECD nations agreed they all should try to "co-ordinate the roles of health and social care systems so that they provide appropriate and integrated care for those with long-term needs" (OECD 1998). We argue that the German and Japanese LTC programs, and those in a few other nations, can be labeled "comprehensive" since they generally satisfy the following criteria. First, they are distinct in following a logic of long-term care rather than being subsumed as an offshoot of health care, social services, or some other policy. Second, they are broad in incorporating and to some extent coordinating a variety of services to meet the needs of frail older people and their caregivers. Third, the LTC programs are inclusive, with most if not all frail older people (and therefore, a substantial portion of the 65-plus population) eligible. In both Germany and Japan, there are no severe means tests, or exclusions because family care is available. Fourth, they are protecting family incomes by covering a reasonably high share of the financial and other costs of caregiving.

Apart from Germany and Japan, we would say that the term "comprehensive LTC" applies to Scandinavian nations, Belgium, the Netherlands, Austria, some provinces of Canada, and perhaps some other nations. While the criteria are a bit fuzzy, we think they do capture the important dimensions and give us a way to look at programs that are quite different in their structure and operation.

Costs

Germany and Japan (and others) would not have moved to a comprehensive LTC system if they expected the economic burdens to be prohibitive. The public and private costs of LTC are difficult to assess for different reasons. First, in all countries—even in Scandinavia—family members provide most care, and public accounting excludes such labor. Lacking exact data, one can assume that the *total* burden of long-term care on a society is largely a function of its old-age population, particularly those over eighty. It should be noted that the level of LTC services actually being provided in each country has no necessary relationship with the model adopted. For example, in the tax-based Scandinavian countries, the safety net is placed quite high so that individuals will be provided with services that are more generous than the German social-insurance system. On the other hand, the German system is more generous than the United Kingdom's current tax-based system.[2]

The second factor is how much formal, paid-for care families receive. Third, how much of formal care is provided in the public and private sectors. Both these factors vary considerably. In a OECD study of long-term care in nineteen rich industrialized nations outside Scandinavia, total formal LTC spending in 2000 varied from 0.6 to 1.6 percent of GDP (OECD 2005).[3] The public share of formal care averaged 79 percent with somewhat less variation.

Averages are harder to interpret than cases, as illustrated by the data on Sweden, Germany, and the United States.[4] Sweden sets the standard for generous care and high public responsibility. In 2000, its total spending on LTC was 2.89 percent of GDP, and 95 percent of that came from public sources.

In the United States, with its very partial coverage, total LTC spending was 1.29 percent of GDP, of which only 57 percent was public. The total amount spent on LTC in the United States was above the OECD average partly because prices are high; the public share was the lowest in the sample. Germany has a comprehensive system, but the out-of-pocket share is relatively high. Total LTC spending is 1.35 percent of GDP, of which 70 percent is public. The German example indicates that comprehensive LTC need not be extremely expensive—as a share of GDP, its spending was only slightly above that of the United States, and the share of its public expenditure in 2000 was only a third that of Sweden. Yet it offered an extensive program.

In the future, the total burden of LTC for society is likely to rise with demographic change. That growth, however, is tempered somewhat by decreasing disability among the elderly.[5] If unpaid (mainly female) family caregivers would be less willing to take on that burden, formal caregiving has to increase at a higher rate than implied by demography alone. What share of caregiving, or the risks of needing or providing care, should be "socialized" rather than left with individuals and families, is an important matter for public policy choice.

The record to date implies that many countries could move toward comprehensive and meaningful LTC by additional public spending of less than 2 percent of GDP. The question of how generous the coverage should be—Sweden versus Germany, say—is a matter of national preference. After the initial start-up period, experience shows that it is relatively easy to keep spending in check. There is little likelihood of a "cost explosion," at least compared with health care.[6]

A point to keep in mind is that at present, someone, in some form, already bears nearly all of these "costs"—a frail older person in the form of substandard care; a daughter or spouse in the form of exhausting work; a family in the form of rapid spend-down of a lifetime of savings; government, health insurers, or providers in the form of inappropriate and often overly expensive substitutes for good long-term care. The proper question for governments is whether overall a distinct, public system for long-term care can sufficiently enhance fairness, effectiveness, and efficiency to warrant the additional cost. The proper answer for rich nations, in our view, is yes.

How to Expand: Via Health Care?

We say no: LTC should be a distinct system, not part of medical care. Medical care aims to cure acute illness, not to manage chronic disability. Putting physicians or medical administrators in charge of long-term care can lead to both overmedicalization (such as at the terminal stage of life) and un-dermedicalization (such as in rehabilitation). A physician's professional opin-ion is vital for medical care decisions but is not so important in choosing among LTC alternatives or evaluating their quality. If professional help is needed, it is more about advice and assistance, where physician self-confidence and patient deference could be a minus.

Locating LTC in the acute care sector thus runs the risk of "infection" by inherently high-cost practices and of the leeching away of resources by more powerful actors. A good (or bad) example of the latter is Canada, where de-mands for post-acute home care, caused by lowering length of stay in hospi-tals, led to reduced spending for the frail or chronically ill elderly (Hollander 1999).

Still more fundamentally, medical care is notoriously hard to ration. After all, withholding treatment may be a life-or-death matter. The tendency is to do whatever is medically necessary (and possible) for the individual patient, whatever the cost. Societies mostly feel that treatment should not be related to the ability to pay. In long-term care, the issue at stake is more the degree of comfort or unpleasantness than life or death, and so spending is easier to constrain.

In many respects, long-term care is part of daily life. The idea that everyone is entitled to some minimum level of care, but those with more money can live more comfortably, is far more acceptable in LTC than in medical care. Thus, reaching consensus on the public-private mix in funding LTC is much more feasible than acute care.[7]

Two Models for Independent, Distinct LTC Systems

A variety of institutional mechanisms around the world serves to fund and provide long-term care. However, when policy makers and the general public become convinced of the need for a major expansion, it is helpful to think in terms of "ideal models." One is to build on existing social services provided by local governments and paid by taxes. The other is the creation of a new, separate, social insurance program for LTC partly funded by social in-surance contributions or earmarked taxation. Although hybrids are possible, characteristics of these two models tend to cluster together.

Scandinavia and the United Kingdom have tax-based models of long-term care. Those systems have developed incrementally from earlier welfare or social services aimed mainly at poor people. Over time, they expanded to provide ser-vices to frail old people (particularly community-based services) and relaxed the means test. Clients usually apply to a local agency, where a caseworker decides what services they need. A local monopoly provider, either a government agency or private organization, delivers the services. Eligibility criteria are flexible and measure each individual's need relative to the rest of the population. The criteria also can include the availability of informal support.

As for the social insurance model, conceivably it can develop incrementally by expanding health insurance. For example, there have been suggestions to expand the coverage of both American and Canadian Medicare by adding LTC, thus broadening eligibility for the current programs.[8] However, for the reasons previously noted, we believe there is a strong logic for establishing an independent system. Public, mandatory LTC insurance receives its funding completely or in part out of designated insurance premiums. Explicit and objective criteria based on the extent of physical or mental disability serve to define the benefits. In the cases of Germany and Japan, eligibility criteria do not include income and availability of informal care. Choice of services and providers is in principle up to the patients and the family since they receive benefits in cash or (in effect) vouchers.

An advantage of the tax-based and means-tested social services model is that the resources are targeted. That way money is not "wasted" on people with higher incomes or families that can provide informal support. Second, it is easier to monitor the quantity and quality of care at the individual and local levels. Third, services can expand or contract incrementally depending on the fiscal situation. For example, in the early 1990s, Swedish municipal governments were able to target home and community-based care on heavier care cases. Consequently, the share of people over sixty-five years old receiving these services dropped from 13.4 percent to 9 percent between 1990 and 1995 (OECD 2005, 41). The changes were mainly "behind the scenes," as municipal care managers dealt with individual cases. There was less opposition than would have been the case with an explicit limitation of eligibility in a social insurance program, where changes are likely to be national and visible.

There are also some disadvantages of tax-based systems. Monopoly providers—public, voluntary, or private—tend to be run for the convenience of the organization and its staff with little incentive for better performance. For example, the charitable organizations that provided community-based services in Germany before it initiated long-term care insurance were famous for not working evenings and weekends. That changed quickly when German patients got to choose providers. Interviews suggest that similar problems occur even in high-provision nations such as Sweden and the Netherlands. In the former, political accountability via elected local officials can be an effective check (more so than contracting out to private organizations with a monopoly position). Also—with the noted exception of Scandinavia, where the norm of entitlement by right seems to be well developed—the stigma of means testing may inhibit both participation and support from the middle class. Finally, bureaucratic provision can be hard to integrate with self-financed care.

The main advantage of the social insurance model rests on making LTC an explicit entitlement for everyone. The model eliminates complicated and sometimes demeaning social and financial eligibility rules and arbitrary bureaucratic decisions. Letting consumers decide what they want, for example, choosing between medical and social services, mitigates turf battles and encourages competition over quality and possibly price. Disadvantages of this model include the "dead-weight cost" of covering people with enough resources of their own, the difficulty of monitoring the appropriateness of services, and lack of flexibility.

As a practical matter, the choice between the two models is usually less a question of philosophical preferences than of institutional legacies. It is no coincidence that social-service-based long-term care (Scandinavia, the United Kingdom, Canada, Australia, and New Zealand) is found in nations where taxes or de facto taxes are main funding sources for health care. The countries that took the social insurance approach for LTC—Israel, Germany, Austria, the Netherlands, and Japan—also provide health care through social insurance. One reason is that the administration and provision of LTC requires a substantial infrastructure. It is easier to build that up from an existing system (both Germany and Japan rely on existing health insurance organizations to collect premiums and manage finances). Another reason is that policy makers and citizens are likely to think in accustomed channels, even about new issues. Institutional path dependency thus explains most of the choice of LTC model.

Still, an institutional legacy is not a predetermined fate. Many countries, including the United States, have experience with both types of social policy. They thus can mix the two (as in Austria and the Netherlands) or make explicit choices. Japan is another example: It was headed toward a tax-based system but changed course and decided on social insurance instead.

Policy Learning in Japan

If any country has shown itself keen to learn from abroad, particularly in a policy area where it is thought to be backward, surely it would be Japan. Much of its early civilization, including its written language, came from China and Korea. In the second half of the nineteenth century the Japanese were renowned for seeking models of constitutions, legal systems, corporations, and railroads in the advanced countries of the West. After the defeat in

World War II, Japan adopted many institutions from the United States—for the imports that took root, the adoption was usually quite willing. Throughout the postwar period, Japan's main policy goal could be characterized as "catching up with the West" in many areas.[9]

Much of its social policy followed this pattern; Japanese policy makers long saw themselves as "behind" Western practice in this area. The government forced a nearly wholesale switch from Oriental to Western medicine in the late nineteenth century. German practices deeply influenced pension and other programs for workers in the prewar period. The American occupation reshaped the Japanese public assistance system, while the most influential official "vision" of future social policy in 1947 was called "Japan's Beveridge Report" after the document that founded the British welfare state. Academics in social policy and social work have long made their reputations from study abroad and translations and adaptations of foreign classics. Time and time again, when an opportunity for social policy change seemed likely, bureaucrats and experts would turn to collecting as much relevant information as they could from the West.

The Development of Long-Term Care Insurance in Japan

Given this background, long-term care policy seems a good place to see how international policy borrowing works. Japan's program started up five years after the similar program in Germany. However, the story is subtler than one might expect, as our analysis of the key decisions will show.

The initial agenda-setting stage of comprehensive long-term care insurance was quite similar in Germany and Japan. In each country, in 1989–90, a leading conservative politician with long involvement in social policy took the initiative. In both cases, they proposed a major initiative for frail older people essentially for electoral appeal. In Germany, the entrepreneur was Norbert Blüm, then Minister of Social Affairs and longtime leader of the progressive or labor wing of the ruling Christian Democratic Union (Christliche Democratische Union Deutschlands, CDU). An election was coming up in December 1990 in the difficult political environment of the German reunification as well as lackluster economic performance. Blüm thought the CDU needed a positive-sounding issue, particularly one that would hold on to its traditional high support rate among the elderly.[10] In Japan, Hashimoto Ryuutarou, long the most influential politician in social policy and powerful enough to become prime minister five years later, had been held responsible for losing one election in the summer of 1989; his party faced another defeat in February 1990. Opposition parties were attacking the government about the lack of concrete policies to back up its claim for the need of a new value-added tax due to rapid aging (Campbell 1992).

German social policy specialists had been debating long-term care since the mid-1970s. They considered market-driven and tax-based solutions, as well as social insurance—either expanding the health insurance system or establishing an independent program. However, the choice of social insurance seemed natural for Germany—the country had practically invented the model under Bismarck. When Blüm brought the idea to the top of the national agenda in 1990, the other alternatives fell by the wayside. The ensuing debate along accustomed lines centered on the level and allocation of costs. The LTCI plan, Pflegeversicherung, passed the German Parliament in 1994 and started in 1995.

Japanese officials had likewise been worried about the frail elderly for years. The first serious suggestion that Japan might take a social insurance approach came from a leading official in the Ministry of Health, Labor and Welfare (MHW) in early 1989 (Okuma 2005). In a more relaxed time, that could have been the start of a long-lasting bureaucratic policy development process. An advisory panel issued a thoughtful and favorable report in December of that year, right about the time that Prime Minister Hashimoto decided a quick and bold policy initiative was needed.

However, if only because the new social insurance proposal was not close to being ready, the new policy came from the Social Affairs Bureau of the MHW. This bureau had jurisdiction in this area. It patched together a list of existing programs plus a few new ideas in the social welfare tradition. Next, it guessed how much these services could be expanded by 1999 and wrote up a "Ten Year Strategy for Health and Welfare of the Elderly," known as the "Gold Plan." The budget process for 1990 was nearly completed at the time, but an intervention by the Liberal Democratic Party (LDP) expanded the funds available for its first year to give the plan some credibility.

The Gold Plan implied a significant expansion of public responsibility. It called for "socialization of caregiving" (*kaigo no shakaika*), meaning that the government would share the burden for ordinary old people, not just those who were poor or did not have children. However, it did not change the system. That is, the new services were to be delivered the same way as the old means-tested and strictly limited programs. Municipal governments ran them directly or contracted them out, and paid for them from their own budgets, with substantial subsidies from the national government.

One might say that Japan had embarked on the road to Scandinavia. In fact, to the extent any foreign models were influential, earlier admiring visits to Sweden and Denmark by academics, activists, and even some MHW officials had helped shape Japanese thinking on social policy. The main story of the Gold Plan, however, was a reach for whatever solutions were nearest to hand, not borrowing from abroad.

The Gold Plan "worked" in the sense that it was the main election promise of the Liberal Democrats in 1990, and they won the election. To the surprise of some conservatives who thought Japanese believed in family care, it also worked in that once these services became available, the public responded with an upsurge in demand. Without that impetus from the public, it is quite possible that the Gold Plan would have shared the fate of many election promises and just withered away. As it was, the government had to draw up a "New Gold Plan" in 1994, with heightened service levels projected for 1999.

Meanwhile, the MHW officials and their allies who favored a social insurance approach continued to talk. Early in 1993, the ministry established another advisory committee behind the scenes, and this bureaucratically sponsored group came up with a proposal for long-term care insurance (Kaigo Hoken). The MHW released this plan with wide publicity in April 1994. Three conditions favored this social insurance alternative.

First, the very success of the Gold Plan was causing worries. Its rapid growth would soon require additional taxes, seen as anathema. Moreover, the management of a broad program for the middle class through an administrative structure designed for a narrow program targeted on the poor and childless caused great strains. For example, there were essentially no criteria for eligibility and few administrative guidelines for service delivery. Decisions about who got care and how much varied enormously from case to case. Local authorities could not easily solve such problems. Unlike Sweden's expansion years earlier, Japan lacked staff trained in social work and other infrastructure for large-scale local administration.[11]

The second condition that favored social insurance was a spirit of reform throughout the Japanese government that can be seen as part of a global trend toward neoliberal ideas. This included New Public Management (NPM) reforms in public administration, American-style health economics, and a general pro-market, anti-government bias. In talking with MHW officials who were involved with developing Kaigo Hoken, we were struck by their intense distaste for the arbitrary and monopolistic bureaucratic mechanisms of Japanese welfare policy (called the *sochisei*). The officials wanted to overthrow these practices by putting decision-making power in the hands of consumers and by fostering competition among providers. The long-term care problem provided an opportunity for a more fundamental application of market-oriented principles (from either American-style health economics or NPM) than any other major policy change in this period.

The third condition was the development of LTCI in Germany. In the early 1990s several MHW officials visited Germany to talk with their counterparts and academic experts. The German example was a source of credibility and legitimacy for a social insurance approach to long-term care.

MHW officials hoped they could move quickly from the Spring 1994 Report to the submission of a draft bill to the legislature in 1995, but politics interrupted the process. The main factors were extraneous to Kaigo Hoken, although some necessary negotiations with interest groups such as local governments, physicians, and social service organizations also took time. These negotiations did not alter the core ideas drawn up by the officials and the handful of experts and enthusiasts around them. In most important respects, the bill as enacted in 1997 was faithful to the ministry's proposal in 1994.

What Accounts for Kaigo Hoken?

Can the development of long-term care insurance in Japan be called a case of cross-national learning? Certainly some features of the new LTCI program came directly from abroad. Alzheimer Group Homes, the fastest growing program in the Kaigo Hoken menu, was a direct import from Denmark. More generally, Yamazaki Shirou, one of the officials who helped develop the idea early in his career (and later became a leading policy maker and spokesman on long-term care in the MHW), is fond of saying that Japan borrowed the best from three countries: social insurance from Germany, care management from England, and structured care plans from the United States.[12]

However, on closer examination this proposition does not explain very much. Take care managers, for example: the name is the same as in the United Kingdom, but the role is actually quite different and unlike anything found in other countries. Care managers in Japan do not work within a budget that is set for all their clients; each client has her own personal budget or benefit allowance, and the care manager's role is to provide advice, offer options, and coordinate services.

More generally, the LTCI case does not look much like the classic "catching-up" model of borrowing. That is, long-term care was hardly a normal item on the welfare state menu where Japan would feel an urge to catch up. Media coverage mostly focused on long-term care problems in Japan, not solutions in foreign countries.[13] Given the prior commitment to "socializing care" in the Gold Plan—which was almost completely homegrown—and the inherent problems of the tax-based approach in the Japanese context, we believe that Japan would have wound up doing pretty much the same thing even without the example of Germany. In fact, even at the level of program details, other than Alzheimer's Group Homes, it is hard to find examples of direct influence.

What about the influence of neoliberalism? In Germany, businessmen and the Free Democratic Party (Freie Demokratische Partei) advanced the private LTCI alternative from the start of the debate over long-term care in the 1970s. A few thousand people signed up for such policies in the 1980s. When it came to real negotiations for a national policy in the early 1990s, however, German policy makers rejected private LTCI as too paltry a solution if voluntary and too complicated if compulsory (Schneider 1999, 36–38). The campaign for private LTCI was perhaps an example of classic opposition to the welfare state rather than neoliberalism, but the public LTCI ultimately reflected newer trends in public management. Clients eligible for home- and community-based services could choose the agency and services they wanted, up to their assessed level of need (they could pay for more out of pocket, but few did). This degree of consumer choice was one new element; the fact that profit-making agencies could compete with established providers was another.

In Japan, the introduction of consumer choice and competition aroused a more fervent discussion than in Germany. For one thing, there was an emotional confrontation between market and social welfare ideologies, or between American and Scandinavian styles. For another, the stakes were higher because the volume of services affected was much higher in Japan (see discussion later in this chapter). Commercial chains, hospitals, and some local entrepreneurs (either commercial or not-for-profit organizations) started new agencies all over the country, sharply challenging traditional providers of home- and community-based services.

To put the story in a nutshell: It was politicians who put LTC on the policy agenda in both countries because they perceived rising public concern and were also aware of the strains LTC was putting on other public programs. The only likely cross-national influence at that early stage was that some other countries, particularly in Scandinavia and the Netherlands, had already established comprehensive long-term care programs. Both Germany and Japan adopted the solutions that fit most naturally into their institutional heritages, social insurance, and the Gold Plan direct services expansion, respectively. The initial solution worked in Germany, but when direct services ran into trouble in Japan, a group of officials were ready to push social insurance as an alternative.

It might be seen as surprising that it was MHW elite officials—who would seem to be most advantaged by a bureaucratic welfare system—who had taken the lead in attacking it. This development was probably because they were the most familiar with its limitations and failings. All had spent some years working at the local government level as part of their career path. As in many other sectors in Japan, it was these officials—not politicians, their staffs, or some interest group—who took the lead in figuring out a workable long-term care system. The idea of using market mechanisms may have been drawn from new public management ideas or the writings of American health economists, but their determination to change the old ways did not come from ideological infection. It came from their diagnosis of Japanese problems.

An analyst trying to explain the similarities in the German and Japanese comprehensive LTC programs would thus not put much emphasis on Japan pulling program ideas directly from other countries' experiences, from Germany or anywhere else. They are more a matter of common problems leading policy makers with somewhat similar orientations to reach common solutions. But explaining differences between the two programs is more complicated.

Germany and Japan Compared

The German and Japanese programs were quite different in several important respects. The following subsections provide brief explanations of the main reasons for the divergent approaches.[14]

AGE AS A CRITERION FOR ELIGIBILITY IN GERMANY AND JAPAN

Defining eligibility by condition and age and collecting contributions from all workers and employers are common in social insurance. In Germany, the question of whether employers should pay was controversial, but the age issue was not. Germany covers disabled of all ages. Japan discussed general eligibility but decided to aim the program mainly at the elderly. It was, after all, the old-age problem that had drawn intense concern for years. Disability groups were wary of the change. Politicians were opposed to making younger workers (and their employers) pay for such a benefit that most beneficiaries would only receive in the distant future.[15]

THE SIZE OF THE LONG-TERM CARE PROGRAM
IN GERMANY AND JAPAN

The Japanese program is bigger and its access threshold is lower. Of Japan's seven eligibility categories, the lowest three would not be eligible in Germany. Of the 65-plus population, about 10 percent are eligible in Germany, compared to over 15 percent in Japan. The benefits are higher in

Japan—even three times higher for community-based care at a similar, moderate level of need. Germany covers 50 percent of need whereas Japan covers 90 percent.

The difference is mainly due to the situations during the time periods that the programs were started. Many people in Japan were getting free or quite low-cost care, often at relatively low levels of need. They received this care from "hospitals" (for all practical purposes nursing homes) covered by health insurance, but also from community-based services. The latter had expanded rapidly under the Gold Plan programs in the 1990s. Japanese policy makers did not dare to worsen these beneficiaries' coverage with the new policy. In Germany, community-based programs had not been well developed, and institutional LTC was being paid out-of-pocket, by charity or by public assistance, not from stigma-free health insurance.

FISCAL CONTROLS OF LONG-TERM CARE IN GERMANY AND JAPAN

One major difference of the long-term care programs is that the German program has tight fiscal controls and Japan does not. Contribution rates and benefit amounts are fixed by law in Germany. After its implementation, the budgets for long-term care were not raised even to adjust for inflation. In Japan, eligibility criteria are fixed by law. Contribution rates have risen accordingly as more people have applied and have come to use more services. In Germany, fiscal conservatives (the Treasury, big business, and conservative politicians) were active and powerful in the process leading to enactment of LTCI. Program advocates had to impose tight controls to gain passage (Rothgang 2005). Opposition to the proposal in Japan mainly came from the left, people worried that the program was insufficiently generous. Fiscal conservatives were not much heard from prior to enactment in Japan. The Treasury actually supported the bill because it justified a long-sought increase in the consumption tax (since half was to be financed by taxes), big business was preoccupied with the unending recession and was overly tempted by alleged savings in their health insurance costs (by transferring LTC hospital care to LTCI), and politicians may have been awed by public opinion polls running strongly in favor of the program.[16]

DETERMINATION OF ELIGIBILITY AND LEVEL OF NEED

In Germany, physicians and nurses working for the LTCI carriers assessed patients' eligibility and needs. This choice was natural for Germany. The process to assess benefit eligibility in health insurance was similar. The carriers (the same for both programs) already employed a "service corps" that could do the work. Japanese health insurance worked differently in that ordinary physicians made decisions about coverage (followed by an expert review of claims). Clearly this approach would be uncontrollable in long-term care, so Japan turned to an "objective" computerized questionnaire reviewed by an independent committee. On the social service side, Japan lacked a trained pool of social workers to make objective and appropriate decisions, as in Sweden. Japan introduced the impersonal, computerized system as a reaction against what was perceived as unfair and ad hoc decisions made by municipal workers. Whether intended or not, employing a staff who could do the assessment gave German insurers a good opportunity to tighten standards behind the scenes to control their spending. Japan did not have this possibility.

THE ROLE OF LOCAL GOVERNMENT

Local governments are key actors in Japan but not in Germany. The sickness funds in Germany manage the LTCI system alongside (but separate from) health insurance. Thus, giving the funds this role was a natural choice—they already had the necessary administrative infrastructure and experience. The sickness funds do not have much real discretion over policy, since the national-level regulation provides a strong framework. They are administrative rather than political organizations.[17] In Japan, municipal governments are the insurance carriers for LTC. They were the logical choice since they were already managing a major health insurance program. Moreover, given the legacy of direct provision of welfare services, policy makers saw the municipal-level governments as most appropriate for taking responsibility for social policy.

In order to meet this goal, local officials gained significant, though limited, authority in planning for LTC services in Japan. They license new providers, monitor quality, and handle complaints. Municipalities also decide what services they offer beyond those specified in the national legislation, such as meals-on-wheels. Most important, based on a formal plan for services and spending over the next three years, they set the level of premiums charged to residents aged sixty-five years and older.[18] Should they overspend, they have to raise revenues by increasing premiums to pay back the deficit in the next period.

Cash Allowances versus Benefits in Kind

Germany offers a cash allowance to support family care of frail older people, while in Japan, benefits are limited to formal services only. Policy makers in Germany, a few dissenting social welfare specialists aside, considered cash payments as normal for social insurance. They also felt that paying (mainly) daughters to stay home and provide care would reward traditional family values and provide good care at low cost.[19] One could expect that this approach would be even more popular in Japan. It is widely seen as a very family-oriented society, and has a much higher propensity for older people to live with adult children than other countries.[20] Japanese policy makers looked at but rejected the German example. As one official remarked at a meeting of the commission preparing the LTCI legislation: "In some cases, by receiving cash, the pattern of family caregiving would become fixed (*koteika*), and in particular there is the danger that women will be tied down (*shibaritsukareru*) to family caregiving. A cash benefit is allowed in German LTCI, but the family situation is different in Japan and Germany" (Kouseishou Koureisha Kaigo Taisaku Honbu Jimukyoku 1996, 129).

Most Germans wanted to recognize the burden on family caregivers and reward them, thus buttressing the traditional model. Japanese policy makers, on the other hand, wanted to remove those burdens and abolish the traditional model, which they saw as oppressing women. The underlying reason why this feminist proposition had resonance in Japan is probably that intergenerational households can generate a lot of tension and resentment, compared to a pattern of daughters who live apart helping their parents, as characteristic of Germany.[21]

FINANCIAL SUSTAINABILITY OF LONG-TERM CARE

By the middle of its first decade, the sustainability of LTCI was threatened by declining benefits in Germany and by cost escalation in Japan. The German LTCI ran for ten years with no change in contribution rates. Its rigid rules even prohibited adjustments for inflation and forced a decline in benefits. The program nonetheless went somewhat into the red because the poor economy led to lower-than-expected revenues. The revenues were not enough to cover mounting expenditure because of increasing numbers of recipients. A second factor pushing up expenditure was an increase in the ratio of beneficiaries choosing services in kind, more expensive than the cash benefits. Complaints about low benefit levels, particularly insufficient consideration of dementia, also mounted over the years. Reform proposals thus centered on obtaining new revenue sources, such as a small private (but mandatory) supplementary LTCI or through widening the tax base by including the 10 percent of the population who are now privately insured and have a much better risk structure (Rothgang 2005). In fact, the grand coalition (CDU/CSU-SPD) could not agree on any of the bolder approaches and so just agreed to raise the contribution from 1.7 to 1.95 percent of income.

In contrast, as participation expanded, spending on long-term care rose more rapidly than had been projected in Japan. Financial reviews are scheduled every three years. The first review led to an increase in premiums of 13 percent. The second review was scheduled for 2006. Originally, experts predicted it would lead to a 28 percent increase. This annual rate of increase of about 6 percent over the entire period, apparently accelerating, was alarming to MHW officials. They came up with a plan to move lighter-care recipients out of the regular program and into a new system of "preventive caregiving." The idea was to delay dependence (arguing that too much reliance on wheelchairs or homemaking services would accelerate decline), but the reform was mainly aimed at saving money. The proposal came as part of a fifth-year review scheduled in the original LTCI legislation; it also included the transfer of some of the "hotel costs" for institutional care to residents and their families. These two reform measures caused a marginal drop in projected contributions for the period 2006–2008.

Legitimacy of a public program largely rests on perceptions of effective performance and reasonable cost. In the eyes of the authorities, Germany's program had become too small and too rigid, while Japan's program started to look too big. Thus, their sustainability appeared to be under threat within each country, and policy makers felt pressure to act.

The more fundamental point from an international perspective, however, is that both programs had clearly become institutionalized within a very short time. In neither case were there serious calls for abandoning or radically restructuring the LTC program. Most everyone concerned had come to see comprehensive long-term care as a reasonable and worthwhile solution to a serious problem, both for individual families and the nation as a whole.

Conclusion

Several countries have established a comprehensive long-term care program as an integral part of their social security system. The motives for doing so range from population aging, declining traditional sources of care, distortions and fiscal strains in programs designed for health, social welfare, and housing, to perceptions of unfairness among the public. To satisfy those needs and demands, comprehensive programs need to satisfy the criteria of being distinct, broad, inclusive, and substantial. The experience shows that the cost for long-term care insurance is likely to be in the range of 1 to 2 percent of GDP. That share is considerably lower than for health care. It is also more controllable because it is easier to ration—benefits pertain to living conditions, not life or death, so topping up by private means is socially acceptable in most countries.

The idea of pursuing a comprehensive solution to the long-term care problem reached the policy agenda in Germany and Japan in similar fashion—an election promise by a conservative politician around 1990. Germany adopted its program in one stage in 1994; Japan took one approach in 1990 and then changed course in 1997. The resulting programs are broadly similar though with important differences. These circumstances make for an interesting case for cross-national policy learning and comparative public policy.

With regard to cross-national learning, we agree with White's argument that the role of cross-national learning in policy change is problematic largely because we do not understand the general process of policy learning very well, and Klein's observation that researchers often erroneously "assume policy makers start off with a set of clearly articulated set of values or goals to guide their steps, and that the choice of possible policy options and instruments is made only after a rigorous analysis of the evidence."[22] What is needed, as this volume's Introduction suggests, is a more realistic general picture of how domestic and foreign ideas, both problems and solutions, interact with politics (interests and power) in policy change.[23]

One point in our analysis is, despite Japan's generally deserved reputation for international "copying" (pejorative for "learning"), the reason the problem of frail elders got onto its agenda had little to do with what Germany or anyone else had done earlier. This was mainly a "parallel" process, in the words of the introductory chapter, where the similarities are due to common pressures and circumstances.[24] And although both the Scandinavian-type solutions adopted in 1990 and the LTCI idea in 1997 owe something to prior examples, with small exceptions (such as Alzheimer Group Homes from Denmark), these two choices were mainly derived from domestic factors.

Still, a prior foreign example can be important on the politics side rather than the ideas side of a policy-change process. Some policy entrepreneurs may come up with solutions on their own, but a good strategy for convincing others is to point to prior foreign experience to cloak the proposal with legitimacy.[25] This strategy was clearly helpful in the case of LTCI in Japan, though it might not have been if there had been more opposition. It is interesting that proponents of the idea of cash allowances for family care mentioned the German precedent, but as previously noted, it was countered by arguing that conditions in the two countries were different.

With regard to comparative analysis, we certainly second the Introduction's observation: "There may be some irony in the fact that the most careful cross-national analyses tend to have reinforced a sense of the contingency and specificity of the way things work out at different times in different places."[26] Even so, cross-national analysis can be helpful in lighting up anomalies that would not be noticed when examining a single country. For example, Germany and Japan contrast sharply on the issue of controlling future costs of LTCI. Germany has been very strict and Japan seems very relaxed, and that should produce pointed questions in both contexts. Asking why the difference occurred leads to a "dog that didn't bark" observation about the Japanese process: The Ministry of Finance, big business, and conservative public finance scholars—all of whom on the basis of past performance would be expected to resist a big new social policy—were nearly absent from the scene. Asking why could well lead to new understandings of the Japanese policy process.

The most startling anomalies are that German LTCI was so much more family-oriented than the plan coming from Japan's famously familistic state, and that LTCI in Japan—the famous welfare laggard—was so much bigger than in Germany's gigantic welfare state. The former observation leads to a seemingly perverse sociocultural factor, namely, that familism (as exemplified by old people living with their children) can produce enough tension to work against strengthening family caregiving. The latter observation leads to a basic institutionalist point that policy change builds on its institutional legacy. Japan built its LTCI on earlier practice.

Japan first went down the Scandinavian road of direct, tax-financed services. LTC policy had already picked up a good deal of momentum when the government later swerved onto the German road of social insurance. This story in itself leads to the important point that institutions are important but are not all-determining. That Germany went for social insurance may have been inevitable, given its historical-institutional heritage. Japan had enough heritage for both direct services and social insurance to be able to chose one and then, after some policy learning, switch to the other.

In this chapter we have only sketched in arguments that deserve a full explication.[27] And we can make no claims for generalizability of any findings because this is, after all, an N=2 study. Still, we have confidence in the importance of those points. Looking specifically at cross-national experience, in the context of policy learning more generally, can add some explanatory power. And when one finds similar policy changes in two (or maybe three or four) countries, comparative analysis can lead to unexpected insights into characteristics both of policy and of political systems. Finally, both kinds of research benefit from a realistic rather than idealistic and abstract model of how policy making works.

Notes

1. Germany passed its LTCI in 1994. In 2005, the contribution rate was 1.95 percent of taxable income. Sick funds administer the scheme, and employ physicians and nurses who assess needs and eligibility for LTC. Insured can choose between services in kind or vouchers. They can spend those vouchers to contract formal home care or pay relatives. The LTCI covers, on average, 50 percent of all costs. Japan's LTCI passed in 1997. Only persons older than 40 contribute, and eligibility is mostly limited to elderly over 65. Local municipalities administer the scheme. They employ case managers who only provide advice and coordinate care as Japan has a nation-wide computerized assessment procedure. Beneficiaries can spend their personal budget on contracting formal services. The LTCI covers 70 percent of the costs.

2. Secondary factors would include cross-national variations in morbidity rates or in the propensity to get upset about serious neglect of frail older people. Presumably such differences would correlate with national income.

3. The average was 1.25 percent (OECD 2005).

4. Japan is not included here because the OECD data are for 2000 when LTCI was not really established. The figures understate Japanese expenditures by not including LTC in hospitals covered by medical insurance. If accurate and current comparative data were available, they would probably put Japan about midway between Sweden and Germany.

5. Some argue that medical and lifestyle advances will produce a "compression of morbidity" and drastically reduce the demand for long-term care: Stephane Jacobzone, Emmanuelle Cambois, Emmanuel Chaplain, and Jean-Marie Robine, "Long Term Care Services to Older People, a Perspective on Future Needs: The Impact of an Improving Health of Older Persons," in *Maintaining Prosperity in an Ageing Society: The OECD Study on the Policy Implications of Ageing,* Working Paper AWP 4.2 (Paris: OECD, 1998). Manton and Gu argue that not only relative but also absolute numbers of elderly needing institutionalization are declining in the United States, and that the rate of "compression" is accelerating. Our guess is that for most countries this effect will not be enough to outweigh the simple increase in numbers of frail elderly. Kenneth G. Manton and XiLiang Gu, "Changes in the Prevalence of Chronic Disability in the United States Black and Nonblack Population above 65 from 1982 to 1999," *Proceedings of the National Academy of Sciences* 91 (2001): 6354–59.

6. "For mature long-term care systems, public spending has remained fairly stable as a share of total public expenditure on health and long-term care" (OECD 2005, 30).

7. In contrast, efforts to prioritize publicly funded health resources have met with dismal results: Aside from cosmetic surgery and a few other procedures, it has proved difficult to categorically exclude certain services. Craig Mitton and Cam Donaldson, *Priority Setting Toolkit* (London: BMJ Publishing, 2004).

8. For the United States, see Jacob Hacker and Harold Pollack, "Health Cuts are the Real 'Death Tax,'" *Los Angeles Times* (August 21, 2005).

9. As Eleanor Westney has warned, it is a mistake to see Japan as a "rational shopper" that picks out the "best model" and adopts it as is. The learning process is more

complicated and should be seen more as adaptation than adoption. *Imitation and Innovation: The Transfer of Western Organizational Patterns to Meiji Japan* (Cambridge, MA: Harvard University Press, 1987).

10. The best analyses of the process in Germany are Ulrike Götting, Karin Haug, and Karl Hinrichs, "The Long Road to Long-Term Care Insurance in Germany," *Journal of Public Policy* 14, no. 3 (1994): 285–309; and Ulrike Schneider (1999).

11. None of the national universities provided undergraduate or graduate training in social work. Only a few of the private universities then offered any clinical training. Many local government officials were assigned to social welfare agencies as part of their career path, some coming directly from the Public Works Department, for example.

12. Yamazaki described Kaigo Hoken in this way to both authors in separate conversations.

13. An impressionistic judgment. There were not a few stories about local Scandinavian innovations, but not about social insurance in Germany, Austria, or the Netherlands.

14. For reasons of space, this chapter does not include much description of the two long-term care insurance programs. See our "Japan's Radical Reform of Long-Term Care," *Journal of Social Policy and Administration* 37, no. 1 (February 2003): 21–34, and the articles on Germany cited above. For somewhat more detailed analysis of most of these differences, see John Creighton Campbell, "How Policies Differ: Long-Term-Care insurance in Japan and Germany," in *Aging and Social Policy: A German-Japanese Comparison,* ed. Harald Conrad and Ralph Lutzeler (Munich: Iudicium, 2002).

15. As a political compromise, Japanese pay premiums starting at age forty, and a small number of people aged forty to sixty-four who have "aging-related" disabilities such as Alzheimer's or Parkinson's disease are eligible for benefits. Less than 5 percent of beneficiaries are younger than sixty-five.

16. Still more mysterious is why conservative public finance scholars, who were very alert to what they saw as waste in pensions and health insurance, paid almost no attention to LTCI. It is true that the program was relatively small. The key point may be that economic journals had not discussed the issue since there were few prior examples and the German debate was too recent for scholarly publication. Conservatives within the LDP voiced criticism shortly before LTCI was implemented, around both fiscal and social issues, but it was quelled with token changes.

17. To avoid competition among funds, which would be impossible to manage without inordinate efforts at risk adjustment, in effect all the funds pool their contributions and their expenditures. Therefore, they all charge the same contribution rate of 1.7 percent of wages up to a ceiling; this is shared equally with employers. Pensioners initially had half their contributions covered by their pension funds, but since 2004 they cover it all themselves.

18. More precisely, the municipality sets the "average" premium level; the actual amounts differ among individuals on a scale by income. Differences among localities, depending on their balance of revenues and services, can be as high as fourfold.

19. The fact that family members who received cash allowances for caregiving had their social insurance premiums paid was an added attraction.

20. Around 80 percent of people 65-plus in 1960 and still almost half today, compared with 10 to 15 percent in most Western countries including Germany.

21. Another reason for the policy difference is that the German system is more purely social insurance, which tends toward cash benefits and is completely supported from premium revenue (which in fact was collected even before benefits began). In Japan, half the revenue comes from ordinary budgets financed from taxes, so it is hard to increase spending suddenly. Everyone would apply for a cash benefit immediately, while demand for formal services would increase more gradually (as turned out to be the case).

22. See Chapters 2 and 12.

23. For example, John W. Kingdon, *Agendas, Alternatives, and Public Policy* (Boston: Little, Brown, 1984); Frank R. Baumgartner and Byron D. Jones, *Agendas and Instability in American Politics* (Chicago: University of Chicago Press, 1993); and especially John C. Campbell, *How Policies Change: The Japanese Government and the Aging Society* (Princeton, NJ: Princeton University Press, 1992).

24. See Marmorin the Introduction to this volume.

25. The fact that citing foreign experience is more often used to attack rather than support new policy ideas in the United States, as White points out, does not make this point any less important in other countries.

26. From Chapter 6. Note that Klein's view of the usefulness of comparative research in Chapter 12 is more dismissive than ironic.

27. Campbell, "How Policies Differ" (see Note 14) has longer analyses of these points, and more will be provided in future publications.

References

Campbell, J. C. 1992. *How policies change: The Japanese government and the aging society.* Princeton, NJ: Princeton University Press.

Hollander, M. J. 1999. Substudy 1: Comparative cost analysis of home care and residential care services; Preliminary findings. *National evaluation of the cost-effectiveness of home care.* Victoria, BC: University of Victoria Centre on Aging and Hollander Analytical Services. http://www.homecarestudy.com/index.html.

Kouseishou Koureisha Kaigo Taisaku Honbu Jimukyoku. 1996. *Koureisha kaigo hoken seido no sousetsu ni tsuite* [Regarding the establishment of the long-term care insurance for the elderly system]. Tokyo: Gyousei.

OECD. *See* Organisation for Economic Co-operation and Development.

Okuma, Y. 2005. Gorudo Puran to otoko wa dokyou sanningumi [The Gold Plan and Three Brave Men]. *Kaigo Hoken Jouhou* 5 (10): 26–29.

Organisation for Economic Co-operation and Development. 1998. *The new social policy agenda for a caring world.* Meeting of the Employment, Labour and Social Affairs Committee at Ministerial Level on Social Policy. Paris, June 23–24. http://www.oecd .org/document/34/0,2340,en_2649_33933_2674146_1_1_1_1,00.html.

Organisation for Economic Co-operation and Development. 2005. *The OECD health project: Long-term care for older people.* Paris: OECD.

Rothgang, H. 2005. Long-term care in Germany. In *Reforming health social security: Proceedings of an international seminar,* 57–84. World Bank Working Paper Series

2005–4. http://www-wds.worldbank.org/external/default/WDSContentServer/WDSP/IB/2006/06/12/000112742_20060612112129/Rendered/PDF/363940REVoKeioo PaperoforoWBoWeb.pdf.

Schneider, U. 1999. Germany's social long-term care insurance: Design, implementation, and evaluation. *International Social Security Review* 52 (2): 31–74.

Sundström, G., and M. Thorslund. 1994. Caring for the frail elderly in Sweden. In *The graying of the world: Who will care for the frail elderly?* ed. L. K. Olson. Binghamton, NY: Haworth Press.

Regulating Private Health Insurance Markets

JÜRGEN WASEM AND STEFAN GREß

Compared to other sources of health care finance, private health insurance (PHI) is of minor importance in Western Europe and Canada. On average, private health insurance contributes less than 10 percent to health expenditures in these countries. However, PHI played a relatively significant role in the Netherlands (15 percent), Canada (11 percent) and Germany (13 percent) in 2000 (Colombo and Tapay 2004).[1] Within the OECD, it is only in the United States that PHI accounts for more than 30 percent of health care expenditure (roughly one-third of all health care expenditures). Some critics argue that the high level of American dissatisfaction with health care (Blendon 1990; Schoen et al. 2000) precisely reflects the relatively large importance of private health insurance in the United States.

On the other hand, adequately regulated PHI markets are appealing alternatives to so-called socialized medicine for market-oriented health economists not only in the United States (Enthoven 1994) but also in Western Europe (Henke 1999). Moreover, a number of Western European politicians want to strengthen the role of the consumer within health care, and part of their strategy is to increase the role of PHI in financing and delivering health care. Since the mid-1980s, the share of PHI in health finance has increased in many countries and some experts expect a further increase in the coming years.

What are then the issues in regulating PHI? The second section of this chapter describes the various functions of PHI. The third section focuses on central problems of regulatory frameworks for private health insurance.[2] The fourth section presents conclusions.

Functions of Private Health Insurance in Health Care Systems

Private health insurance covers a wide variety of arrangements. The distinction between private insurance and self-insurance arrangements (for example, self-insured plans by employers) is not always clear. On the supply side, PHI covers commercial insurance firms (both stockholder and mutual; among them also insurers owned by the state) as well as not-for-profit agencies. Insurance business can be run by conventional indemnity insurers, which (only) reimburse costs, as well as by more expansive insurers, which provide some form of managed care.[3] On the demand side of PHI markets, individuals as well as groups or corporate actors (for example, employers, professional organizations) may seek insurance. Typical of PHI markets are voluntary contracts for both sides. However, some countries have imposed (or have discussed the option) mandatory contracts (for one or both sides). Risk spreading between the parties involved (insurer, insured, health care providers, employers) varies considerably between the different types of PHI contracts.

The scale and shaping of PHI regulation varies greatly across different countries. This variation results from country-specific historical developments as well as international trends.[4] But it also reflects the particular function of PHI in the nations' systems of social and health care politics. Basically, PHI fulfills three functions in health care systems (Wasem, Greß, and Okma 2004):

First, for parts of a country's population, PHI may be the only coverage available, as when those parts do not have access to public schemes. PHI thus functions as an *alternative* to public arrangements.[5] This alternative is particularly the case in countries with large means-tested public health benefit schemes (United States) or in systems where the eligibility for social health insurance depends on income or employment status (for example, Germany or the Netherlands until 2006) or age (U.S. Medicare). In Germany, people at a certain point in time have had the right to choose between participation in the public or in the private health insurance scheme. But, once they have chosen PHI, they are no longer eligible for the public system (Germany). The need for regulating the rules of the game of alternative PHI is particularly large because an unregulated market cannot guarantee that those without entitlement to the public system will have access to adequate insurance.

The second function of PHI is to *supplement* public schemes. *Supplementary* PHI can offer coverage for services not insured in the public system (for example, dental care for adults in the Netherlands as well as dental care and pharmaceuticals in Canada, but also upgraded hospital services such as private or semiprivate rooms in almost every country). Supplementary PHI can also reduce out-of-pocket payments (for example, "Medigap" insurance in the United States, coverage for co-payments in France and Belgium, dental care in Germany). Health economists sometimes argue that optional, supplemental insurance should not be a matter of social concern (Shmueli 2001). This argument is one reason why EU member states since 1994 may regulate supplemental insurance to only a very limited extent. However, the need for regulation of supplemental insurance increases if the coverage of public schemes decreases. If public benefit schemes are rather comprehensive and of good quality, supplementary PHI basically covers luxury goods (for example, more comfortable board and lodging in hospitals). As a consequence, a smaller degree of regulation for supplementary PHI than for alternative PHI is more justifiable in terms of social acceptability.[6] Sometimes not only private health insurers but also social health insurers or their subsidiaries offer supplemental PHI (as for instance in Switzerland, Belgium, and the Netherlands). If this is the case, government has to design a regulatory framework for competition between private and social health insurers. There the rationale is to make sure that social health insurers do not use supplementary PHI as a tool for risk selection in the public sector.[7]

The third function of PHI is to *complement* public schemes. *Complementary* PHI provides *double cover*: Those entitled to benefits of the public system might buy private insurance to cover at least partly the same benefits as the public system. People purchase such private insurance for a variety of reasons. They seek to get services quicker than in the public system (queue jumping), they want better or more comfortable services, or they want treatment from health care providers who are excluded from delivering services within the public system. Complementary PHI seems to occur primarily in tax-financed health care systems (for example, the United Kingdom), but may play a modest role in systems with a compulsory social health insurance.

To draw a borderline between *complementary* PHI and *supplementary* PHI is often a bit arbitrary. In Germany, for instance, treatment by junior doctors employed in hospitals is part of the sickness funds' benefit schemes. Sickness fund members may buy additional PHI coverage for treatment by hospitals' senior doctors—but as they do not get any premium reduction (and sickness funds do not get any reduction of hospital bills in these cases), this arrangement is a kind of double coverage. Sometimes it is also difficult to draw a line between *complementary* PHI and *alternative* PHI. The closer in fact *complementary* PHI is to *alternative* PHI, the higher is the need for extensive regulation in order to obtain a socially desirable outcome.

Because of differences in health care systems, the relative importance of the three functions in the United States, Canada, the Netherlands, and Germany varies widely. In Germany and the United States complementary PHI is irrelevant. Due to waiting times in the public system, complementary PHI increasingly became an issue in the Netherlands in the 1990s (Brouwer and Hermans 1999) and Canada (Flood, Sossin, and Roach 2005). Due to the limited extent of public schemes in the United States, PHI primarily serves as an alternative for the majority of the population not entitled to one of the public schemes. About forty-five million U.S. residents, or almost 16 percent of the population, have no health insurance at all (U.S. Census Bureau 2004). About 74 percent of the nonelderly population is covered by alternative PHI. This is mostly provided through group coverage by an employer (68 percent).[8] The benefits covered vary considerably. There is also supplementary PHI for those entitled to public schemes. About 70 percent of Medicare-insured have access to supplementary PHI; half of those are employer-sponsored, though there is a declining trend in employer-sponsored health benefits for retirees (U.S. Census Bureau 2001).

In the Netherlands, alternative private health insurance disappeared from the market in 2006.[9] Before 2006, employees and self-employed persons with incomes above the eligibility ceiling had to leave social health insurance. They could take out private health insurance as an alternative—although they did not have to. The Dutch legislature undertook a major health care reform in 2005 that lead to an obligation for every Dutch resident to take out health insurance for acute care (Den Exter 2005; see Chapter 5). The Dutch government did market its reform under the headline "privatization of social health insurance." In fact, however, the reform introduces universal health insurance for acute care, run by health insurers that are privately owned but have to follow the rules of social health insurance.[10] These rules include premium restrictions, open enrollment and risk adjustment. Since 2006, conventional private health insurance in the Netherlands is thus mostly confined to supplemental coverage. Supplementary PHI finances less than 5 percent of total health care expenditures, but around 95 percent of the population has some kind of supplemental coverage. It includes mostly dental services for adults and some other services that the government had delisted from the public benefits package in the 1990s.

In Germany, less than 10 percent of the population (7.5 million persons) is covered by alternative PHI, half of them civil servants.[11] In contrast to the Netherlands before 2006, employees above the income ceiling are allowed to choose between social and private health insurance. They are not obliged to leave social health insurance. When becoming self-employed, people can choose between staying in social health insurance or opting out to have private health insurance. Group contracts are of minor importance. Slightly more than 10 percent of persons covered in social health insurance have supplementary insurance (7.5 million persons). By law, sickness funds or their subsidiaries cannot offer such coverage. Supplementary PHI has a share of around 14 percent of total private health insurance in terms of premium income (Verband der privaten Krankenversicherung e.V. 2000).

In Canada, it is well known that 100 percent of the population has access to the public health insurance scheme run by the provinces. Most provinces prohibit private insurers from offering complementary PHI for the entitlements of the Canada Health Act. However, the Supreme Court challenged this regulation in June 2005. In a narrow four-to-three decision, the Supreme Court of Canada struck down Quebec laws prohibiting the sale of complementary PHI on the basis that they violate Quebec's Charter of Human Rights and Freedoms. This result may evoke further charter challenges to similar laws in other provinces, but the question of whether they will succeed remains unanswered for the time being (Flood, Sossin, and Roach 2005).

So far, PHI in Canada is mostly supplementary. Around fifteen million people in Canada have some kind of supplementary PHI, mostly for pharmaceuticals and dental care. Employers usually provide PHI, although they often require employees to contribute to the premiums. The percentage of health care expenses covered by PHI in Canada has grown since the late 90s, as government has excluded some services from the public scheme and costs of pharmaceuticals—which are not covered by the public scheme at all—are growing faster than average costs (Jost 2001).

Central Problems of Regulating Private Health Insurance

There is a widespread consensus amongst politicians in the field of health and health economists that unregulated private health insurance markets would result in markets failures and not lead to socially desirable outcomes (Arrow 1963). However, regulation will interfere with the autonomy of health insurers (and to a lesser extent of at least some insured). Consequently, there is a trade-off between the autonomy of market actors and the density of regulation. Collective self-regulation by insurance companies may sometimes be possible and sufficient. However, the experience of all countries with PHI shows that the dynamics of health insurance markets and diverging interests between competing health insurers sooner or later require legal intervention.[12] In this section we analyze the central problems and possible solutions for the regulation of (mostly alternative) private health insurance.

ASSURING ADEQUATE PHI ACCESS FOR UNFAVORABLE RISKS

Perhaps the most important problem of unregulated private health insurance markets is their tendency to exclude unfavorable risks (such as individuals with preexisting conditions) from adequate access to insurance contracts. In most of Europe and in Canada, there is a broad societal consensus that every citizen should be entitled to health care. However, in competitive insurance markets private health insurers who do not differentiate between good and unfavorable risks will face a disproportionately higher share of applications for insurance contracts from unfavorable risks and would not be able to compete with discriminating insurers. Therefore, as a private business, it is entirely rational for health insurance companies to discriminate against higher-risk persons. They will either deny access for unfavorable risks altogether; they will provide coverage only with a nonstandard, preexisting condition limitation; or charge a risk-related extra premium for unfavorable risks. This rational behavior of insurers does not lead to outcomes regarded as desirable in societies that place a high priority on access to health according to need. The results are noninsurance or underinsurance. Experiences from the Netherlands (Schut 1995; Okma 1997) as well as from the United States (Jost 2001) show that in competitive health insurance markets voluntary renunciation of discrimination against unfavorable risks is not possible in the long run.[13] In practice, unfavorable risks will find it difficult to get adequate access to PHI.

To ensure access to health insurance for persons with unfavorable risks, countries have tried a variety of approaches during the last 30 years. Most of them applied to alternative PHI or (in the case of Ireland) complementary PHI. Discrimination against unfavorable risks in supplementary PHI is widespread. As public schemes limit entitlements, however, this may become less acceptable. The attempt of the French government to increase access for low-income persons to supplementary PHI by providing means-tested subsidies (Turquet 2004) and the initiative of the European Parliament for the revision of European regulation for supplementary PHI (Rocard 2000) are first indicators of more regulation in that particular area of PHI.

One possible way to safeguard access to health insurance for those rejected by private health insurers (or unable to pay expensive premiums) is to offer such high-risk groups access to public schemes. Another way is to offer access to a special (quasi-)public scheme for those people. Public health insurance programs thus compensate for the deficiencies of the risk pooling capabilities of competitive PHI markets.

Several states in the United States use this type of approach. Twenty-nine states have established (quasi-) public schemes for otherwise medically uninsurable individuals (Achman and Chollet 2001). Those persons are entitled to enter a contract with one of the high-risk insurance programs provided that they have not been accepted for a normal PHI contract and/or have received treatment for some specific diseases since the 1990s. The state governments set maximum premium rates. They set the rate some 25 percent or so above the index rate in the individual market with comparable benefit packages, which is already very expensive, given the purchasers negotiating power and loading fee. For eligible individuals, who often have serious chronic illnesses, the premiums are generally high relative to income and include significant deductibles and co-payments. Still, premium income generally covers only about half of the schemes' expenditures, and state budgets cover the deficit. Although in principle this approach might be effective in compensating for PHI's tendency to discriminate against unfavorable risks, its quantitative scale in the United States is rather limited. In the early 1990s, about one million out of thirty-seven million uninsured did not have insurance primarily because of their health conditions. Less than 150,000 individuals are enrolled in one of the above high-risks schemes (Achman and Chollet 2001).

Instead of implementing a separate public scheme for medically uninsurable individuals, government can impose regulation to reduce or prevent this kind of risk selection within PHI. For example, government can enforce mandatory open enrollment; prohibit the exclusion of coverage for nonstandard, preexisting conditions; prohibit or limit risk-related extra premiums; and mandate community-rated premiums. Moreover, it can create rules for rate bands or rate approval. Like the first approach, most of these measures imply a subsidization of unfavorable risks. But instead of taxes, the "good risks" insured with PHI provide cross-subsidy.

In 1986, the Netherlands implemented such an approach for all insured not eligible for public health insurance and not able to get access to alternative private health insurance. In this case, all privately insured paid a surcharge over their regular premium. This surcharge served as a funding source for the excess cost of the high-risk groups of insured under the scheme (Okma 1997). This specific arrangement disappeared in 2006 as all residents were required to obtain access to the new health insurance. Germany has applied similar regulations to its private long-term care insurance. The United States has implemented federal legislation in order to increase access for unfavorable risks, especially for small group and individual contracts. Since 1996 they also have limited the extent to which private health insurers may impose preexisting condition restraints. Furthermore, private health insurers in the United States cannot discriminate against unfavorable risks in group contracts, and they have to renew contracts with small employers (two to fifty employees) who seek coverage. Some states have more restrictive regulation. All these measures in the United States, however, had only very limited effects on coverage. And some insurance companies have left the small group market altogether (Jost 2001).

Government-imposed measures—such as mandatory open enrollment, prohibition of preexisting condition limitations, and prohibiting or limiting of extra-premiums—face the problem of adverse selection and free-rider behavior. If insurers are under obligation to accept everybody who applies for contracts, applicants could decide not to join the insurance before they think they will need it. Good risks could seek very low coverage first and switch to more comprehensive coverage when they fall ill. This can lead to a chain reaction of more and more good risks not seeking comprehensive insurance and may finally result in a breakdown of the health insurance market (Akerlof 1970; Rothschild and Stiglitz 1976).[14]

To avoid problems of adverse selection, the Dutch WTZ scheme offered a standardized benefits package (Standard Package Policy) to certain high-risk groups. In order to reduce adverse selection even further, people were only entitled to enter the system if they applied for the Standard Package Policy within one year after leaving the public system. In Ireland, similar regulation minimizes adverse selection by requiring waiting periods for all benefits as well as special waiting periods for benefits with respect to a medical condition existing before enrolling; the same applies to switching from schemes with a low level of benefits to those with a higher benefit level. In Germany's private long-term care insurance the following measures are confined to a minimum benefit package as well: mandatory open enrollment; renunciation of nonstandard, preexisting condition limitations; and limiting of extra premiums. To avoid adverse selection, the minimum benefit package for long-term care is compulsory for almost everybody not insured in the public scheme.

Assuring access to PHI for unfavorable risks by regulating the private market does not only produce problems of adverse selection. It might also create incentives for risk selection (cream skimming) by competing health insurers. If insurers have to accept everyone seeking insurance at the same rate, they cannot exclude unfavorable risks or charge an extra premium reflecting unfavorable health status. Insurers thus benefit (or lose) because of the unequal distribution of risk. Germany's private long-term care insurance regulation (like the Irish private health insurance) includes a risk-adjustment scheme. Risk-adjustment schemes aim to compensate insurers with a higher share of high-risk insured in their portfolio. In a way, this reduces incentives for efficiency. The more insurers can pool actual expenditures, the less they have a stake in cost containment. Paradoxically, the Dutch public sick funds were facing more risk than the private insurers as the latter received financial compensation for their high-risk insured. The sick funds thus had more incentives to improve efficiency than private health insurers. The use of risk-adjustment methods has evoked extensive debate. More intelligent schemes of risk adjustment using risk adjusters such as diagnostic and cost information are possible but very costly and difficult to implement and to administer. Some health economists argue that such risk adjustment is the most effective way to combine competition, increase incentives for efficiency, and reduce incentives for cream skimming (Van de Ven and Ellis 2000). In some PHI markets they are established already—for instance in the U.S. Medicare Managed Care Market, where participating HMOs receive risk-adjusted capitation payments (Health Care Financing Administration 1999). Still, such regulation has not improved access to health insurance.

ASSURING LIFETIME COVERAGE IN PHI AND AFFORDABLE PREMIUMS FOR AGING INSURED

On average, health status declines with rising age. Unregulated health insurance markets might not guarantee lifetime insurance coverage because insurers would profit from dropping their elderly insured or charge unaffordable premiums. The fate of individual and small group PHI in the United States illustrates that rising premiums, when risk has worsened in current contracts, are likely if market power on the demand side is small (Jost 2001).

This result might be unacceptable. Some European countries have regulations to safeguard contract renewal for alternative PHI. In other countries, the regulation applies to supplementary PHI as well.

To address the problem of cost escalation due to aging, several countries allow privately insured elderly access to public health cover programs or have designed public health coverage especially for the aged (United States).[15] However, this solution may produce unwanted distributional effects. Public programs that work on a pay-as-you-go basis are financed implicitly according to the principle of intergenerational solidarity. At any point of time, working adults subsidize health care for the old. If privately insured aged persons were allowed to (re)enter a public program, the result would be unfair in terms of intergenerational solidarity—especially when one part of the young population is privately insured while the other is enrolled in public programs. Privately insured young persons would not contribute to intergenerational solidarity within the public system but would profit from this solidarity when old.[16]

Another way to safeguard access to health insurance for the elderly people is regulation that assures *lifetime coverage within PHI.* At a minimum, it could prohibit insurers from canceling insurance contracts. Unfortunately, this regulation by itself would not prevent premiums from becoming unaffordable for the old insured. On average, as noted, health care costs percapita rise with age. Risk-related premium calculation can ultimately lead to risk-equivalent premiums for each age cohort. For the elderly insured this would normally mean that premiums increase as income decreases in retirement. Although one might argue that the rational insured should be aware of this development and voluntarily accumulate savings before retirement to pay for higher premiums after retirement, reliance on individual voluntary solutions clearly creates a problem.

Instead of relying on voluntary initiative by the individuals, government basically can intervene with two instruments. First, it can impose some kind of *intergenerational solidarity* to make sure that privately insured young people contribute to the higher costs of privately insured elderly persons. Ireland, for instance, has opted for intergenerational solidarity by regulating premium calculation. Insurers have to charge premiums based on community rating, regardless of the age of the insured. Since the distribution of old people may vary between the insurers, the Irish government has had to make a provision for risk equalization. Similarly, until 2006, the Netherlands had cross-subsidies within private insurance. High-risk groups who were not eligible for social health insurance could opt for the Standard Package Policy previously mentioned—and a large majority of retirees did so. Since the government-set premiums did not cover costs, all other private insured paid a surcharge to cover the deficit of the Standard Package Policy.[17]

As a second instrument, regulation compels private health insurers to apply elements of annuity calculation of life insurance (capital-funded PHI). In this model the premiums paid by young cohorts will be saved and used when they have grown old (*intrapersonal, intertemporal reallocation*). This approach means redistribution between young and old insured is avoided, and the functioning of insurance is relatively independent of the ratio of old to young insured. It has been used in Germany's regulation of PHI calculation since the 1950s. However, health care inflation as well as increases in life expectancy resulted in a savings shortfall of the annuities. This led to premiums rising sharply for the elderly (Wasem 1996). Therefore, legislation in 2000 added obligatory elements of intergenerational solidarity to PHI calculation.[18] If insurers were given leeway on how to handle these mechanisms, their rules might well become difficult to understand for the consumer. If so, detailed regulation would be necessary so that potential subscribers could have a basis for a rational insurance decision.

ASSURING COST-EFFECTIVE HEALTH CARE FOR PRIVATELY INSURED

Private health insurance in competitive markets, it is widely assumed, not only should keep administrative costs low, but also control the costs of its insured. Otherwise, ceteris paribus, private insurers would risk losing market shares to more cost-conscious competitors. In reality, however, the cost-consciousness of private health insurers depends on several variables. First, the incentive to control costs will fall if they have a higher share of insured who in fact cannot switch to another insurer because of age or health status. For example, competitive pressure for German insurers in alternative PHI is quite low, since elderly insured cannot transfer the savings component of the premium they paid at an earlier age. Due to the high age-related premium for new contracts, it is doubly unattractive to switch. Cost-consciousness will also be limited if insurers pool expenditures via risk-adjustment schemes that do not accurately reflect costs. This situation turned out to be one of the problems both the Dutch Standard Policy Scheme and the German Private Long-Term Care Insurance faced.

Private health insurers are not only expected to "manage costs," they also are expected to realize value for money. Most insured attach great importance to the quality of health care services. From an economic point of view, costs and quality of health care services depend to a large extent on the incentives health care providers face. However, traditionally, private health insurers did not try to influence incentives on the supply side, such as remuneration systems for physicians. Policy makers considered free choice of providers a guarantee for high quality. To influence costs (reduce consumption), private health insurers used instruments at the demand side of health care. Insurance contracts included mechanisms such as co-payments and deductibles to increase cost consciousness of consumers. These mechanisms in turn are supposed to put indirect pressure on the behavior of providers.

Instead of trying to actively influence the supply of health care delivery, private health insurers in Europe primarily rely on government intervention. This reliance reflects the fact that governments in those countries regulate the structure of health care supply in both public and private schemes. In many cases, the market power of private health insurers is too small to play an active role in influencing health care provision.

Consequently, a regulatory framework of health care supply is normally required to effectively control costs of PHI. Key components of such a framework are payment modes for providers treating privately insured. Providers may be required to charge the same amount to public and private insured (as in the Netherlands until 2006) or may be allowed to charge higher amounts to PHI patients, within certain limits (Germany).

Policy makers (in most of Europe and in Canada) are first of all interested in the viability of public schemes. Thus, they want to contain the growth rates of these systems. Cost containment of private expenditure is of secondary importance. Therefore, we often see that attempts to contain costs in the public sector encourage cost shifting toward the private sector (both PHI and out-of-pocket spending). Health care providers commonly compensate for global budgets, spending cuts, and other cost controls in the public sector by raising volume or price for their services in the private sector.[19] Governments sometimes shift costs to private schemes by allowing higher fees to compensate providers for cost-containment measures in the public sector.[20]

In contrast to most of Europe, private health insurers in the United States have increasingly influenced the structure of health care supply. Most of them adapted some kind of "managed care" and fee negotiations with providers. Thus, they have contractual relations not only with their insured but with health care providers as well. Managed care has become a common feature of competing private health insurers in the United States. This development led to some success in cost containment. However, it is still unclear to some whether this success was based on a one-time gain at times of competition for market share or whether managed care strategies truly introduced cost discipline into the market. (See Chapter 2 for a fuller treatment of this issue.)

How successful can PHI be, as far as cost containment and cost-effective delivery of care are concerned? For many health economists, a competitive pluralistic health insurance system with a significant share of PHI offering a variety of managed care plans is the key requirement for more value for money in health care. For others, the very fact that health care expenditures in the United States correlate with a high share of PHI proves that less fragmentation, less competition, and more public regulation are needed (Reinhardt 1999; Rice 1998). Empirical evidence is scarce, although it is quite clear that PHI has higher administrative costs than public schemes due to high costs for marketing and underwriting.

Conclusions

Private health insurance and public arrangements follow different principles. Public schemes such as social health insurance are explicitly designed to fulfill political goals, such as financing according to ability to pay and access to health care according to need. Economic incentives to improve efficiency of health care are not inherent parts of these schemes, although some countries have tried some kind of regulated competition between public carriers of insurance (Greß 2004). In contrast, private health insurers act in competitive markets and react to market forces. The outcome of this process is not necessarily socially acceptable. Private health insurance markets thus can be (and in fact often are) regulated in order to produce more socially acceptable results. Self-regulation of private health insurers is not likely to work properly. Intervention by the legislature, we argue, will be needed.

The extent and form of regulation varies. It depends on the specific function PHI performs in health care systems. Regulation seems to follow a progression—beginning with restraints on pre-existing conditions exclusion clauses and minimal coverage mandates through community rating requirements, to other bans on risk underwriting and ending up with mandated risk pooling. We have shown that there are different forms of regulation to assure access to PHI for unfavorable risks and to keep PHI affordable for the sick and the old. Public regulation can prevent health care costs for the privately insured from growing faster than costs in the public sector—although policy makers might prefer to compensate health care providers for cost containment in the public sector by allowing growing costs in the private sector. However, the assumed benefits of private health insurance—its flexibility, potential for innovation, and consumer autonomy—are crippled as government increasingly dictates the terms of insurance contracts. To their already considerable administrative costs, private health insurers now must add regulatory compliance costs. This inevitably leads to the question: Where is the added value that justifies the added costs of private health insurance (Jost 2001)?

Regulating private insurers in order to decrease competitive forces while at the same time increasing regulation in the public sector may, in fact, lead to convergence of both systems. The introduction of universal ("privatized") social health insurance in the Netherlands in 2006 is an example of this trend. In Germany, the discussion on convergence of the two systems has been ongoing for a decade or more (Wasem 1995). In the long run, this route might be the way to go for other countries, too.

Notes

The authors gratefully acknowledge comments to an earlier version of this paper by Stefan Gildemeister.

1. Of course we are aware of methodological problems of comparing such parameters across countries. Thus, these figures are only rough indicators of the importance of private health insurance in individual countries

2. Unfortunately, politicians responsible for health policy are not always responsible for PHI regulation as well. For instance, in Germany the Ministry of Finance and the Ministry of Justice are responsible for private insurance regulation, including private *health* insurance. In most states of the United States, technically there are three types of regulatory entities: elected insurance commissioners, appointed insurance commissioners, and "other," including Departments of Commerce.

3. The degree of innovation amongst insurers differs very much across countries. In the United States, there is hardly any insurance company that does not employ some kind of managed care strategy, but in Germany there is hardly any company that does.

4. Thus far, international developments have not affected PHI regulation much. However, in Europe, E.U. regulation is of increasing importance. The third E.U. directive on Non-Life Insurance (that applies to the banking and private insurance sector) has forced several member states to adjust their regulatory framework for PHI.

5. Some U.S. analysts consider public arrangements the exception rather than the rule. However, for reasons of analytical clarity, we ignore this point of view.

6. Public coverage in E.U. member countries has decreased as countries delisted entitlements from social insurance coverage. The European Commission has commissioned a study on that topic to assess possible consequences for European regulation of supplementary PHI (Rocard 2000). The French government introduced a public scheme to increase coverage of supplementary PHI with tax subsidy for low-income people at the beginning of 2000.

7. There is evidence that this is the case in Switzerland (Colombo 2001).

8. Only 6.5 percent of individuals under the age of sixty-five in the United States rely on individual coverage as their primary means of health insurance (Buntin, Marquis, and Yegian 2004).

9. Every resident in the Netherlands is insured in the obligatory public AWBZ scheme for coverage of catastrophic risks and long-term care.

10. It is not yet clear whether the new insurance scheme is, in fact, public or private (see Chapter 5).

11. Civil servants are entitled to subsidies by their employer.

12. In the Netherlands and Germany, interests of traditional insurers and those founded less than 20 years ago—who do not insure many elderly—diverge significantly. That divergence also makes effective voluntary regulation to prevent risk selection hard if not impossible.

13. The Irish example demonstrates that voluntary regulation of discrimination against unfavorable risks is possible—if there is a monopoly on the supply side of the insurance market. In Germany, all private health insurers voluntarily agreed to limit discrimination against unfavorable risks among young civil servants. Basically they fear provoking political discussion on the insurance scheme for civil servants, which might also lead to reforms unfavorable for insurance companies. The German private insurers do not agree on more controversial issues. The Association of Private Health Insurers sometimes seeks legal support to obtain regulation that it considers necessary in terms of social acceptability of PHI, but which it cannot achieve through self-regulation.

14. Research of public high-risk insurance schemes in the United States found that some insured "gamble that they could get by without purchasing health insurance until they became ill" as well (Zellner et al. 1993, 173–74). However, due to the separation of public high-risk schemes from PHI markets, this adverse selection did not affect the functioning of these markets.

15. In the Netherlands, as well as in Germany, privately insured retirees were entitled to join public health insurance until the end of the 1980s.

16. Inequity is the main reason that reentry to the public systems has been abolished in both Germany and the Netherlands.

17. In Germany, too, all private health insurers have to offer a Standard Policy to privately insured persons older than sixty-five years with ten years of pre-insurance in alternative PHI and for insured older than fifty-five with private pre-insurance and income below the income ceiling. The benefit level is comparable to that of the sickness funds, and the premium may not exceed the maximum premium of the public schemes. In case of a deficit, those having PHI in regular schemes have to contribute. The demand for the Standard Package Policy, however, is quite low (3,000 contracts in the year 2000), since maximum premiums are quite substantial.

18. According to this legislation, insurers have to use part of the annuity savings of young insured to subsidize the premiums of the elderly. Furthermore, since 2000, private health insurers have to add a flat 10 percent on individual premiums for new contracts to compensate for increasing health care expenditures.

19. This form of cost shifting has become less common in the United States as managed care organizations have imposed tighter controls over contracts and utilization. Where providers used cost shifting in order to support care for the uninsured, they now find themselves less able to do so. In Germany, physicians in ambulatory care are paid fee-for-service for patients with PHI. They have reacted to global budgets in the public sector by increasing the volume of service for the privately insured..

20. Since persons with PHI usually have higher incomes than those insured in public schemes, informal cross-subsidies from the private to the public sector might be justified in terms of socially desirable redistribution. However, formal direct transfers are more transparent.

References

Achman, L., and D. Chollet. 2001. *High risk pools of limited help to the uninsurable.* New York: Commonwealth Fund.

Akerlof, G. A. 1970. The market for "lemons": Quality uncertainty and the market mechanism. *Quarterly Journal of Economics* 84: 488–500.

Arrow, K. J. 1963. Uncertainty and the welfare economics of medical care. *American Economic Review* 53: 941–73.

Blendon, R. J. 1990. Satisfaction with health systems in ten nations. *Health Affairs* 9 (2): 185–92.

Brouwer, W., and H. Hermans. 1999. Private clinics for employees as a Dutch solution for waiting lists: Economic and legal arguments. *Health Policy* 47 (1): 1–17.

Buntin, M. B., M. S. Marquis, and J. M. Yegian. 2004. The role of the individual health insurance market and prospects for change. *Health Affairs* 23 (6): 79–90.

Colombo, F. 2001. *Towards more choice in social protection? Individual choice of insurer in basic mandatory health insurance in Switzerland.* Labour Market and Social Policy Occasional Papers, No. 53. Paris: OECD.

Colombo, F., and N. Tapay. 2004. *Private health insurance in OECD countries: The benefits and costs for individuals and health systems.* Health Working Paper, No. 15. Paris: OECD.

den Exter, A. 2005. Blending private and social health insurance in the Netherlands: Challenges posed by the EU. In *Access to care, access to justice: The legal debate over private health insurance in Canada,* ed. C. Flood, L. Sossin and K. Roach. Toronto: University of Toronto Press.

Enthoven, A. 1994. On the ideal market structure for third-party purchasing of health care. *Social Science and Medicine* 39: 1413–24.

Flood, C., L. Sossin, and K. Roach, eds. 2005. *Access to care, access to justice: The legal debate over private health insurance in Canada.* Toronto: University of Toronto Press.

Greß, S. 2004. *Competition in social health insurance: A three-country comparison.* Diskussionsbeitrag Nr. 135, Fachbereich Wirtschaftswissenschaften der Universität Duisburg-Essen, Campus Essen, DE.

Health Care Financing Administration. 1999. Proposed method of incorporating health status risk adjusters into Medicare+Choice Payments. Prepared by the Health Care Financing Administration, Office of Strategic Planning, Research and Evaluation Group, Division of Payment Research. Washington: Health Care Financing Administration.

Henke, K. 1999. Socially bounded competition in Germany. *Health Affairs* 18 (4): 203–06.

Jost, T. S. 2001. Private or public approaches to insuring the uninsured: Lessons from international experience with private insurance. *New York University Law Review* 76 (2): 419–93.

Okma, K. G. H. 1997. *Studies on Dutch health politics, policies and law.* PhD diss., University of Utrecht, NL.

Reinhardt, U. 1999. The predictable managed care kvetch on the rocky road from adolescence to adulthood. *Journal of Health Politics, Policy and Law* 24 (5): 897–910.

Rice, T. 1998. *The economics of health reconsidered.* Chicago: Health Administration Press.

Rocard, M. 2000. *Report on supplementary health insurance (A5–0266/2000).* Brussels: European Parliament.

Rothschild, M., and J. E. Stiglitz. 1976. Equilibrium in competitive insurance markets: An essay on the economics of imperfect information. *Quarterly Journal of Economics* 90: 629–49.

Schoen, C., K. Davis, C. DesRoches, K. Donelan, and R. J. Blendon. 2000. Health insurance markets and income inequality: Findings from an international health policy survey. *Health Policy* 51: 67–85.

Schut, F. T. 1995. *Competition in the Dutch health care sector.* Ridderkerk, NL: Ridderprint.

Shmueli, A. 2001. The effect of health on acute care supplemental insurance ownership: An empirical analysis. *Health Economics* 10: 341–50.

Turquet, P. 2004. A stronger role for the private sector in France's health insurance? *International Social Security Review* 57 (4): 67–90.

U.S. Census Bureau. 2001. *Health Insurance Coverage 2000: Current Population Reports.* Washington DC: U.S. Census Bureau.

Van de Ven, W. P. M. M., and R. P. Ellis. 2000. Risk adjustment in competitive health plan markets. In *Handbook of health economics,* A. J. Culyer and J. P. Newhouse, eds. Amsterdam: Elsevier.

Verband der privaten Krankenversicherung e. V. 2000. *Private health insurance: Facts and figures 1999/2000.* Cologne: Association of private health insurance companies.

Wasem, J. 1995. Gesetzliche und private Krankenversicherung—auf dem Weg zur Konvergenz? [Public and Private Health Insurance – on their way to convergence] *Sozialer Fortschritt* 4: 89–96.

Wasem, J. 1996. Private Krankenversicherung und ältere Versicherte. In *Alter und Gesundheit,* [Private Health Insurance and Aged Insured. In: Age and Health] ed. P. Oberender. Baden-Baden: Nomos.

Wasem, J., S. Greß, and K. G. H. Okma. 2004. The role of private health insurance in social health insurance countries. In *Social health insurance in Western Europe,* ed. R. Saltman, R. Busse, and J. Figueras. London: Open University Press.

Zellner, B. B., D. Haugen, and B. Dowd. 1993. A study of Minnesota's high risk health insurance pool. *Inquiry* 30 (Summer):170-9.

12

Learning from Others and Learning from Mistakes
Reflections on Health Policy Making

RUDOLF KLEIN

Learning about other countries is rather like breathing: Only the brain-dead are likely to avoid the experience. None of us can escape the bombardment of information about what is happening in other countries. The process of learning takes many forms. There is the kind of face-to-face exchange of experience that characterizes conferences and similar meetings. There is the systematic diffusion of information by the Organisation for Economic Co-operation and Development (OECD) and other international organizations. There is the annual pilgrimage of academics from conference to conference. There are the formal contacts between politicians and civil servants within the framework of the European Union and informal contacts in other settings. At least as far as the countries represented in this study are concerned, there is a series of overlapping health care policy networks. No one belongs to all of them, but almost everyone in the health care policy business belongs to at least some of them. There is even a common language: English. Learning about other countries must, of course, be sharply distinguished from learning from their experience. The former activity is about collecting information; the latter is about reflecting on that information. Still, even allowing for this distinction, lesson drawing is an expanding industry.

And yet, despite the availability of so much information about what other countries are doing and the speed of its diffusion, we worry about our capacity to learn from the experience of others and search for ways of improving our ability to do so. Rather like health care itself, supply creates its own demand: The appetite for learning seems to grow as the menu of information expands. In what follows, this essay will reflect on this paradox. It is not intended to be, in any way, a systematic analysis of policy learning but instead seeks to identify some of the issues and questions that may—implicitly or explicitly—come up during the course of an international exchange.

Why Do We Want to Learn?

There is something extremely seductive about the notion of policy learning.[1] Given the limited scope for policy experiment in any one country (and the considerable costs, political as well as economic, often involved), what could be more sensible than to draw on the experience of other nations. From this perspective, other countries are to policy makers what laboratories are to scientists: places where policy theories or techniques are tested out. Depending on the success or failure of the experiment, the theories or techniques can then be tried out in one's own country. So, at least, runs the naive version of policy learning. But, of course, the metaphor of scientific experiments is misleading. In the health care policy field, no two laboratories are the same. No two experiments can therefore be replicated with anything even remotely approaching exactitude. The simplistic utopian model of policy learning therefore leads to a nihilistic conclusion: If health care policy making is indeed contingent on its institutional, political, and social context—that is, the national laboratory—then teaming, seen as the transfer of ideas and techniques, would seem to be a recipe for disaster. If a particular technique of cost control is contingent on the cooperation of the medical profession in a corporatist system (as in Germany), there is no point in exporting it to a country (like the United States) that totally lacks such a system.

As this last example suggests, policy learning—if it is to be successful—is at least as much about the analysis of the *circumstances* in which particular innovations succeed (or fail) as about the innovations themselves. To argue that health care policy making is contingent on the national context is therefore not to conclude that the transfer of experience is impossible but that an understanding of that context is a necessary condition for drawing any transnational conclusions about the exportability (or otherwise) of any lessons learned. Before transplanting any policies, we have to make sure that there is institutional compatibility between donor and recipient. So, for instance, the ability to implement policy changes depends on political institutions such as electoral systems: It will be much higher in countries such as

Britain where the executive commands an automatic majority in the legislature than in countries such as the Netherlands where coalition politics greatly complicate the task of implementation. Again, policy notions deeply embedded in a century-old culture of social solidarity (as in Germany) will not be easily transferrable to countries (such as the United States) lacking such a tradition.

All these points would suggest that an analysis of the environment of health policy—by which I mean taking account not just of political institutions but civic traditions, tax systems, and administrative resources—must have priority over the analysis of specific health care policy issues in any teaming process. The test of any model of health care is its appropriateness to a particular setting; consequently, the challenge to improving our capacity to learn from the experience of other countries is to deepen our understanding of the respects in which they differ or are similar. The point would seem obvious enough, but for the fact that there are a variety of institutions such as the World Bank that seem to be in the business of huckstering all-purpose models (usually designed by economists) supposedly applicable to all countries. Real learning, I would argue, is about *distinguishing:* about knowing when a particular model is relevant or irrelevant to the specific circumstances of a country.

Policy learning, I would further suggest, is as much a process of self-examination—of reflecting on the characteristics of one's own country and health care system—as of looking at the experience of others. Indeed the experience of other countries is largely valuable insofar as it prompts such a process of critical introspection by enlarging our sense of what is possible and adding to our repertory of possible policy tools. For policy learning in practice is not about the *transfer* of ideas or techniques—in this respect the transplantation metaphor is misleading—but about their *adaptation* to local circumstances. The experience of other countries stimulates the policy imagination and nudges policy makers in particular directions. But the process of naturalizing foreign experience tends also to translate it into forms that are suitable for the national environment. The case of competition in health care illustrates the point well. The meaning given to this notion (inherently many-layered) has been very different in the various countries that have seemingly embraced it: If the vocabulary is international, the way in which it is translated into policy remains national. So, for example, the health care system that emerged in the United Kingdom under the flag of the internal market is very different from that contemplated in the Netherlands. Similarly, many European countries have flirted with the idea of importing diagnosis-related groups (DRGs) as a policy tool from the United States, but they have done so in very different ways and with different purposes in mind, depending on local circumstances (Kimberly and Pouvourville 1993). Translation often means transformation.

Above all, cross-national learning is not pursued for its own sake. First, it presupposes a coincidence of concerns in the exporting and importing countries. Interest in the experience of other countries is a function of discontent or anxiety about conditions in one's own country. Second, cross-national curiosity is not a neutral intellectual exercise. Receptivity to foreign ideas is a function of the extent to which they reinforce or fit in with existing policy predilections and prejudices. The experience of other countries may be used in domestic policy debate to inspire either emulation or repudiation. As Marmor and Plowden have argued, "ideas are elements in policy warfare whose take-up is determined not by their intrinsic validity but by the local setting—its present moods and circumstances, and structures" (Marmor and Plowden 1991). Thus in Britain the experience of the United States is often invoked in political debate to elicit a knee-jerk repudiation of anything that looks remotely like a market, while conversely in the United States the experience of Britain's NHS is invoked to provoke horror at the very idea of "socialized medicine" (Klein 1991).

For learning from other countries is not just about adopting or adapting new ideas. Negative learning—avoiding the mistakes of others—may be just as important as positive learning. But in either instance, the experience of other countries serves—as Marmor and Plowden suggest—to provide ammunition for domestic conflicts. They are battles to impose a particular view of the world in a universe of multiple versions of the truth. Some policies or techniques are unambiguous failures or successes. But in most cases there are complex balance sheets, and success or failure may be contingent on particular local conditions. Not surprisingly, therefore, selective perception and disputes about the interpretation of evidence characterize cross-national comparisons. Even if we are driven by shared problems and anxieties to examine the experience of other countries, what we find will be viewed through the prism of national values and presented in the rhetoric of politics.

Learning about What from Whom?

So far this essay has used the notion of cross-national teaming in an undifferentiated and rather promiscuous way. Now the time has come to unpackage it and to define the specific characteristics of what is being learned more precisely. For, as I will argue in this section, the various dimensions of cross-national learning may differ in important respects. In particular, the teaming circuits—the networks of people involved in the process of acquiring and interpreting information about what is happening in other countries—will differ, as will the audiences involved. Deciding *whom* to learn from may also decide *what* we learn.

The most comprehensive form of cross-national learning is when we compare systems of health care provision—that is, the way in which they are financed and organized—in the search for that elusive formula that will allow us to reconcile cost containment, efficiency, equity, and effectiveness. However, much of policy learning is more limited in its ambition and more narrowly focused on specific problems or programs. So, for example, the onset of AIDS in Britain sent politicians and civil servants scurrying to the United States to discover what could be learned from American experience. Similarly, the Oregon approach to limiting the menu of health care attracted a long procession of international tourists. Again, there may be much interest in comparing experience about the impact of introducing charges for services on patterns of use. In all these instances, the focus of attention is on policy issues. But much of cross-national learning may be about organizational processes or managerial techniques: The introduction and international marketing of DRGs provide one obvious example. Lastly, there is the continual frenzy of cross-national learning that characterizes the delivery of medical care itself: the rapid transfer of new technology (in its widest sense) from country to country. Finally, it must be stressed that policy teaming is as much about the past as about the present. That is, although it is easy to get excited about policy innovation, and to focus on what is new, some of the most policy-relevant questions can only be answered by looking at the experience of different countries over decades.

There are, therefore, different worlds of cross-national learning within the health care arena. And one of the explanations for the paradox noted at the start of this essay—that the appetite for the exchange of information grows as the supply increases—may well be that there is too little contact between these worlds. The introduction of new management tools has clear implications for public policy: Should DRGs, for example, be used simply in order to prompt critical self-examination by managers and clinicians or as a reimbursement mechanism? The transfer of medical technology, similarly, has very obvious implications for health care budgets—but the policy makers who will pick up the bill (or seek ways of restraining its growth) are not involved in the process of cross-national learning. So it may well be that *controlling* cross-national learning—constraining the adoption of imported ideas—is at least as important as promoting free trade in information. Perhaps we should be putting more emphasis on studying the way in which different countries test and make use of imported ideas and techniques to see what we can learn from their successes (or failures) in preventing the adoption of half-baked or untried notions or technologies—a point discussed further in the next, and final, section of this essay.

If we accept that cross-national learning is rather like a multi-ring circus with different actors performing in each of them—then some other implications may follow as well. In particular, it may be that the problems of such learning—the evaluation of what is happening in another country—are compounded by the fact that different actors use different languages and have different perspectives. Practical policy makers—by which I mean both civil servants and politicians—do not, for example, have the same agenda as academics. Neither do they necessarily draw on the same kind of knowledge (Lindblom and Cohen 1979). They may both operate in the field of health policy, but their concerns and questions will be rather different. Civil servants may perhaps be more concerned with questions of feasibility and implementability than academics. Just as among academics, political scientists will pay more attention to this dimension of policy making than economists. There may well also be differences in their views about who counts as authoritative interpreters of reality. Just as academics will naturally look to their peers, so will civil servants. And, of course, both policy makers and academics will differ—in turn—from medical practitioners and managers.

The papers collected in this volume are, in effect, a declaration of faith in the possibility of a common language between people from different countries bringing different perspectives to bear. I would go one step further and argue that the testing of ideas depends precisely on having a confrontation of perspectives: occupational and disciplinary as well as national. However, it may be helpful to acknowledge and to identify explicitly what the differences are between the various groups, rather than attempting to reduce them to a bland Esperanto. Precisely because learning from other countries is such a value-laden exercise, precisely because there are so many different reasons for wanting to look at the experience of other countries, it is important to know who wants to know what and why rather than assuming that a common interest in comparisons necessarily involves a commonality of purpose or a shared assumptive world.

How Do We Know When to Learn?

There is another factor in cross-national learning that has so far not been considered: the time dimension. During what stage in the policy cycle and at what point in the life history of a program or technical innovation should we start getting interested and seeking out any lessons? The obvious temptation is to rush in as quickly as possible. Policy making (and even more so, the academic study of policy making) has a lot in common with the fashion industry. No one likes to be caught wearing yesterday's ideas.

The adoption of new policy models, new programs, or new techniques commands attention and generates intellectual excitement. The searchlight of academic inquiry—and the consequent flow of information to the policy community—therefore tends to focus disproportionately on what is new. And, to an extent, this focus is only right. If one of the most important roles of policy learning is—as argued earlier—to stir up our own ideas and to stretch our imagination, then the shock of the new provides an appropriate stimulus.

But there is also a case for arguing that policy learning should only take place when the new models, programs, and techniques have been tested and evaluated over time in their country of origin. What, after all, is the point of rushing in to study a new experiment—far less to adopt a new model— before there is any evidence about its outcome? If no policy is better than its implementability, then why not wait to see how it works out in practice? After all, the durability of an institutional innovation or program may be one of the most important tests of its desirability; there seems little point in rushing in to adopt something that may ultimately be abandoned by the originating country. And if we accept this line of argument, the real beneficiaries of cross-national teaming will be those countries who come last in the queue of would-be adaptors.

There is a further twist to this argument. A cautious approach to the import of foreign models might even suggest waiting until several countries have tried out a particular policy or program model in order to test its robustness and its sensitivity to different institutional environments. A careful analysis of the life cycles of policy experiments in a variety of countries might help to identify the common elements that characterize the most successful models. In other words, the most valuable form of cross-national policy learning may be the study of the patterns of success and failure over time, not in any single country but in a whole population of countries: the intellectual model being not the laboratory experiment but historical epidemiology.

It is an argument that, on balance, I find convincing. It cannot be swallowed whole, however. It applies much more strongly to policy learning about health care systems as a whole than to policy learning about the design of programs to handle crises. If policy makers are in a situation where they must take immediate action, as they were in the case of AIDS, then it is futile to argue that learning should be delayed until there has been an opportunity to study evaluation reports on what has been done in a range of other countries. There is, in any case, a problem about the notion that cross-national learning should be filtered through evaluation studies. One of the characteristics of many programs is that they change over their life cycle, that is, there is a constant process of adjustment in the light of experience. The same is even more true of the introduction of new models for the organization or financing of health care systems. So, for example, Britain's National Health Service has become an institution that is constantly reinventing itself: It is a car that is being reengineered even while it is roaring round the test track. Evaluating what happened in the past might thus be a poor guide to the model's likely future performance.

But the example of the NHS suggests that there may be another dimension to cross-national learning. So far in this essay the emphasis has been on learning about the substance of new models, programs, or techniques, and asking the question: Are they successful (whatever that may mean) or not? But there is another question, which is about the process of introducing change.

Random Uncontrolled Trials and Fluffy Balls of Wool

Most policy making in the field of health care is only rarely about designing new blueprints based on first principles. The very fact that the countries represented in this volume (even the United States) have developed complex health care systems means that the scope for policy maneuver and the available options for change are constrained by the institutions and the interests that were created by the process of developing those systems. Rather, policy making is all about dealing with discomfort and reducing dissonance. It represents an exercise in narrowing the gap between the actual and the desirable, in reducing the tension produced by conflicting signals, and in taking action to minimize prospective risks within the constraints of the historic legacy.

It follows from this view that models of the policy process that assume policy makers start off with a set of clearly articulated values or goals to guide their steps, and that the choice of possible policy options and instruments is made only after a rigorous analysis of the evidence, are actively misleading. And it is misleading not only as a description of what actually happens in policy making—that is fairly self-evident—but also as a prescription for what ought to happen.

The rational model of policy making in the textbooks (which is what we are talking about) is in fact profoundly irrational, as well as naïve in its assumption that if only we were clear about our values—the objectives we are trying to achieve—and if only we could mobilize enough knowledge-based evidence, we could avoid the disappointments and problems that now afflict the search for better ways of running our health care systems.

In practice, it is impossible to separate values and facts. Policy making—as Sir Geoffrey Vickers pointed out a long time ago in his classic study of decision making (Vickers 1965)—is about dialogue between the two. "Facts are relevant only in relation to some judgment of value," he argued, "and judgments of value are operative only in relation to some configuration of facts." Further, our values may often be in conflict with each other: The real art of policy lies in striking an acceptable balance between competing objectives. Finally, our knowledge will always be inadequate. Policy making is a voyage of discovery with incomplete or inaccurate maps and often faulty compasses: Indeed it is often only the process of exploration that allows us to start constructing accurate maps.

So what? All those engaged in policy making or analysis know that they are engaged in a messy business: that policy making is the art of the possible, not the science of optimizing national well-being. But I think we can draw some positive conclusions from this unexciting—rather platitudinous—observation. A helpful starting point is to look at what health care policy making has in common with the practice of medicine, following a seminal article that Amitai Etzioni published some years ago (Etzioni 1985). Like the process of making a diagnosis and moving on to prescribing remedies, policy making involves an iterative process of trial and error in conditions of uncertainty. In the case of medicine, it has been argued that there is no scientific evidence about the effectiveness (or otherwise) of something like 80 percent of medical interventions. And even where there is such evidence, there may still be a large area of uncertainty about what works in the case of individual patients, particularly in the case of those presenting complex problems with multiple symptoms.

Let us apply this model to health care policy making. No one has tried to estimate what proportion of policy instruments can be "scientifically" demonstrated to be effective. We have no randomized controlled trials (RCTs). All we have are international comparisons that are, in effect, randomized uncontrolled trials (RUTs), and therefore do not allow for contingent circumstances (in this case, the specific context of national institutions and cultures). These RUTs may be highly suggestive: They may indicate, for example, that single-payer systems are more likely to control costs successfully than multiple-payer systems. But overall, I suspect that the knowledge base of health policy making is even narrower—and more precarious—than that of medicine. Often we have solutions in search of problems. Consider, for example, the case of decentralization. What problem is this supposed to address? Is it an answer to the problems of governments in hard times, who having centralized credit when budgets were expanding, now want to diffuse blame for unpopular decisions that may flow from budget cuts? Or is it supposed to be the answer to problems of bureaucratic rigidity and a consequent lack of responsiveness to consumer preferences?

One reaction to such skepticism is, of course, to argue for expanding the knowledge base of policy making: to systematically test policy instruments. And who can be against that? But a word of warning: The policy cycle is not the same as the research cycle. By the time that research delivers its verdict, the policy agenda is apt to have changed. So, too, may the context of decision making. More important still, policy instruments tend to be contingent on specific, local circumstances—hence, of course, the difficulty of testing policy instruments experimentally or using the experience of other countries. If competition works in California (as it appears to do), does it follow that it will work in the Netherlands or Germany or Canada? Here the important thing may be to use local experience to clearly define the conditions necessary for either failure or success.

So what of "fluffy balls of wool"? It was John Maynard Keynes who observed that ideas were apt to be like fluffy balls of wool (Cairncross 1996). They tend to be clearly articulated and defined only in the process of arguing about them and applying them. So one danger—all the greater because of the acceleration in the rate at which ideas are now transmitted across the globe—is that ideas may pass into common currency while still at the fluffy-ball-of-wool stage: before they have been properly unpicked. One such example might be "managed care": a concept whose persuasive power depends crucially on the fact that it is so fluffy that everyone can read into it what he or she wants.

So we come back to the central problem of policy making in the health care field: How do we devise better policies for resource distribution, for promoting consumer choice (or whatever) in conditions of uncertainty? One way forward is to compare the way in which different countries address the problem of uncertainty in policy making, that is, to shift the focus of comparison from the specific instruments used or solutions adopted, to the different national strategies for changing systems. Which are the most successful strategies for managing change? Which are best calculated to avoid the pitfalls involved in implementing policies in the absence, usually, of solid evidence about what works best?

Dealing with Uncertainty

A word of warning before I expand on this theme. I realize, of course, that national strategies of change are not, as a rule, the product of explicit decisions. They tend to be a by-product of the institutional arrangements, political configurations, and the constellation of interests in individual countries. The policy process is inevitably constrained by, and reflects, national circumstances. So it would be naïve to think of the various models that I am about to describe as representing free choice by decision makers. Still, always bearing this reservation in mind, I think it is instructive to look at the models of policy process that comparative experience offers. Oversimplifying heroically, I suggest that there are three basic models.

First, there is the "big-bang" model, that is, comprehensively redesigning the system in one go. Here the classic examples are Britain's 1991 health care reforms (although even these did not involve a fundamental redesign of the financial and organizational structure) and President Clinton's abortive attempt to do the same in the United States. Second, there is the model of incremental or evolutionary reform: a cumulative, step-by-step process. Here the best example is perhaps the way in which Germany has tackled health care reform over the years by introducing a series of measures that gradually expanded the realm of the politically acceptable. Third, there is the model of pluralistic reform. Here the best example is Sweden, where different counties have adopted somewhat different approaches to widening consumer choice and introducing elements of competition. Similarly, it might be argued that in the United States, the various reforms introduced by individual states offer an experiment in pluralistic change. And there is some evidence that Canada may move in the same way.

All this may be a touch overneat. Certainly, the experience of some countries suggests that, in practice, the models may be rather mixed. The Netherlands started out with big-bang ambitions, and then fell back on an incremental approach with a final lurch into radical reform. Britain's NHS turned out to be a self-inventing institution, in that the 1991 blueprint was considerably modified during the process of implementation and in the light of experience but subsequently provided the springboard for Labour policies that echoed many of the original Conservative aspirations.

So what are the strengths and weaknesses of these different models of change? What can we learn from the experience of different countries? Let me suggest some tentative conclusions.

First, the incremental and pluralistic models seem to score rather well on coping with uncertainty. Incrementalism can be seen as a way of testing the ground, with each step in the policy process being an experiment, as it were, and allowing scope for policies to be modified in the light of experience. It fits comfortably with the medical model of step-by-step exploration, of moving toward diagnosis and prescription by a process of dialogue. Similarly, the pluralistic model seems to offer opportunities for testing options: for having local experiments that may subsequently be adopted by others.

Second, these two models appear to have the advantage in terms of political feasibility. Whereas the big-bang approach tends to mobilize strong coalitions of opposing interests, the incremental and pluralistic strategies may be able to divide the opposition. And by avoiding all-out confrontation, they may also avoid a legacy of bitterness, so facilitating implementation. In the case of Britain's big-bang reforms, for example, the legacy of bitterness left by the strategy used to introduce them—overriding the objections of the medical profession—was certainly one of the factors that made their subsequent history so stormy.

Third, the big-bang strategy does have the great advantage that, if successful, it actually delivers. In theory, too, it might be expected to have greater coherence than changes introduced piecemeal over time. It may, however, score less well on stability and "stickability," that is, the ability to survive a regime change, since it tends to accentuate divisions rather than creating consensus.

All three models require critical scrutiny. "Incrementalism" is an ambiguous word. It may simply represent a series of compromises and desperate expedients that end in fudges and muddles: a surrender, in effect, to the power of interest groups. Alternatively, incrementalism may mean a step-by-step approach to problem solving, a process of inquiry and discovery designed to achieve specific goals, even though both means and ends may be modified or adapted in light of the knowledge generated by the process itself.

Similarly, while the evolutionary or pluralistic models provide, in theory, opportunities for learning from experience and readjusting policies accordingly, it does not necessarily follow that those opportunities will be taken. How, in practice, do different countries evaluate change? Do they have the appropriate mechanisms for learning from experience, and what are they? Finally, we have to ask how far, if we adopt a pluralist strategy—if we decentralize the ability to experiment—are we prepared to accept differences within any given national system of health care? And again, how effective are the mechanisms for evaluating and disseminating the effects of local experiments?

In this regard, one of the principal benefits of cross-national learning may be to provide more knowledge about how best to cope with a lack of knowledge in health care policy making: how to maximize our ability to learn from, and redress, the mistakes that we inevitably will make. From this perspective we should perhaps be at least as interested in policy failures as in policy successes.

Note

1. The best and most comprehensive review of this topic, to which I am greatly indebted, is provided by Richard Rose, *Lesson-Drawing in Public Policy* (Chatham, NJ: Chatham House, 1993).

References

Cairncross, A. 1996. Keynes the man. *Economist,* April 20, 99–100.
Etzioni, A. 1985. Making policy for complex systems: A medical model for economics. *Journal of Policy Analysis* 4 (3): 383–95.
Kimberly, John R., and Gerard de Pouvourville. 1993. *The migration of managerial innovation: Diagnosis-related groups and health care administration in Western Europe.* San Francisco: Jossey-Bass.
Klein, R. 1991. Risks and benefits of comparative studies. *Milbank Quarterly* 69 (2): 275–91.
Lindblom, C. E., and D. K. Cohen. 1979. *Usable knowledge.* New Haven, CT: Yale University Press.
Marmor, T. R., and W. Plowden. 1991. Rhetoric and reality in the intellectual jet stream: The export to Britain from America of questionable ideas. *Journal of Health Politics, Policy and Law* 16 (4): 807–12.
Vickers, G. 1965. *The art of judgment.* London: Chapman Fr Hall.

Appendix
National Health Accounts: A Tool for International Comparison of Health Spending

MARKUS SCHNEIDER

Since early 1960s, international organizations have promoted the development of national health accounts (NHAs) as a statistical tool for depicting national health expenditure and for international macroeconomic analysis of health systems. NHAs are a systematic description of financial flows related to health. Information derived from NHAs has been used to study the potential determinants of growth of health care, the public-private mix of health financing, and the relation to income growth. Both the methodology and the statistics of the national accounts, developed under the auspices of the United Nations in 1953, with subsequent revisions in 1968 and 1993, have facilitated the formation of standards for international comparisons. In contrast to national accounts, most NHAs do not aim to present a full set of accounts of production, income generation, and expenditures, but to inform about the structure of resources devoted to health care.

The collection of economic information about financial and economic transactions in health systems has made enormous progress since the late 1970s when the Organization for Economic Co-operation and Development (OECD) regularly started to collect data about its member states health systems. The World Bank and the World Health Organization (WHO) stimulated the compilation of NHAs by several international studies as the World Development Report 1993 *Investing in Health* and the World Health Report 2000 *Health Systems: Improving Performance*. The later tried to benchmark the performance of 191 health systems using health expenditures as input variable. National and international organizations including the OECD, EUROSTAT, the

WHO, the World Bank, and the Pan American Health Organization (PAHO) joined efforts to guide national accountants to adhere to internationally developed manuals (OECD 2000; WHO 2003; PAHO 2005). This effort has helped provide better insight into the economic structure of health systems. It has also enriched international health policy discussions with accurate and reliable estimates of economic transactions within health systems. At the same time, however, NHAs still face methodological problems including a lack of consistent and comparable data about financing and providing health care, and the role of NHAs in health policy analysis is still modest.

The presentation of the health expenditure accounts in the five countries of this book starts with a historical flashback, followed by a discussion of conceptual issues. The third section presents the basic pillars of health expenditure accounts: (1) who pays (2) whom (3) for what. The fourth section discusses statistical realization of NHAs. Differences in institutional structures and other reasons have led to divergent health data. In some cases, such conceptual issues combined with national definitions of data offer space for "data gambling" that allow the use of data in a contradicting way. Therefore, the fifth section deals with the main indicators derived from health expenditure accounts. The sixth and seventh sections present health expenditure accounts for the United States, Canada, Germany, the Netherlands, and the United Kingdom. Finally, the eighth section discusses issues in the future development of NHAs.

History

The earliest effort to present internationally comparative data on health care was *The Cost of Medical Care,* published by the International Labor Office in 1959 (Maxwell 1981). The study presents data for fourteen countries spanning the period 1945–1955. In those countries, total costs of medical care per person covered varied little, from around 1.75 to around 2.0 percent of national income at factor cost per person, regardless of the method of providing medical care. The next major initiative to compare health accounts took place under auspices of the World Health Organization (WHO). Professor Brian Abel-Smith (1963, 1967) developed in two studies the first standardized framework for international health expenditure accounting. One main finding was that in the 1950s, all high-income countries, except the United Kingdom, had seen a rise in their health expenditures as a proportion of national income. This rate of increase implied that an additional 1 percent of gross national product (GNP) was likely to be absorbed in health services every ten years. If this trend continued, some countries would be devoting more than 10 percent of the GNP to health care before the end of the century. In fact, the United States reached this threshold already in 1982, Germany in 1995, and Canada in 2004.

International comparisons have stimulated both national efforts to improve accuracy as well as the methodology of expenditure estimates. As national health expenditure accounts heavily depend on national definitions, international organizations took a leading role in the standardization of definitions. The OECD took the lead to gather and publish health accounts annually. This was a major step forward to make the data available for health system analysis by a wider audience. Next, the System of National Accounts (SNA) set rules for reporting economic transactions in the economy as a whole with the aim to measure the total income produced by a country. This also benefited the development of health expenditures accounts. National accounts consider the health care industry and the consumption and production of health services and goods more or less as satellite accounts.

The United States has maintained detailed expenditure accounts for health care since the early 1960s, with time series on health expenditure tracing back to the 1920s (Berman 1999). The Centers for Medicare and Medicaid Services (CMS) annually publish health expenditure data including a forecast and special analysis. The work is tied to article 702 of the Social Security Act: to study and make recommendations relating to social insurance and matters of administrative policy (Fetter 2006). The U.S. health accounts, named National Health Expenditure Accounts (NHEA), differ from the OECD approach in their definitions of borderlines and classifications for health care and other sectors. For example, NHEA includes research spending, while the OECD puts that activity outside the total health expenditure boundary.

Not only the borderline—What is inside and what is outside the health accounts?—but also the breakdown of health spending has been a permanent issue for discussion of health accounts. One interesting subject of spending analysis is the impact of different diseases. The standardized reporting of diseases based on the International Classification of Diseases supported the implementation of cost-of-illness accounts. Since the pioneering work of Dorothy Rice 1996, cost-of-illness accounts have been developed for several countries, among others Australia, Canada, Germany, and The Netherlands.

In Canada, the Department of National Health and Welfare (DNHW) initiated the National Health Accounts in the early 1960s, around the time all provinces implemented their publicly financed programs of hospital insurance. They compiled expenditure data by source of finance for five categories of personal health care: hospitals, prescription drugs, physicians, dentists, and other health professionals. The DNHW established 1953 as the base year as this was the earliest year with comparable data among provinces. In the 1970s and 1980s, the DNHW added other expenditure categories such as nursing homes, nonprescription drugs, medical aids, home care, ambulance services, occupational health, voluntary health organizations, training of health workers, and a broad category of "other health expenditure" (Fortin 2004). The latter included public health, capital expenditures, administration of insurance programs, and research funding. Health Canada (the successor of DNHW) maintained the National Health Accounts until 1995 when the newly established Canadian Institute for Health Information (CIHI) took over responsibility. CIHI further refined and improved data collection and estimation methods. It revised back time series to 1975 to incorporate these enhancements (CIHI 2008).

Germany started its health accounts in the 1970s inspired by the rising contribution rates for Statutory Health Insurance (SHI). The first report by the Federal Ministry of Labor and Social Affairs (then the supervisory body of SHI) covered the period 1970–1975 (Statistisches Bundesamt 1978). Until the mid-1990s, the estimates included cash benefits in the case of sickness and disability. Since 1995, the health transactions focus on type of services, health care providers, and financing agents. Furthermore, the ministry has linked the accounts to the cost of illness and health labor accounts. In 2006, Germany published the first fully consistent health accounts defined by the OECD standard, the SHA 1.0 (Statistisches Bundesamt 2006). Detailed additional information in the German health accounts are given about cost-of-illness and human resources by professions, age, gender, full-time and part-time jobs, and health industries (Statistisches Bundesamt 2008).

In the Netherlands, the Central Bureau of Statistics published the first comprehensive accounts in the 1960s (CBS 1994). The compilations distinguished outpatient and inpatient care providers. CBS sought to revise its method with the so-called CCP "common and comparable package" project to define and measure a common and comparable package of health care services between six countries (Van Mosseveld and Van Son 1999). In a further effort, CBS tried to integrated health and social care in the data (Van Mosseveld and Smit 2005). In the Netherlands, one question of health spending analysis has always been the impact of different diseases. In 1979, a first attempt was made with an allocation of health care to diagnosis groups, resulting in the calculation of the cost of heart and vascular diseases in the Netherlands over the year 1976. Due to lack of appropriate data only estimates were presented (Kauling and Oosterhof 1982). Further studies divided the total costs of health care using four dimensions: health care provider, diagnosis, age-group, and gender. It appeared that the 10 most costly diseases together made up about 40 percent of total Dutch health care costs (Polder and Achterberg 2004).

Compared with the other countries of this study, health accounting in the United Kingdom is still in an experimental phase (Lee, Wallis, and Heasman 2004). The U.K. National Accounts include information on the main components of health expenditure up to 2005. These estimates are consistent with data SNA published in the *Blue Book 2006* (Office of National Statistics [ONS] 2006). The data provide information on major changes in health expenditure between 1997 and 2005 but are not ideal for comparing the level of health expenditure across countries (ONS 2007). Therefore, the Office of Health Economics publishes its own estimates of total health expenditures with a time series going back to 1973 (Yuen 2004; Hawe 2007).

The OECD health database serves as a reference system for many international comparative studies. Over the years, OECD experts have harmonized many concepts and definitions. OECD gatherings served as meeting grounds for experts to discuss data collection, methodology, and interpretations. In 2000, after numerous discussions, especially on the methodological framework, the OECD published a manual for compiling health accounts (SHA, version 1.0). Together with the "Producer Guide" published by WHO and the World Bank in 2003, the SHA sets the standards since 2005 for the routine data collection by EUROSTAT, OECD, and WHO. These three international organizations gather accounts data by the Joint Health Accounts Questionnaire (JHAQ) using the classifications defined by the SHA Manual Version 1.0 (OECD 2000). The JHAQ aims to reduce the burden of the national data suppliers, to increase the possibilities of international analysis of data, and to facilitate the use of the data. All data are checked in a validation process. First results of the JHAQ are published for the years 2003, 2004, and 2005 at the EUROSTAT web-site.

To enhance comparability further, meanwhile, the three organizations started a consultation process for the revision of the SHA Manual with the aim to present by 2011 the SHA Version 2.0. They engaged in efforts to revise and harmonize the SHA with the Producer Guide for health accounts in developing countries and clarify rules of compilation, definitions, and classifications. However, full harmonization of data collection across the globe will not be easy. There is wide variation in national health policies and national (and international) data reporting methods.

The data presented in this appendix cover the United States, Canada, Germany, the Netherlands, and the United Kingdom and use definitions and data of the OECD SHA (version 1.0). As the five countries have developed different accounting frameworks, this overview has reclassified the data to the SHA standards in broad functional categories. This reclassification does not mean that the five countries have compiled all data in the same way from 1975–2005; but the remaining differences are small enough to allow for a reasonably reliable overview.

Conceptual Issues

There are several reasons why policy makers need health expenditure accounts, even while there are competing (and sometimes conflicting) policy goals of equity, economic growth, and sustainability. The answer to "What is the best approach to health expenditure estimates?" depends very much on the question: "What do we want to answer with those estimates?"

Many of the concepts and definitions that underlie national economic accounts also serve as a base for national health accounts developed in the United States and elsewhere. Economists, statisticians, and other experts in public finance might be inclined to link the NHA to the SNA. In fact, this is more or less the approach of Satellite Account to the SNA. Without going into a full discussion about the satellite accounting methodology, however, there are pitfalls. For example, critics point to shortcomings of using GDP as a welfare measure (U.N. 1993). Next, national accounts usually do not include home production of health care. SHA has expanded to include paid home care to relatives, but it still excludes unpaid home care. Another question is whether health accounts should explicitly measure health capital as a basic part of human capital. One can observe a growing demand to broaden health expenditure accounts toward a health satellite account of national accounts including changes in health outputs (Abraham and Mackie 2005; Aizcorbe et al. 2008).

HEALTH CARE MODEL

Health expenditure accounts track the resources of the health system. Who pays, how much, and for what are described in a set of accounts. At the country level, the following macroeconomic equation of Poullier, Hernandez, and Kawabata (2002) holds:

Production of health care = consumption of health care = cost of health care = income from health care

This equation assumes that the items in the equation do balance, but the data compilations start from different areas in health care. Total expenditure (as defined by the OECD SHA manual) is the sum of expenditure on activities that through application of medical, paramedical and nursing knowledge, and technology have the following goals: to promote health and prevent disease; to cure illness and reduce premature mortality; to care for persons affected by chronic illness who require nursing care; to care for persons with health-related impairments and disabilities who require nursing care; to assist patients to die with dignity; and to provide and to administer public health, health programs, health insurance, and other funding arrangements. Activities dealing with food and hygiene control, health research and development, or training of health workers may be health-related, but are not included in the SHA definition of health expenditure.

National definitions and classification of health care expenditures follow national traditions, institutions, and perceptions of what is health care. Total health expenditure—measured as the sum of all health care activities as defined above—is derived from bundling various statistics of health care financing and consumption. As health is produced by many activities in different locations (at home, health care institutions, environment), this collection requires different sources of information.

Because of the variation in institutional frameworks of national health systems, health accounts require agreement over the empirical measurement of certain fixed analytical elements in all comparator countries. These elements are the types of transactions of financing, provision, and consumption of health care services.

To reach international comparability, all countries have to apply the same system boundary and classifications. Furthermore, they have to use a common accounting methodology and statistical procedure. They also have to apply internationally accepted classification of transactions in meaningful categories that share common characteristics. Thus the question is: How can the elements of international classifications be defined and grouped to allow for systematic structuring and meaningful interpretation of national data?

METHODOLOGICAL DIFFERENCES OF COMPILATIONS

The system of health accounts provides a methodology to estimate financial transactions between financing agents, health care providers, and consumers. SHA's main characteristics are (1) total spending is defined by the nature of the activities related to health and health care, and (2) total national spending for a defined period of time consists of the aggregated transactions between financing agents and health care providers. A matrix method is used to ensure reliability of three-dimensional estimates.

Table A.1 National health expenditure accounts approaches

Country	Organization	Approach	Geography	Revisions	Time series
US	CMS	NHEA	Federal/States	2006	1960–2005
CA	CIHI	HEA	Federal/States	2005, 1995	1975–2005
DE	Destatis	GAR	Federal	2006, 1998	1992–2005; 1970–1997
NL	CBS	CA	Federal	2001, 1998	1998–2005; 1972–1992; 1993–1997
UK	ONS	NHA	Federal	2003	1997–2005
	OHE	NHA	Federal	2006	1973–2006

The United States, Canada, Germany, the Netherlands, and the United Kingdom are still using different approaches for health expenditures accounts (see Table A.1). The breakdown of expenditures varies, depending on national institutional patterns and statistical sources. It requires a reclassification for international purposes. To secure comparability, data sometimes have to be aggregated and as a consequence, the breakdown for international comparison is often less detailed. For example, the SHA manual and Producer Guide mention "curative medical services." National statistics may contain more detailed data on primary and nonprimary care.

Statistical Realization and Data

Compiling NHAs fit for international comparison means linking national statistical systems on health care based on a common framework. Health accountants code, classify, transform, and assemble different types of administrative data, from business and households surveys and other sources. Next they aggregate data and finally present them in tables. There is no generally agreed-upon process for standardizing the compilation process and only a few rules of best practice exist. As a consequence, the compilation of health expenditures accounts could lead, with the same input data, to different results. But international comparison requires consistency of data compilation over time and across countries (Schneider 1995). There is no reason to believe that countries will soon unify benefit catalogs or payment systems, which determine administrative data to settle bills and monitor service delivery.

Health expenditure accounts aim to deliver a quantification of the different structures of health care financing and delivery over time. As a consequence of the medical technical progress and changes of the benefit catalogs, new types of transactions appear but also disappear. The income and expenditure statement of Canadian Medicare, the German SHI, or the Dutch social health insurance need regular adjustment, often on an annual basis. Over longer periods of time the national classifications bundle millions of different transactions into groups like "care delivered by hospitals." But—as we have seen in earlier chapters in this book—hospitals might fulfill quite different tasks across countries. For example, hospitals in the Netherlands and Canada, provide the both inpatient and outpatient specialist care, but German hospitals focus mainly on inpatient care (see Chapter 8).

Despite the Common Market policy of the European Union (E.U.), the responsibility for finance, delivery and regulation of health care is at the level of the individual E.U. member states. There is no Europe-wide program comparable to U.S. Medicare. All twenty-seven E.U. member states gather information about their national health care transactions. Comparing NHA data between the countries of this study (or others) still requires some ex-post recompilations. For example, in 2005, the U.S. total health spending was $2.0 trillion as defined by NHA and $1.96 trillion defined by SHA because the SHA excludes research spending (OECD 2008).

Indicators

NHA manuals give the following reasons for compiling health accounts: (1) provide basic financial information on health systems; (2) provide information on how health funds are distributed across the different services, interventions, and activities in the health system; (3) facilitate valid spatial and temporal comparisons of health expenditure; (4) show who benefits from health expenditure in terms of its financial value and fairness in distribution; and (5) inform health policy and help to improve the performance of health systems. The most prominent indicators are the following: total health expenditures per capita in national currency and in international purchasing power parities (PPP), total health expenditures as a share of GDP, public and private health expenditures as percent of GDP, and public health expenditures as share of government spending.

Except for the first indicator (health expenditure in national currency), all indicators can be used in international comparisons, as they are independent of currency. The major problem with these indicators is the interpretation. What does the higher ratio of health expenditure to GDP of Country A as compared to County B mean? Total health spending share of GDP is cited as a measure of the ability and willingness of a society to purchase health care. The GDP ratio is also used to measure the input cost of health care provision (WHO 2000), which might encourage some governments to engage in "gambling" of statistical compilations.

In many countries, NHAs are limited with respect to information on outputs and outcomes of the health system, in particular as to patient information such as disease prevalence and incidence, or the volume of services or unit costs. The data do not reveal much about determinants of health and health expenditures.

Divergent Spending Developments

The availability of comparable international data on health expenditures has made clear that there is no convergence in health care spending among countries. In fact, in the period considered, health spending grew quite differently among the five countries investigated.

HEALTH SPENDING AS GDP RATIO

Health expenditures, described both as percent of GDP and expenditure per capita, diverged between the United States on the one hand and Canada, Germany, the Netherlands, and the United Kingdom on the other hand. In the United States, for almost all years since 1965, growth in health care spending outpaced economic growth. Consequently, health spending as a share of GDP more than doubled between 1975 and 2005, from 8.0 to 15.7 percent of GDP (CMS 2008).

In Canada, total health expenditures as a share of GDP were 7.0 percent in 1975. In the following years, total health expenditures expanded almost as rapidly as GDP, but in the early 1980s, the two rates of growth started to diverge. The ratio of total health expenditures to GDP increased significantly during the period 1988–1992, reaching 9.9 percent for the first time in 1992. Real health expenditures then grew more slowly than GDP between 1993 and 1997; consequently, the health expenditures to GDP ratio fell again to 8.8 percent in 1997. Real health expenditures grew faster than GDP between 1998 and 2005, with the result that the health expenditures to GDP ratio reached 10.0 percent in 2003. Compilations for 2005 show a GDP ratio of 10.1 percent. This ratio is forecast to be 10.4 percent in 2007 and 10.5 percent in 2008 as defined by the international standards of health expenditures by the OECD (CIHI 2008).

In Germany, the year 1975 marks the start of a period of extensive cost-containment debate (Schneider 1991). The former minister of social affairs in the State of Rhineland-Palatinate, Heiner Geissler, forecasted that with continued high growth rates of health care expenditures, half of the GNP would be devoted for health expenditures by the year 2000 (Geissler 1976). In fact, successive governments enacted a series of cost-containment acts in the period 1975–1990. This led to a modest increase of the health expenditures to GDP ratio from 8.4 to 9.2 percent. After reunification in 1989, the health expenditures to GDP ratio increased significantly, mostly due to the cost of upgrading of the East German health system and the introduction of statutory long-term care insurance in the period 1995–1997. The ratio reached 10.7 percent in 2005 for the whole of Germany, due largely to the lower per-capita income in East Germany. However, when viewed separately, the West German health system grew to only 10.1 percent of GDP as compared to 14.3 percent in East Germany (despite lower health expenditures per capita for East Germans). As can be seen, reunification led to a structural break in the time series of health expenditures for whole Germany (OECD 2008). The comparison in this subsection is therefore focusing on West Germany.

The Netherlands has devoted much less of its GDP to health compared to West Germany over the period 1975–2005. Until the end of the 1990s, it had the second lowest health expenditures to GDP ratio of the five countries examined in this volume. As in Germany, the Netherlands faced many health reforms that tried to stabilize contribution rates (Okma 2001). It is difficult, however, to follow all these changes over the period 1975–2005, because the Dutch Central Bureau of Statistics (CBS) does not provide historical time series. The compilations made by the author have linked the data from various sources following the rules of OECD SHA (CBS 1994; Van Mosseveld and Smit 2005; Smit et al. 2006). According to these compilations, the health expenditures to GDP ratio rose from 6.9 percent to 9.2 percent in the period 1975–2005, about the same increase as observed for Canada, but higher than in West Germany over the whole time span.

The United Kingdom closed up with the Netherlands at the end of the 1990s. It devotes about the same amount, 9.2 percent of its GDP, to health care as defined by the international definitions of health care boundary of SHA. Although this figure is the same as for the the Netherlands, it still means the lowest health spending per capita of the five countries in 2005. The British government has definitely reached its objective to close up with the other European countries. In January 2000, Tony Blair committed to matching European levels of spending on health, or approximately 9 percent of GDP, by 2008 (King's Fund 2005). Since then, the NHS budget has been growing at around 10 percent a year, or about 7.5 percent in real terms. This high growth rate reflects a political judgment about the kind and quality of health care the United Kingdom should have, which has been based on reports by Sir Derek Wanless and his team within the U.K. Treasury (Wanless 2002, 2004; Appleby and Harrison 2006).

One should mention that the Labour government has used OECD figures for the international comparison. The OECD is still publishing lower GDP ratios for the United Kingdom based on ONS data that exclude occupational health care and most spending on long-term care, which is labeled "social care" in Britain (Lee, Wallis, and Heasman 2004).

HEALTH SPENDING PER CAPITA

Health spending is often compared internationally on the basis of expenditure per capita of the population. To do this, national health expenditures need to be converted into a common currency. Purchasing power parities are often used for this purpose, as official exchange rates do not reflect price level differences between countries. PPPs are exchange rates of currencies intended to remove the price-level differences between currencies, thus allowing monetary values to be compared in a common currency. There is a broad discussion how to compile PPPs to be able to make this comparison. OECD compiles general PPPs for the comparison of the GDP per capita in U.S. dollars. These GDP PPPs are used for the comparison of health spending per capita.

In 2005, the United States spent approximately twice as much for medical treatment per capita than the other four countries. What is the reason for this difference? Spending patterns of the United States exhibit higher outlays for all type of services: medical services, long-term care services, pharmaceutical consumption, and administration. There are three exceptions: expenditures for public health per capita (measured at GDP PPP in U.S. dollars) are about the same amount in Canada as in the United States; expenditures for dental care in Germany were until recently higher than in the United States; and expenditures for other services in the United Kingdom, which include expenditure items that cannot be properly allocated to medical care, were also higher than in the United States.

It is remarkable to note the different spending patterns of Canada, West Germany, and the Netherlands in 2005 despite the equivalent level of total health expenditures per capita in these countries as shown in Table A.2. The Dutch are spending less for pharmaceuticals and medical devices than Germans and Canadians but more for medical services. Germans pay more for dental services and Canadians more for public health. The British system has by far the lowest administrative spending.

In 1975, West Germans spent almost the same for health care as U.S. citizens. But in the United States, health spending per capita grew 8.3 percent annually

Table A.2 Per-capita health expenditures as compared to the United States

	1975	1980	1985	1990	1995	2000	2005
				Canada (US = 100)			
Total	80	73	70	62	55	54	52
Medical services	82	70	67	58	48	46	43
Dental services	80	97	95	95	92	86	80
Other services	77	59	65	64	52	49	42
LTC	112	104	90	71	58	63	65
Medical goods	72	73	81	81	87	77	76
Public health	114	107	103	77	80	89	101
Administration	59	34	29	30	31	31	29
Investment	52	56	56	44	37	46	49
				West Germany (US = 100)			
Total	92	90	78	66	60	58	49
Medical services	74	69	59	51	48	48	40
Dental services	192	218	167	135	103	106	87
Other services	189	165	158	100	60	48	24
LTC	45	53	60	57	61	71	69
Medical goods	136	155	144	122	111	87	75
Public health	112	90	75	62	76	60	64
Administration	150	105	80	71	56	49	36
Investment	58	60	51	39	47	43	40
				The Netherlands (US = 100)			
Total	74	68	54	49	46	48	50
Medical services	65	58	45	39	38	42	46
Dental services	69	70	56	52	42	40	43
Other services	169	154	99	84	63	69	73
LTC	134	108	89	70	61	66	76
Medical goods	67	62	58	58	67	55	51
Public health	118	110	79	65	61	47	48
Administration	82	61	48	45	37	36	31
Investment	61	62	50	60	62	58	65
				United Kingdom (US = 100)			
Total	55	48	42	41	43	45	48
Medical services	59	46	41	36	38	41	46
Dental services	41	37	38	48	47	44	45
Other services	112	172	92	127	70	81	112

(continued)

Table A.2 (continued)

	1975	1980	1985	1990	1995	2000	2005
LTC	49	44	42	45	47	49	53
Medical goods	53	61	59	50	67	58	50
Public health	45	39	30	33	30	32	42
Administration	35	25	15	16	19	20	13
Investment	46	36	36	34	44	40	30

over the whole period 1975–2005. Germany's total health expenditures, on the other hand, increased annually only about 6 percent on average. At the end of the period, German health expenditures fell to 50 percent of the U.S. level.

The growth rate of the West German health care system is the lowest of the five countries. In the Netherlands, total health expenditures per capita increased 6.8 percent annually, and in Canada 6.9 percent. As a consequence, the spending levels also diverged between these two countries and the United States.

The NHA estimates can show winners and losers of health expenditure growths. For example, medical goods spending grew faster than medical services in all countries over the whole span of thirty years. Further analysis might link the estimates to the incomes of health professions and human resource developments.

Primary Care and Nonprimary Care

One particular aspect of analysis in this volume is the different role of primary care within the health system. Primary care is seen by many as the key to improving the quality of health arrangements, saving costs, and making health systems more cost-efficient (Saltman, Rico, and Boerma 2006). However, there is a significant difference between stated policy goals, actual program changes, and outcomes. This subsection focuses on the expenditures for primary care and provides some estimates on primary care for the five countries, showing the divergent levels and trends in expenditures.

As the definition of primary care varies among countries, for the purposes of this appendix, the primary care sector is classified by four subcomponents: public health, primary care delivered by doctors, primary care delivered by other professionals, and home care (see Table A.3).

The nonprimary care portion of health spending includes the other health care services: secondary outpatient and inpatient care, tertiary care, inpatient

Table A.3 Classification of primary care and nonprimary care

Primary care	
Public health	Public health activities
Primary care by doctors	Outpatient activities and home visits of general practitioners including family medicine, etc., depending on national classification
Primary care by other professionals	Physiotherapy, psychology, ergotherapy, services proved by midwives
Home care	Home care services except personal care
Secondary care	
Specialist care	Ambulatory activities by specialists and dentists, hospital inpatient acute and chronic care, inpatient rehabilitation, day and night hospital clinics, institutional mental care, rescue services, and patient transport
Dental care	Dental care, prophylactic services by dental practitioners, periodontal services, and dentures
Long-term care	Care in nursing homes and institutional long-term care units
Medical goods	Prescription drugs, OTC, medical devices
Other activities	Administration and investments

medical rehabilitation, long-term care, and mental care. Administration and investments are classified separately as well as drugs, medical nondurables, and durables.

As previously mentioned, the NHAs of the five countries do not explicitly show primary care expenses. It can only be derived using additional information about medical and dental services. There are principally two approaches: (1) taking the primary care services as the starting point, or (2) taking primary care professionals as the starting point. In the first approach, primary care is then compiled from the aggregates of these services multiplied by the respective unit cost. Using the second approach, primary care is compiled from the expenses for these primary care professionals. Ideally one would take the first approach because specialists also provide primary medical care services and would be neglected under the second approach.

Table A.4 Primary care and nonprimary care expenditures, 1975–2005

	1975	1980	1985	1990	1995	2000	2005
				United States			
Primary care	9.1	9.6	11.6	12.5	14.2	13.9	13.6
Secondary care	68.0	69.3	66.9	66.4	65.2	62.4	61.3
Medical goods	12.0	10.3	10.3	10.5	10.2	12.8	13.3
Other expenditures	10.8	10.8	11.1	10.5	10.4	10.9	11.8
Total	100.0	100.0	100.0	100.0	100.0	100.0	100.0
				Canada			
Primary care	11.9	12.8	13.3	15.0	16.1	16.5	16.4
Secondary care	70.1	70.0	68.1	65.0	61.3	57.6	55.8
Medical goods	10.8	10.4	12.0	13.8	16.2	18.3	19.6
Other expenditures	7.3	6.8	6.6	6.3	6.4	7.6	8.3
Total	100.0	100.0	100.0	100.0	100.0	100.0	100.0
				West Germany			
Primary care	14.3	13.2	15.6	16.2	16.5	15.9	16.7
Secondary care	57.3	57.8	55.7	55.4	55.8	56.2	53.7
Medical goods	17.8	17.8	19.1	19.5	18.8	19.2	20.5
Other expenditures	10.7	11.3	9.6	8.9	8.9	8.6	9.1
Total	100.0	100.0	100.0	100.0	100.0	100.0	100.0
				The Netherlands			
Primary care	15.3	16.2	16.0	16.4	15.8	16.9	15.4
Secondary care	65.8	66.4	64.5	61.3	60.7	60.6	63.6
Medical goods	10.8	9.4	11.0	12.6	14.6	14.7	13.5
Other expenditures	8.2	8.0	8.5	9.7	8.9	7.8	7.5
Total	100.0	100.0	100.0	100.0	100.0	100.0	100.0
				United Kingdom			
Primary care	14.2	13.2	13.9	13.7	14.7	15.3	17.0
Secondary care	66.2	66.9	65.2	67.2	62.0	61.2	64.3
Medical goods	11.4	13.0	14.3	12.8	16.1	16.6	13.9
Other expenditures	8.2	6.9	6.5	6.3	7.2	6.9	4.8
Total	100.0	100.0	100.0	100.0	100.0	100.0	100.0

Table A.4 exhibits the compilations based on the second approach. For the five countries, the definition of primary care doctors followed the national definitions, as there is no commonly used international standard. For example in the case of the United States, doctors in the specialties of general practitioner, family medicine, and internal medicine were classified as primary care doctors, which encompasses about 24 percent of all physicians. This percentage has been quite stable during the period 1997–2005. As a consequence, other factors are contributing to the observed growing share of health expenditures for primary health care in the United States, such as the growth of home health services and expenses for other health professionals.

A growing trend in primary care services can be observed in the three countries—United States, Canada, and Germany—but not in the the the Netherlands and the United Kingdom. In contrast to the other countries, the relative supply of physicians working in primary care decreased in the Netherlands and the United Kingdom. Although more information is needed to tease out the reasons for the allocation of resources between the different levels of health care among the five countries, the evidence to date suggests at least one common development over the thirty year period 1975–2005: an increase in the share of health expenditures devoted to medical goods. But there is not a universal development in the share of health expenditures devoted to either primary care or secondary and specialized care.

Estimates of health expenditures based on functional breakdowns are an essential precondition for the analysis of the differences between health systems. However, the compilation of internationally comparable functional breakdowns of health expenditures is still in its infancy. CMS recently made a feasibility study to produce U.S. health spending estimates by function in a single year, consistent with the guidelines set forth in SHA (Cowan, Sisko, and Cylus 2007). Attempts at producing functional estimates for the majority of provider categories have revealed extensive conceptual issues and data gaps between the SHA functions and the U.S. data system, which significantly inhibit the compilation of health care spending by function in the United States. The same holds for the United Kingdom and many other countries.

Further Development

There are several dazzling questions, including the current methodology to be applied for compiling health care expenditures; the issue of health outcomes versus the health care output when measuring prices and productivity of health services; the prevalence of diseases and the cost of illness; the measurement of prevention; investments in medical technologies, research, and human resources developments; and the inclusion of production of health by individuals.

Although international comparison forces countries to improve their accounts, one should not overestimate the role of the NHAs as a tool for health policy development as long as this tool is not commonly used in the national health policy. In fact, the real challenge of health expenditure accounts is the provision of time-consistent figures for national purposes. And here the most important question is: What are the contributions of alternative public spending and health financing patterns to the health development of the population and the increase of productivity of health services?

Improvements in health outcomes are best measured as reduction of mortality and morbidity. Morbidity can be integrated into NHAs, which serve as basis for Cost-of-Illness Accounts (COI). Approaches in this direction also include accounts for particular diseases such as HIV/AIDS. However, presently NHAs fails to include improvements in health outcomes for the whole population. As Berman (1999) mentioned, the term "health accounting" is misleading. Most efforts estimate expenditures for a set of economically defined activities of production and consumption that are better referred to as "health care." Nevertheless, NHAs provide comprehensive information about economic transactions and health system structures based on improved international standards, and are therefore an indispensable tool for health system analysis.

References

Abel-Smith, B. 1963. *Paying for health services: a study of the costs and sources of finance in six countries*. Public Health Papers, no. 17. Geneva: WHO.

Abel-Smith, B. 1967. *An international study of health expenditure and its relevance for health planning*. Public Health Papers, no. 32. Geneva: WHO.

Abraham, K. G. II., and C.D. Mackie (ed.). 2005. *Beyond the market: Designing nonmarket accounts for the United States*, Washington, DC: The National Academic Press.

Aizcorbe, A.M., B. A. Retus, and S. Smith. 2008. Toward a health care satellite account, *BEA Briefing* May 2008: 24–30.

Appleby, J., and A. Harrison. 2006. *Spending on health care: How much is enough?* London: King's Fund.

Berman, P. 1999. What can the US learn from national health accounting elsewhere? *Health Care Financing Review* 21 (2): 47–63.

Canadian Institute for Health Information. 2008. *National health expenditure trends, 1975–2008*. Ottawa: Canadian Institute for Health Information.

CBS. *See* Central Bureau of Statistics.

Centers for Medicare & Medicare Services. 2008. *National Health Expenditures 1960–2007*. Office of the Actuary: National Health Statistics Group.

Central Bureau of Statistics. 1994. *Kosten en Financiering van de Gezondheidszorg* [Costs and financing of health care] *1972–1992*. Voorburg/Heerlen: Statistics Netherlands.

CIHI. *See* Canadian Institute for Health Information.

Cowan, C., A. Sisko, and J. Cylus. 2007. Developing US health spending estimates by function: Experiences and recommendations. Paper presented at the Ninth Meeting of Health Accounts Experts and Correspondents for Health Expenditure Data, Paris, October 8–9.

CMS. See Centers for Medicare & Medicare Services.

Fetter, B. 2006. Origins and elaborations of the National Health Accounts, 1926–2006. *Health Care Financing Review* 28 (1): 53–67.

Fortin, G. 2004. SHA-based health accounts in thirteen OECD countries: Country studies; Canada. *OECD Health Technical Papers*, no. 2.

Geissler, H. 1976. *Krankenversicherungsbudget '80 (Health insurance budget 1980)*. Mainz: Ministerium für Soziales, Gesundheit und Sport.

Hawe, E. 2007. *Compendium of health statistics 2007*. 18th Edition. London: OHE.

International Labor Office. 1959. *The cost of medical care*. Geneva: ILO.

Kauling, R. H. C. M., and W.G. Oosterhof. 1982. Health accounts: An approach to an infrastructure. In *Accounting for health: an international survey*, ed. Levy. E. Paris: Economica: 41–54.

King's Fund. 2005. *An independent audit of the NHS under Labour (1997–2005)*. London: King's Fund Publications.

Lee, P., G. Wallis, D. Heasman. 2004. Total UK health expenditures, 1997–2002. *Economic Trends*, no. 606: 39–45.

Maxwell, R. J. 1981. *Health and wealth*. Lexington, Massachusetts: Lexington Books.

OECD. *See* Organisation for Economic Co-operation and Development.

Office of National Statistics. 2006. *UK national accounts blue book 2006*. London: ONS.

Office of National Statistics. 2007. Expenditure on health in the UK. *National Statistics*. London: ONS.

Organisation for Economic Co-operation and Development. 2000. *A system of health accounts version 1.0*. Paris: OECD.

Organisation for Economic Co-operation and Development. 2008. *OECD health data 2008: Statistics and indicators for 30 countries*. Paris: OECD.

Okma, K. 2001. Health care, health policies and health reforms in the Netherlands. *International Publication Series Health, Welfare and Sport*. No. 7. The Hague: Ministry of Health, Welfare and Sport (VWS).

ONS. *See* Office of National Statistics.

PAHO. *See* Pan American Health Organization.

Pan American Health Organization. 2005. Manual de Cuenta Satélite de Salud (CSS), Version 1.

Polder, J. J., and P.W. Achterberg. 2004. *Cost of illness in the Netherlands—Highlights*. Bilthoven: National Institute for Public Health and the Environment, RIVM Rapport 270751006.

Poullier, J. P., P. Hernandez, and K. Kawabata. 2002. *National health accounts: Concepts, data sources and methodology*. Geneva: WHO.

Rice, D. 1996. *Estimating the cost of illness*. Rockville: Department of Health, Education and Welfare, Health Economic Series no. 6, DHEW pub no (PHS) 947–956. Washington D.C.: U.S. Govt. Printing Office.

Saltman, R. B., A. Rico, and W. G. W. Boerma, eds. 2006. *Primary care in the driver's seat? Organizational reform in European primary care*. Maidenhead, UK: Open University Press.

Schneider, M. 1991. Health care cost containment in the Federal Republic of Germany. *Health Care Financing Review* 12 (3): 87–101.

Schneider, M. 1995. Framework for the international comparison of health expenditures and financing. In *International comparison of health care data, methodology development and application,* ed. C. Van Mosseveld and P. Van Son. Dordrecht, NE: Kluwer Academic Publishers: 263–78.

Smit, J. M., V. C. A. van Polanen Petel, J. van Groen, and A. Jardini. 2006. *Health and social care accounts 1998–2003.* Working paper. Voorburg: Statistics Netherlands.

Smith, C., C. Cowan, S. Heffler, et al. 2006. The national health accounts team: Trends; National health spending in 2005. *Health Affairs* 26 (1): 142–53.

Statistisches Bundesamt. 1978. *Die Struktur der Ausgaben im Gesundheitsbereich und ihre Entwicklung seit 1970: Vertiefende Untersuchung zur Aussagefähigkeit der amtlichen Statistik.* Wiesbaden: Forschungsbericht.

Statistisches Bundesamt. 2006. *Ausgaben, Krankheitskosten und Personal 2004 (Expenditure, cost of illness, human resources).* Presseexemplar. Wiesbaden: Statistisches Bundesamt.

Statistisches Bundesamt. 2008. *Gesundheit—Krankheitskosten 2002, 2004 und 2006 (Health—cost of illness).* Wiesbaden: Statistisches Bundesamt.

U.N. *See* United Nations.

United Nations. 1993. *System of national accounts 1993.* New York: U.N.

Van Mosseveld, C. 2003. *International comparison of health care expenditure, existing frameworks, innovations and data use.* Voorburg: Statistics Netherlands.

Van Mosseveld, C., and P. van Son. 1999. *International comparison of health care data.* Dordrecht: Kluwer Academic Publishers.

Van Mosseveld, C., and J. M. Smit. 2005. *Health and social care accounts 1998–2003.* Working paper. Voorburg: Statistics Netherlands.

Wanless, D. 2002. *Securing our future health: Taking a long-term view.* Final report. London: HM Treasury.

Wanless, D. 2004. *Securing good health for the whole population.* Final report. London: HM Treasury.

WHO. *See* World Health Organization.

World Bank. 1993. *World Development Report 1993: Investing in Health.* Washington D.C.

World Health Organization. 2000. *The world health report 2000: Health systems: Improving performance.* Geneva: WHO.

World Health Organization, U.S. Agency for International Development, and World Bank. 2003. *Guide to producing national health accounts with special applications for low-income and middle-income countries.* Geneva: WHO.

Yuen, P. 2004. *Compendium of health statistics 2004 -2005, 16th Edition.* London: Office of Health Economics.

Table A.5 Per-capita health expenditures as compared to the United States

	1975	1980	1985	1990	1995	2000	2005
			Canada (US = 100)				
Total	84	76	74	67	59	58	52
Medical services	82	70	67	58	48	46	43
Dental services	80	97	95	95	92	86	80
Other services	77	59	65	64	52	49	42
LTC	112	104	90	71	58	63	65
Medical goods	72	73	81	81	87	77	76
Public health	114	107	103	77	80	89	101
Administration	59	34	29	30	31	31	29
Investment	52	56	56	44	37	46	49
			West Germany (US = 100)				
Total	97	95	82	70	65	62	49
Medical services	74	69	59	51	48	48	40
Dental services	192	218	167	135	103	106	90
Other services	189	165	158	100	60	48	22
LTC	45	53	60	57	61	71	69
Medical goods	136	155	144	122	111	87	75
Public health	112	90	75	62	76	60	64
Administration	150	105	80	71	56	49	36
Investment	58	60	51	39	47	43	40
			The Netherlands (US = 100)				
Total	78	71	57	52	50	52	50
Medical services	65	58	45	39	38	42	46
Dental services	69	70	56	52	42	40	43
Other services	169	154	99	84	63	69	73
LTC	134	108	89	70	61	66	76
Medical goods	67	62	58	58	67	55	51
Public health	118	110	79	65	61	47	48
Administration	82	61	48	45	37	36	31
Investment	61	62	50	60	62	58	65

Table A.6 Health expenditures, 1975–2005: United States

	1975	1980	1985	1990	1995	2000	2005
	Millions in national currency						
Total	123.9	236.7	407.8	654.2	927.6	1,233.2	1,947.6
Medical services	76.7	148.1	255.2	409.1	561.3	705.6	1,032.7
Dental services	8.0	13.3	21.7	31.5	44.5	62.0	86.6
Other services	3.3	6.9	13.8	27.7	51.5	76.1	113.9
LTC	9.1	21.4	37.3	65.2	104.6	125.8	169.3
Medical goods	15.6	25.7	44.4	74.0	101.8	170.3	258.8
Public health	3.1	6.4	11.2	20.0	31.0	43.4	56.6
Administration	5.1	12.2	25.7	39.2	58.4	81.2	143.0
Investment	9.0	14.5	22.5	34.7	45.4	63.2	86.8
	Percent of GDP						
Total	7.7	8.5	9.8	11.4	12.5	12.6	15.6
Medical services	4.7	5.3	6.1	7.1	7.6	7.2	8.3
Dental services	0.5	0.5	0.5	0.5	0.6	0.6	0.7
Other services	0.2	0.2	0.3	0.5	0.7	0.8	0.9
LTC	0.6	0.8	0.9	1.1	1.4	1.3	1.4
Medical goods	1.0	0.9	1.1	1.3	1.4	1.7	2.1
Public health	0.2	0.2	0.3	0.3	0.4	0.4	0.5
Administration	0.3	0.4	0.6	0.7	0.8	0.8	1.1
Investment	0.6	0.5	0.5	0.6	0.6	0.6	0.7
	Per capita US$						
Total	574	1,039	1,714	2,621	3,480	4,370	6,591
Medical services	355	650	1,073	1,639	2,106	2,501	3,495
Dental services	37	59	91	126	167	220	293
Other services	15	30	58	111	193	270	385
LTC	42	94	157	261	392	446	573
Medical goods	72	113	187	296	382	604	876
Public health	14	28	47	80	116	154	191
Administration	23	54	108	157	219	288	484
Investment	41	64	94	139	170	224	294

Table A.7 Health Expenditures, 1975–2005: Canada

	1975	1980	1985	1990	1995	2000	2005
	Millions in national currency						
Total	129.7	248.5	431.6	701.3	998.4	1,327.6	1,947.6
Medical services	76.7	148.1	255.2	409.1	561.3	705.6	1,032.7
Dental services	8.0	13.3	21.7	31.5	44.5	62.0	86.6
Other services	3.3	6.9	13.8	27.7	51.5	76.1	113.9
LTC	9.1	21.4	37.3	65.2	104.6	125.8	169.3
Medical goods	15.6	25.7	44.4	74.0	101.8	170.3	258.8
Public health	3.1	6.4	11.2	20.0	31.0	43.4	56.6
Administration	5.1	12.2	25.7	39.2	58.4	81.2	143.0
Investment	9.0	14.5	22.5	34.7	45.4	63.2	86.8
	Percent of GDP						
Total	8.0	9.0	10.3	12.2	13.5	13.6	15.6
Medical services	4.7	5.3	6.1	7.1	7.6	7.2	8.3
Dental services	0.5	0.5	0.5	0.5	0.6	0.6	0.7
Other services	0.2	0.2	0.3	0.5	0.7	0.8	0.9
LTC	0.6	0.8	0.9	1.1	1.4	1.3	1.4
Medical goods	1.0	0.9	1.1	1.3	1.4	1.7	2.1
Public health	0.2	0.2	0.3	0.3	0.4	0.4	0.5
Administration	0.3	0.4	0.6	0.7	0.8	0.8	1.1
Investment	0.6	0.5	0.5	0.6	0.6	0.6	0.7
	Per capita US$ (PPP)						
Total	600	1,091	1,814	2,810	3,746	4,705	6,591
Medical services	355	650	1,073	1,639	2,106	2,501	3,495
Dental services	37	59	91	126	167	220	293
Other services	15	30	58	111	193	270	385
LTC	42	94	157	261	392	446	573
Medical goods	72	113	187	296	382	604	876
Public health	14	28	47	80	116	154	191
Administration	23	54	108	157	219	288	484
Investment	41	64	94	139	170	224	294

Table A.8 Health expenditures, 1975–2005: West Germany

	1975	1980	1985	1990	1995	2000	2005
	Millions in national currency						
Total	44,871	67,983	87,663	114,514	156,700	182,689	201,480
Medical services	21,225	30,803	39,285	52,219	70,604	80,177	87,395
Dental services	5,740	8,792	9,459	10,527	11,928	15,598	16,029
Other services	2,316	3,434	5,682	6,864	8,056	8,717	5,853
LTC	1,529	3,445	5,861	9,259	16,571	21,119	24,798
Medical goods	7,967	12,075	16,772	22,338	29,434	35,146	41,282
Public health	1,288	1,757	2,199	3,068	6,169	6,151	7,748
Administration	2,850	3,882	5,384	6,913	8,526	9,426	11,003
Investment	1,955	2,618	3,021	3,327	5,533	6,408	7,372
	Percent of GDP						
Total	8.4	9.0	9.4	9.2	9.6	10.0	10.1
Medical services	4.0	4.1	4.2	4.2	4.3	4.4	4.4
Dental services	1.1	1.2	1.0	0.8	0.7	0.9	0.8
Other services	0.4	0.5	0.6	0.6	0.5	0.5	0.3
LTC	0.3	0.5	0.6	0.7	1.0	1.2	1.2
Medical goods	1.5	1.6	1.8	1.8	1.8	1.9	2.1
Public health	0.2	0.2	0.2	0.2	0.4	0.3	0.4
Administration	0.5	0.5	0.6	0.6	0.5	0.5	0.6
Investment	0.4	0.3	0.3	0.3	0.3	0.4	0.4
	Per capita US$ (PPP)						
Total	554	986	1,408	1,847	2,255	2,730	3,208
Medical services	262	447	631	842	1,016	1,198	1,391
Dental services	71	128	152	170	172	233	255
Other services	29	50	91	111	116	130	93
LTC	19	50	94	149	239	316	395
Medical goods	98	175	269	360	424	525	657
Public health	16	25	35	49	89	92	123
Administration	35	56	87	112	123	141	175
Investment	24	38	49	54	80	96	117

Table A.9 Health expenditures, 1975–2005: The Netherlands

	1975	1980	1985	1990	1995	2000	2005
	Millions in national currency						
Total	7,334	11,848	14,542	18,573	24,227	33,351	48,720
Medical services	3,776	6,065	7,225	8,771	11,060	15,495	23,476
Dental services	417	653	763	888	983	1,297	1,857
Other services	418	742	852	1,273	1,700	2,748	4,119
LTC	928	1,620	2,072	2,488	3,355	4,390	6,393
Medical goods	790	1,114	1,602	2,339	3,546	4,897	6,570
Public health	274	496	558	711	984	1,077	1,347
Administration	314	523	771	969	1,137	1,525	2,173
Investment	417	635	700	1,134	1,462	1,922	2,784
	Percent of GDP						
Total	6.9	7.3	7.2	7.6	7.9	8.0	9.6
Medical services	3.6	3.8	3.6	3.6	3.6	3.7	4.6
Dental services	0.4	0.4	0.4	0.4	0.3	0.3	0.4
Other services	0.4	0.5	0.4	0.5	0.6	0.7	0.8
LTC	0.9	1.0	1.0	1.0	1.1	1.1	1.3
Medical goods	0.7	0.7	0.8	1.0	1.2	1.2	1.3
Public health	0.3	0.3	0.3	0.3	0.3	0.3	0.3
Administration	0.3	0.3	0.4	0.4	0.4	0.4	0.4
Investment	0.4	0.4	0.3	0.5	0.5	0.5	0.6
	Per capita US$ (PPP)						
Total	447	741	974	1,365	1,741	2,252	3,318
Medical services	230	379	484	645	795	1,046	1,599
Dental services	25	41	51	65	71	88	126
Other services	25	46	57	94	122	186	281
LTC	57	101	139	183	241	297	435
Medical goods	48	70	107	172	255	331	447
Public health	17	31	37	52	71	73	92
Administration	19	33	52	71	82	103	148
Investment	25	40	47	83	105	130	190

Table A.10 Health expenditures, 1975–2005: United Kingdom

	1975	1980	1985	1990	1995	2000	2005
	Millions in national currency						
Total	6,363	14,288	22,672	39,257	57,684	77,323	116,901
Medical services	3,985	8,045	12,973	19,978	28,748	38,110	57,535
Dental services	289	593	1,026	2,054	2,803	3,615	4,971
Other services	324	1,402	1,573	4,801	5,243	8,791	18,173
LTC	396	1,119	1,950	4,008	6,572	8,183	11,429
Medical goods	725	1,853	3,245	5,035	8,904	11,412	16,175
Public health	121	295	423	903	1,238	1,805	2,967
Administration	157	365	473	855	1,473	2,084	2,395
Investment	366	616	1,009	1,623	2,703	3,323	3,256
	Percent of GDP						
Total	6.0	6.2	6.4	7.0	8.0	8.1	9.5
Medical services	3.8	3.5	3.7	3.6	4.0	4.0	4.7
Dental services	0.3	0.3	0.3	0.4	0.4	0.4	0.4
Other services	0.3	0.6	0.4	0.9	0.7	0.9	1.5
LTC	0.4	0.5	0.5	0.7	0.9	0.9	0.9
Medical goods	0.7	0.8	0.9	0.9	1.2	1.2	1.3
Public health	0.1	0.1	0.1	0.2	0.2	0.2	0.2
Administration	0.1	0.2	0.1	0.2	0.2	0.2	0.2
Investment	0.3	0.3	0.3	0.3	0.4	0.3	0.3
	Per capita US$ (PPP)						
Total	333	529	769	1,156	1,604	2,084	3,131
Medical services	208	298	440	588	799	1,027	1,541
Dental services	15	22	35	60	78	97	133
Other services	17	52	53	141	146	237	487
LTC	21	41	66	118	183	221	306
Medical goods	38	69	110	148	248	308	433
Public health	6	11	14	27	34	49	79
Administration	8	14	16	25	41	56	64
Investment	19	23	34	48	75	90	87

Table A.11 Purchasing power parities (PPPs), 1975–2005

	1975	1980	1985	1990	1995	2000	2005
	Conversation rates GDP PPP in US$						
United States	1.00	1.00	1.00	1.00	1.00	1.00	1.00
Canada	1.08	1.15	1.21	1.25	1.22	1.23	1.25
West Germany	1.31	1.12	1.02	0.98	1.03	0.98	0.91
The Netherlands	1.20	1.13	1.03	0.91	0.90	0.93	0.90
United Kingdom	0.34	0.48	0.52	0.59	0.62	0.63	0.62

Example: In 1975, 0.34 British Pound = 1 US$ (GDP PPP).

Source: OECD 2006.

Abbreviations

CA	Care Accounts (NL)
CBS	Central Bureau of Statistics (NL)
CIHI	Canadian Institute for Health Information (CA)
CMS	Centers for Medicare & Medicaid Services (US)
Destatis	German Federal Statistical Office (DE)
GNP	Gross National Product
LTC	Long-term Care Expenditures
NHA	National Health Accounts
NHEA	National Health Expenditure Accounts (US)
OECD	Organisation for Economic Co-operation and Development
OHE	Office of Health Economics (UK)
ONS	Office of National Statistics (UK)
PAHO	The Pan American Health Organization
PPP	Purchasing Power Parities
SHA	System of National Health Accounts
SNA	System of National Accounts
WHO	World Health Organisation

Contributors

John Creighton Campbell
Professor Emeritus of Political Science, University of Michigan

Michael B. Decter
Chair, Cancer Quality Council of Ontario

Aad A. de Roo
Professor of Strategic Healthcare Management, Tilburg University
Director of the Executive MBA–Health Programme, Erasmus University at
  Rotterdam

Mark Exworthy
Reader in Public Management and Policy, School of Management, Royal
  Holloway–University of London

Richard Freeman
Senior Lecturer, School of Social and Political Studies, University of Edinburgh

Stefan Greß
Associate Professor for Health Services Research and Health Economics,
  University of Applied Sciences, Fulda

Naoki Ikegami
Professor and Chair, Department of Health Policy and Management, School of
  Medicine, Keio University

Rudolf Klein
Visiting Professor, London School of Economics

Theodore R. Marmor
Emeritus Professor of Public Policy School of Management, Yale University

Kieke G. H. Okma
Adjunct Associate Professor, Wagner School of Public Service, New York University
Visiting Professor, Catholic University, Leuven

Martin Pfaff
Emeritus Professor of Economics, University of Augsburg

Markus Schneider
BASYS Beratungsgesellschaft für angewandte Systemforschung mbH, Bavaria

Carolyn Hughes Tuohy
Professor Emeritus of Political Science and Senior Fellow, School of Public Policy
  and Governance, University of Toronto

Jürgen Wasem
Professor and Director of the Institute for Health Services Management, University of Duisburg-Essen

Joseph White
Luxenberg Family Professor of Public Policy, Department of Political Science, Case Western Reserve University

Index

Aaron, Henry, 31, 32, 37
Aetna, 40, 41, 44, 46
Alma–Ata Declaration, 199, 205, 232
American Medical Association (AMA),
   196, 211

Bevan, Aneurin, 158
Beveridge, Lord, economic model and
   report, 17, 109, 115, 123, 204
Bismarck, model of social insurance, 88,
   92, 107, 108, 109, 115, 123, 204, 273
Blair, Prime Minister, 28, 54
Blüm, Norbert, 272, 273

Canada, health care system of
   (Medicare), 2, 3, 34; Alberta,
   hospitals, 217, 218; Alberta, province
   of, 68, 69, 77, 80, 82, 217–218;
   British Columbia Medical Association
   (BCMA), 68; Canada Health Act
   of 1984 (CHA), 31, 65, 67, 215,
   234–235; Chaoulli case, 79, 81, 216,
   218, 234; community control, 33;
   Comparison to NHS (United
   Kingdom), 63, 64, 68, 74; comparison
   to US Health model, 51, 85;

Conservative Party, 70, 80, 85; cost
   sharing, 31, 34, 35; decentralization,
   28, 31, 33; establishing framework,
   63, 64; GDP spending, 9, 25, 79, 321,
   341; LaLonde Report, 205; Liberal
   Party Government, 67, 80, 81, 82, 85;
   Mazankowski Report, 217; medical
   schools, 71; Ontario Medical
   Association (OMA), 68, 82; private
   sector growth, 72, 73; projected costs,
   79, 80; provincial government's role,
   68, 69, 70, 72, 84, 217; public
   opinion surveys, 68, 69, 71, 72, 75;
   public spending, 61, 62, 65, 84;
   Quebec party, 76, 78, 79, 80, 81, 85;
   reform debates involving US model, 4,
   5, 12, 19; restructuring act of 1996,
   70, 71; Romanow Report, 78, 85;
   single-payer, 64, 77, 82; surgery,
   waiting times, 62, 71, 77, 78
Center for Studying Health System
   Change, 39, 44, 45, 49
Chaoulli case, 79, 81, 216, 218, 234
Clinton, President Bill, health reform
   plan, ix, 7, 18, 30, 31, 32, 37, 54,
   211, 315

Community health centers: in Canada, 69, 71; in the United States, 39

Congressional Budget Office (CBO), 28, 32

Consumer choice: in Canada, 65, 69, 71, 74; in Germany, 92, 105, 110, 111, 187, 220, 276, 298; in Japan, 276; in the Netherlands, 123, 130, 140, 145–148, 198, 228; in the United Kingdom, 164, 170, 192, 230; in the United States, 30, 31, 34, 43, 48, 55, 195

Cross-national analysis: barriers to learning, x, 4, 5, 8, 310, 311, 314; the challenges of, vii, ix, 4, 5, 7, 316, 317; failures of, 6–7, 10–12, 14, 309, 311–312; methodological issues, 1, 2, 5, 6, 7, 15, 171, 300n1, 309; policy learning, x, 2, 3, 6, 15, 170, 173n4, 260, 265, 275, 282–283, 308, 314; promises of, 2, 3, 6–7, 10–12; US and UK exchange, 4, 17, 26, 30, 83, 155, 170, 308

Dekker, Wisse, Commission and Plan, 31, 33, 127, 128, 130, 132, 133*tab*, 148

Demographics: aging population, 266, 268; boomer generation, 208; in Germany, 266

Diagnosis related groups (DRGs): in Germany, 93, 108, 222, 237; importing the model from the United States, 108, 309; in the Netherlands, 224, 237, 238; in the United Kingdom, 159, 212, 231; in the United States, 37, 212, 234, 307, 309

Elderly care, in United States. *See* United States, health care system of: Medicare

Enthoven, Alain, 33, 148

Evidence-based medicine: in Germany, x, 88, 91, 99, 100–107, 113; in the United Kingdom, 159

Germany, health care system of: Agenda 2010, 97; Bundesrat (2nd chamber of Parliament), 91, 95; cost containment, 96, 97, 110; Cost Containment Acts: Health Insurance Cost Containment Act in 1977, 92, 93; cost-sharing, 31; disease management programs, 105, 106; evidence-based policy making, 99, 100, 101–103, 105–106; family care givers, 266, 268, 280; funding of health care, 27; GDP spending, 9, 25, 83, 95, 321, 329, 342; GDP spending, on long-term care, 186, 187; governing parties, on cost containing, 96, 97, 110; Health Care Reform Act of 1989, 93, 94, 95; Health Care Structure Act of 1993, 95, 96, 105, 110, 111; Health Insurance Restructuring Acts of 1997, 96; Health Reform Act of 2000, 96, 106, 110; Health System Modernization Act of 2004, 93, 96, 107, 110; Hospital Cost Containment Act of 1981, 92; influence of other OECD reforms, 105, 106; influence of US reforms, 107; learning from other countries, 107–109; Liberal-Conservative coalition parties, 95; long-term care, 123, 186, 187, 221, 235; model of health care, 50, 88, 89; neocorporatist model, 235, 237, 306; origins of system, 88; pharmaceuticals, control of, 90, 91; private insurance, 88, 92; private-public health spending, 95; public opinion survey, 71; Red-Green Coalition, 96, 110; Risk Structure Compensation Act of 2002, 105; sick fund financing, xi, 50, 72, 89, 97, 186, 253, 279, 284, 290, 292, 302; sick fund, mandated insurance, 204, 219, 235; similarities with the Netherlands, 123, 147n5, 223, 224; Strengthening Competition Health Insurance Act of 2007, 97

Griffiths, Roy, 156

Gross Domestic Product (GDP)
spending: health spending as ratio,
328; in OECD countries, 321, 324,
327, 328, 330. *See also* separately
under Canada, health care system of
(Medicare); Germany, health care
system of; The Netherlands, health
care system of; United Kingdom,
health care system of; and United
States, health care system of

Hashimoto, Ryuutarou, Prime Minister
of Japan, 271, 273
Health care reform: debates in Canada,
ix, 75, 78, 82, 83n5; debates in
Germany, x, 91, 92, 94, 96, 98, 105,
112; debates in OECD countries,
1, 2, 8, 9, 11, 92; debates regarding
markets, 96, 107, 118; reform acts,
93; terminology, 17n2, 92
Health Maintenance Organizations
(HMOs): backlash, 211, 234;
containing pharmaceutical costs, 254;
in the Netherlands, 138; Kaiser
Permanente model, 40, 42, 44, 194; in
the US, 26, 27, 34, 39–45, 199
Hospital associations: Canada, 75;
Germany, 90; the Netherlands, 128,
146
Hospitals: for elderly patients in
Canada, 205; for elderly patients in
Germany, 205; length of stay (LOS),
205, 206, 211, 212, 221, 225, 230;
mergers, 220; origins, 203, 208;
teaching hospitals in Canada, 217,
218; teaching hospitals in Germany,
220; teaching hospitals in the
Netherlands, 128; teaching hospitals
in the United Kingdom, 204; Tenet
case (US), 213–214; in the United
States, 26, 39, 209, 233

Iglehart, John, 42
Illich, Ivan, 205

Japan: health care model, 266; long-term
care model, 265–267, 272; paying
family caregivers, 280; policy learning
from the West, 272; Prime Minister
Hashimoto, 272, 273

Kaiser Family Foundation Report, 32
Kaiser Permanente, 40, 42, 44, 163,
170, 194

Lalonde Report, 205
Long-term care (LTC): aging
demographics, 266, 268; boomer
generation, 208; in Canada, 218, 270;
family care givers, in Germany and
Japan, 266, 268, 280; GDP spending,
267, 268, 281; in Germany, 123, 186,
187, 221, 235; insurance (LTCI),
265, 275–283; in the Netherlands,
128, 130, 139, 143–144; in OECD
countries, 266–268; in the United
Kingdom, 236

Managed care: in Canada, 72; Europe's
interest in, 5, 16, 17n3, 195, 196, 314;
in the United States: discussion of,
30–33, 38, 40–44, 50–52, 200n15; in
US hospitals, 211, 234; in US Medicare,
55, 211; in US pharmaceutical costs,
254; in US primary care, 194
Medicaid. *See* United States, health care
system of
Medical Savings Accounts (MSAs), 31,
53, 77
Medical technology, 232, 233, 309; cost
of, 208; in Dutch hospitals, 225; in
German hospitals, 220; measure of
performance, 209
Medicare. *See* Canada, health care
system of; Elderly care; United States,
health care system of

National Health Service (NHS). *See*
United Kingdom, health care system of

The Netherlands, health care system of:
characteristics of, 124, 127, 128;
covenants in Dutch social policy,
127; covenants with hospitals, 128;
covenants with pharmacists, 128;
Dekker Commission and Plan, 31, 33,
127, 128, 130, 148; GDP spending,
329, 343; Health Insurance Law of
2006, 127, 132, 134; Health Reform
of 2006 (Zorgverzekeringswet [Zvw]),
124–125; long-term care, 128, 130,
139, 143–144; Maastricht Treaty
(1991), 134; market reforms, 120,
122, 126, 127, 146; neocorporatist
model, 120, 122, 126, 227, 236,
237; Polder model, 120, 124, 126;
primary care, GPs as gatekeepers,
188, 196–198; private clinics, rise of,
138; private insurance, 124, 125, 137,
138, 149; private treatment centers,
139; private treatment, specialists'
role, 189; Purple Coalition, 131, 133;
reforms, in 1980s and 1990s, 122,
126, 127; sick fund, demise of, 136,
137; sick fund, financing, 125, 130,
134–135, 143, 147, 223, 296; sick
fund, regional boundaries, 130, 132,
133, 137, 143; similarities with
Germany, 123, 147n5, 223, 224;
uninsured, 136, 137, 145; Wassenaar
Agreement of 1982, 7
Newhouse, Joseph, 31

Osler, William, 208

Pharmaceutical industry: in Canada,
73, 248; GDP spending, 246, 247;
generics, 250, 252–255, 261n5; in
Germany, 33, 90, 91, 200; inflation
costs, 84; international companies,
245; in OECD countries, 244–248;
patient co-payments, 248–249; pricing,
6, 251–252; regulation, 245, 251, 254,
256; safety criteria, 248; supranational
regulation, discussion of, 257–259; in

United States, 26; in US Medicare
coverage, 25, 234; in US research, 30
Preferred Providers Organizations
(PPOs), in the United States, 43, 44
Primary care: categories of, 184, 185;
community approach, 182, 183, 185,
187, 197; cost reduction, 183, 184;
definitions of, 182, 196, 199; as
entry point, 182, 196; expenditures,
332–335; GYNs as primary care
physicians, 184, 185; patient–centered,
183; physicians as gatekeepers, 183,
184, 186, 187, 194, 195; physicians
as managers, 166, 186; self-referral,
187
Primary care in Canada, 35, 65, 71, 74;
capitation of costs, 190; reform, 77,
78, 82
Primary care in Germany: *Hausärtzte*
idea, 186, 220; specialists' role, 186,
187
Primary care in the Netherlands: Dutch
model, 108; GPs as gatekeeper, 188,
196, 197, 198; specialists' role, 189
Primary care in the United Kingdom:
capitation of costs, 193; cost control
on secondary and tertiary care, 193,
199; fundholding practices, 157, 167,
168, 191, 192, 195, 212, 230; GPs
as gatekeepers, 193, 198; GPs as
managers, 166, 191; service shortages,
197, 199
Primary care in the United States:
fundholding practices, 194;
gatekeepers, physicians as, 194, 195;
managed care backlash, 195, 196;
managed care and primary care,
194–196; nurse practitioners role, 194;
specialists, 194, 196
Private Health Insurance (PHI): in
Canada, 78, 79; in Germany, 88, 92,
219; in the Netherlands, 124, 125,
137, 138, 149, 224; PHI markets in
OECD countries, discussion of,
288–290; in Quebec, 81; in the United

Kingdom, 162; in the United States, 26, 29, 48, 215; vs. US Medicare spending, 32, 38

Rand Experiment, 31
Reischauer, Robert, 31, 32, 37

Single-payer system, 313; in Canada, 64–69, 77, 82

United Kingdom, health care system of: Acheson Review, 158; Anglo-American learning, 155, 170; clinical monitoring (QOF), 166; devolution of NHS, 160, 161; elective surgery, waiting time, 163, 164, 230; GDP spending, 192, 329, 330, 344; GPs, role of, 155, 167, 172; information technology, discussion of, 168; "internal market" initiatives, 68, 74, 229, 230, 236, 307; Labour Party, new, 157, 159, 163, 167, 168, 192, 200n10, 230, 330; Labour Party, old, 158, 167; Millan Commission, 161; Modernization Agency, 157; National Health Insurance (NHS), establishment of, 153, 155, 204; National Institute for Clinical Excellence (NICE), 108, 159, 231, 256, 260; NHS in international policy debates, 154; NHS model, 147n5, 148n8, 154, 155, 156; primary care groups (PCGs later PCTs), 157, 158, 172; Reorganization of 1974, 156, 158, 165; Scottish Nationalist Party (SNP), 161; Thatcher government reform, 156, 170, 236; Wanless Report of 2002, 171, 230, 330

United States General Accountability Office (GAO), 30, 48
United States, health care system of: Balanced Budget Act of 1997, 37; Clinton plan, 31; comparisons to other democracies, 24; employer-based coverage, 25, 28, 34, 38–39, 43–49; GDP spending, 9, 25, 28, 36*tab*, 37, 321, 340; Gynecologists as primary care,184, 185; Health Maintenance Organizations (HMOs), 26, 27, 34, 39–45, 195; Health Savings Accounts (HSAs), 29, 31; HMO backlash, 211, 214; managed care backlash, 43, 195, 196; managed care, in primary care, 194, 195, 196; Medicaid (low-income population), 26, 28, 32, 39, 54, 210, 321; Medicaid enrollment, 38; Medicaid premiums, 46, 48; Medicare, costs of, 28, 35–38, 44, 53n14, 54n25; Medicare, cost-sharing, 52n5; Medicare, coverage of elderly, 25, 26, 31, 32, 36, 210; Medicare, hospital coverage, 210, 215; Medicare, long-term care, 36–38; Medicare Modernization Act of 2003, 54n23; Medicare, privatization of, 30, 31, 32, 38, 44, 53n15, 54n23, 291, 296; public view of health care system, 68–69; risk shifting, 42; uninsured, hospital treatment of, 34, 212; uninsured population, 39, 294; Veterans Health Administration, 26, 51, 170, 199, 210

Wanless Report of 2002, 171, 230, 330

Advance praise for *The Adventures of Cancer Girl and God*

"Having had melanoma in my thirties, I am so grateful for this piercingly honest, encouraging, real, and straightforward book. Courie offers her readers the open invitation to tell the truth of their experience of cancer, and to carry that experience into sustained prayer through reflection and journaling. Highly recommended."

—Mary C. Earle, author of *Days of Grace: Meditations and Practices for Living with Illness*

"Anna Fitch Courie writes with a brutal honesty that's refreshing and disturbing all at the same time. As a 'cancer boy' myself, I was there with her through every sentence of her book. There is no redemptive quality in having cancer. It's not a God-induced opportunity to witness to our faith. As Anna writes, it just plain 'sucks.' So, cancer can never give us a hyphenated identity, because our full identity, as Anna attests, is already grounded in the God who wonderfully created us and more wonderfully redeemed us in Jesus Christ."

—The Rt. Rev. Scott Anson Benhase, Bishop of Georgia

"There is so much to love about *The Adventures of Cancer Girl and God*! Imagine a memoir that is also a retrospective, accompanied by a playful workbook where the reader is invited to reflect on his or her own life alongside the author. Anna takes our hand and guides us through every nook and cranny of her diagnosis—from denial, to anger, to gratitude, to denial, to faith, to denial, to joy. Along the way, we reflect with her on our closest relationships, on our own anger or sadness, on our favorite swear words and deepest prayers. I found reading this book was like reading through the Psalms; all human emotions are present, and are of God. Honest, raw, and courageous, the author's story is at once intensely personal and universal. Her experiences along her journey, even when solitary, remind her to reach out to those around her, and to God. You will find yourself journeying beside her and cheering her on, while leaning more deeply into your own life and faith."

—The Rev. Cricket Cooper, author of *Chemo Pilgrim*

"In *Christ Walk* Anna Fitch Courie invited us all on a journey, a Lenten walk with Jesus. Now she takes us on a hero's quest, with an honesty and tenacity like no other. Whether you have felt betrayed by your body, gone through the illness of a loved one, or simply strive each day to be a follower of Jesus, *Cancer Girl* inspires, challenges, motivates, and empowers all of us toward a closer relationship with God."

—The Rev. Benjamin Gildas of *Priest Pulse* podcast

THE ADVENTURES OF
CANCER GIRL
AND GOD

A JOURNEY OF FAITH, HEALTH, AND HEALING

ANNA FITCH COURIE

FOREWORD BY BEN EMANUEL, MD

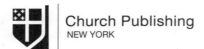

Church Publishing
NEW YORK

For Treb

Church Publishing
19 East 34th Street
New York, NY 10016
www.churchpublishing.org

Cover design by Marc Whitaker/MTWdesign.net
Typeset by Rose Design

Library of Congress Cataloging-in-Publication Data

Names: Fitch Courie, Anna, author.
Title: The adventures of cancer girl and God : a journey of faith, health, and healing / Anna Fitch Courie.
Description: New York, NY : Church Publishing, [2018]
Identifiers: LCCN 2017053796 (print) | LCCN 2018011806 (ebook) | ISBN 9781640650114 (ebook) | ISBN 9781640650107 (pbk.)
Subjects: LCSH: Cancer—Patients—Religious life. | Fitch Courie, Anna.
Classification: LCC BV4910.33 (ebook) | LCC BV4910.33 .F58 2018 (print) | DDC 248.8/6196994—dc23
LC record available at https://lccn.loc.gov/2017053796

Printed in Canada

Contents

Foreword   vii

Prologue   ix

1. Day 1: I Am So Very Angry with God   1
2. Day 2: The Anxiety Is Overwhelming   5
3. Day 3: Coming Out of the Cancer Closet   8
4. Day 4: A Litany of "God Bless"   12
5. Day 5: In Sickness and in Health   19
6. Day 6: Today I Felt Normal   25
7. Day 8: Answer This *One* Question   31
8. Day 11: The Whispers of God at Midnight   36
9. Day 12: Don't Play the Gambling Game   41
10. Day ?: What Pain Will Do to You   46
11. Day 13: Humor   51
12. Day 15: Goonies Never Say Die   54
13. Day 18: We Are Groot   60
14. Day 20: You've Got Your Good Days and Your Bad Days   64
15. Day 21: Three Weeks. I Want My Mama   69
16. Day 23: David and Goliath   77
17. Day 30: One Month In   82
18. Multiple Days: The Number One "No-No"   87
19. Day 32: Making Bad Good   93
20. Day 39: "So, How Are You?"   99
21. Day 42: Crazy Things That Happen When You Have Cancer (or Other Diagnosis)   106
22. Day 49: God Advertises in Neon Signs   113

23. Happy Thanksgiving!   123

24. Day 57: Wearing Yourself Thin: What Not to Do   127

25. Day ????: Where Is My Breaking Point?   131

26. Another Day Has Passed: Ten Bits of Advice
    to the Healthcare Industry   138

27. Day 70: You Will *Never* Believe What I Have Chosen   143

28. On the First Day of Christmas . . .   152

29. Saying Good-Bye   157

30. Day 125: Another Day with Cancer,
    or Just Another Day?   164

31. It's World Cancer Day   169

32. My Six-Month Cancerversary   174

33. Somewhere around Nine Months . . .   180

34. Day 365: A Year with Cancer   186

35. Forty Things I've Learned Since Turning Forty   193

Epilogue   203

Acknowledgments   205

Foreword

As this book goes to press, it is estimated that over 1.6 million people will be diagnosed with cancer and over 600 thousand will die of cancer this year. As shocking as the numbers are in aggregate, they do not tell the whole story because the entire story is composed of millions of individual stories, with each representing a unique person, their family, friends, and everyone with whom they interact. The ultimate reach of these diseases that we collectively call cancer is millions of people at any one time. And yet, each patient, though surrounded by loved ones and support systems, is still alone in their feelings in a way that others cannot quite comprehend.

In this book, Anna Fitch Courie gives us some insight into the effects that cancer has at the personal level. Beyond the statistics, this book allows the reader to see up close the thoughts and fears, challenges and concerns that are all but universal as each person faces their disease. Thought-provoking, frank, and uncompromisingly honest, the words on these pages reflect the truth as faced by a woman confronting this difficult ordeal. And though we in medicine are beginning to have great success in many areas where we battle cancer, the hard and frightening work of these battles is being waged by Anna and millions like her who must confront this enemy.

This book will have familiar tones for those who are facing or have faced such an ordeal themselves. As such, it can serve as a valuable resource for those patients who are looking for answers in areas where even the questions are not easily formed. Sharing in Anna's journey can provide a comfort to other patients in knowing that they are not alone in their questions of medicine, life, and even faith.

For caregivers, family, and loved ones, this book serves as an indispensable guide to let us see beyond the diagnosis, beyond the treatment options, beyond the prognosis. Indeed, through Anna's generosity and sharing, the reader sees the person who must deal with all the issues that this disease brings. Though her journey is personal and unique, Anna's questions, struggles, and even answers will resonate with others who have trod their own difficult paths. This universality of emotions gives these words applicability in other lives.

The book is not always easy to read—the subject matter is difficult and frightening by definition. But the struggle that Anna wages ultimately is ennobling and gives the reader a sense of hope even in the dark times. I recommend this book to all who are personally or peripherally confronted with cancer as a means to share in the humanity of these experiences and better understand what each patient faces in their own personal struggle.

Dr. Ben Emanuel
Anatomic Pathology & Clinical Pathology
Anderson, South Carolina

Prologue

I am a nerd. I love epic stories. I love fantasy, science fiction, action, and adventure. Upon reflection, it is not necessarily the genre itself that calls to me—it is the plot formation where the good guy (or gal) wins the battle. I like heroes and heroines. I like good versus evil, and I love "happy endings."

When I sat down to write *The Adventures of Cancer Girl and God*, I wanted more than anything to be the hero of my own story. I want desperately to win out over cancer and beat the snot out of this evil disease. That wasn't in the cards I was dealt. I have a type of cancer that is chronic. I don't get to get rid of it. It's a part of me. My wellness depends completely on how well I take care of myself and manage my disease on a day-to-day basis. Sometimes I rock my cancer world, and other days, it gets the better part of me. Through my journey, I've learned tricks for dealing with living with disease; one of those tricks is visioning how I want to see myself.

I picture myself in a cape, powerful and fierce. It brings a smile to my face to think of smashing cancer cells under my feet. It is a *positive* vision of where I wanted to go on my journey and it keeps me fighting the good fight. I want *you* to find a heroic vision of yourself as well.

Most heroes have superpowers. My superpower is my faith in God. I would not be here to tell you this story, and attempt to provide you with a vision of hope for your own journey, without God. In ways I cannot begin to articulate, or even fully comprehend, God has blessed my life and given me the strength to see illness in a different light. My hope is to help others see their illness or disease differently too. It is incredibly difficult to be hopeful in the middle of crisis. It is uniquely challenging to find grace in the midst of death, illness, and disease. I feel fiercely that grace is there. Grace is an amazing superpower. I believe you have that superpower too.

My story originally unfolded on my blog: *www.christwalk40day.blog spot.com*. Many of the feelings I expressed there were written in real time, as my cancer story unfolded. I have since gone back to those writings to both remember how I felt in that moment and provide clarity as to how I feel now, in the hopes that I might turn it into a lesson for others. If I help one cancer patient (or another person struggling with illness and disease) feel that they are understood, and hold true to the fear, the anger, the anxiety, and the personal growth that can occur because of illness, then every word in this book was worth writing.

There are parts of the story that are incredibly raw. Breathe through them.

There are parts of the story that are my own only. You may not feel the same way. Be with me in them.

There are parts of the story that have yet to be completed. Pray with me through them.

I will do the same for you. We do not take journeys in a vacuum. You are not alone. I am not alone. So please, join me on my quest of health, faith, fitness, humor, and healing, as Cancer Girl and God go on a journey together.

With love, —*Anna*

I Am So Very Angry with God

My God, My God, why have you forsaken me? (Ps. 22:1)

How I Felt . . .

I just found out I have cancer. My body, as usual, has betrayed me. An angry fire lives under my skin and I fight the tears that try to leak out. I am hot. I am cold. I am sweating. I shiver. I feel like I may throw up.

I am so pissed right now. I will ask your forgiveness for my crudity later, but this is a raw wound. I am angry, furious with God, furious with my body, and furious with life.

What did I ever do to deserve this? I do not understand how living a clean life, following the Good Book, and trying my damnedest leads me to this. I try so hard. I have more questions than answers. I am in a stage. I hate being in a stage. I am a statistic. I hate being a statistic.

I do not want cancer. Moreover, with all apologies to my friends with cancer, I do not want to be labeled a cancer patient. I can say with 100 percent confidence that I am sure they don't or did not want to be seen as patients either. This cancer business is seriously inconvenient.

I do not want a litany of doctors or visits. I have been there, done that. I lost my hearing when I was twelve to an autoimmune disease; I have had multiple surgeries and been through many autoimmune disease therapies. I've lost my hair, been in the hospital on holidays, had my body scarred, and gone through the rehabilitation phase. Been there, done that. I hate being sick. I hate the experience of being subjected to the medical arena. I do not want this journey that is set before me. I do not want this season.

I want a normal life. I want to raise my children. Grow old with my husband. I want to travel and eat good food. I want to see my grandchildren and watch my kids graduate from college, get married, become successful. I want a normal body. I have had an abnormal body my entire life. I hate my abnormal body.

I do not want to hear that I am a warrior, or a conqueror, or how tough I am. I am more comfortable with a drama-free life. I am ok with the status quo. I am ok with the boring.

I feel utterly betrayed by God. In part of my brain I realize how silly this is but this is how I feel. I feel like I have done something wrong and I'm being punished for some unknown deed.

I am pissed. My cheeks feel like frying pans are sitting on the hard shelf of my cheekbones and my head throbs. I am not ready for this. I have follicular lymphoma. As far as cancers go, it is probably the "right" one to have. It is treatable, but noncurable—what does that mean? It is malignant, but nonaggressive. What does that mean? It sure feels like an aggressive intrusion on my life. That does not make me want it more. I wish I could turn back the clock and not pick up the phone when my surgeon called. I am not ready for this.

But I will be. Let me grieve. Let me get angry and let me find my fighting spirit. I will win this war against cancer. I will find my spiritual equilibrium. I will see the glass half-full.

But until then, I will grieve and I will be angry.

God? Why have you done this to me?

What I Learned . . .

Finding out you have cancer sucks. It does not matter what form it is, how aggressive it is, where it is located, or how far it has spread, or not spread. The word "cancer" in and of itself is a horrible, hate-filled, fear-filled word. The word "cancer" can literally steal the breath from your body. Cancer is probably one of the number one words that people never want to hear from their doctor.

Cancer happens to so many people, and yet each experience is unique. The approaches to cancer treatment are manifold and very specific to the type of cancer you have, what stage it is at, how symptomatic you are (or are not), and a myriad of other factors that need to be understood with thorough conversations with your doctor. The word "cancer" is used as an umbrella word to describe a disease that is very different depending on the *type* of cancer you have. No two cancers are the same.

The problem is that when you hear the word "cancer," it is hard to hear anything else or absorb any information. Life stops in your head. The shock of the word "cancer" takes a *long* time to heal. Give yourself permission to be angry (it is normal), grieve (it is normal), break something (it is normal), hurt (it is normal), or whatever it is that you feel or need during this time. Make sure you take someone with you to your next doctor's appointment; you may not hear things well right now and you'll need a second set of ears moving forward. You have a lot of thoughts, feelings, concerns, fears, and anxieties that are swirling around in your head. Get yourself a wingman. Even superheroes have sidekicks. Find one, and make sure they take their role seriously.

Your Story . . .

What is your disease? Give it a name:

_____

_____

_____

_____

_____

_____

_____

_____

_____

_____

_____

How do you feel? Let it out:

_____

_____

_____

_____

_____

_____

_____

_____

_____

DAY

2

The Anxiety Is Overwhelming

Why are you so far from helping me, from the words of my groaning? (Ps. 22:1)

How I Felt . . .

The anxiety continues to leave me breathless. It is several days before I can see my doctor. They are booked it seems. I don't know why. I just know I have to wait. I am nauseous. I can barely eat. I do not know what to say to my children. I do not know how to look at my husband. I do not know how to show up at work.

I am weak. I need medication. I have called for a prescription of Xanax to cope. I cannot seem to find the words to pray for this. My faith has been hijacked and I don't know what to do. I don't know what to do. I know I should pray, but I don't know the words to use. I am so very, very scared.

Failure does not even begin to cover how I feel. I feel like I should know what to do. I feel like I should know what to pray. I feel that my body has failed me, and that I have done something wrong. I hate myself. I hate my body. I honestly hate God. I am paralyzed.

What I Learned . . .

The diagnosis is not going to go away the next day when you get up. It will still be there looming over your head. I felt this way, and I am pretty sure that most people with illnesses feel this way as well. You hope when you wake up the day after finding out this kind of news that it was all a bad dream.

I thought I could pray through my fear and anxiety, except I was truly still angry at God, and so had nothing to say. I had no words to share; nothing was breaking through the anger of being thirty-eight and having my life come to a screeching halt. There were so many feelings jockeying for space in my mind. I was angry to be in this position. I felt I took good care of myself and should not be afflicted with this disease. I believed I lived a "godly, righteous, and sober" life and should be spared of this indignity. I did everything right. I played life by the book. The shame I felt was as though I did something wrong. My fear shook at what the unknown future held. All these emotions create a brick wall between you and prayer at first.

This is normal. The anxiety is normal. The anger is normal. The fear that is overwhelming is also normal. Your diagnosis has presented you with a world of the unknown that looms ahead on the horizon and you cannot see the sun. You will be breathing normally one moment, and the next second anxiety will inexplicably seize your breath and freeze your lungs. You will think that the oxygen in the air you breathe has suddenly dropped. You will look around wildly, wondering how you got here. It will wake you in the middle of the night for no apparent reason. Your fight-or-flight response has been triggered and your body is attempting to deal with it. You will be angry at God for a while.

Guess what? God gets it. God is there, even if you do not feel like you can talk to God, pray to God, or even think of God in this moment. God is not going anywhere. God will be there when you are ready to talk to God. God is very patient.

Taking medication is not a failure. You may feel much like me. While I felt like I was a derelict for needing a prescription for my anxiety, it was a lifesaver. It took the edge off so I could think clearly again. Do not punish yourself for needing help. It also is normal. There is a gift in allowing medication to mitigate your anxiety so you can think more clearly. It helps your body deal with that fight-or-flight response that has been triggered. It will help you sleep, which helps your body to heal. You are not a disappointment for needing medicine or a professional ear to discuss your overwhelming emotions. I do know that if you do *not* deal with those emotions, they can come back to haunt you for a long time. Do *not* be afraid to get help. I promise it is okay. Taking medications is part of a holistic approach to managing *your* health so that *you* can be successful on this illness journey. Medication, prayer, meditation, yoga, acupuncture, massage, physical therapy, and so on are all a part of the plan to get you well again. It is absolutely okay to need help when you have a disease.

Remember that how you feel each day is not the end of the story. One day, or two days, is not the whole scope of what your life will be like. It *is* a season. It will pass. Give yourself permission to do what you need to do to get through to the fighting stage.

Your Story . . .

On a scale of 1–10 (or 100), how would you rate your anxiety?

_____

_____

_____

_____

_____

_____

_____

_____

How does that make you feel?

_____

_____

_____

_____

_____

_____

_____

_____

Coming Out of the Cancer Closet

But as for me, my prayer is to you, O Lord. At an acceptable time, O God, in the abundance of your steadfast love, answer me. (Ps. 69:13)

How I Felt . . .

Day three: yesterday I came out of the closet; the cancer closet with my friends and family. I was not sure how it would be received. I know sometimes that my writing can get to be too much for people. It is okay. I get that. However, I find writing therapeutic and this is my time to chronicle the good, the bad, the ugly, and the beautiful.

My aunt used to tell me I cried so prettily. If only she saw me yesterday as I scrolled through the overwhelming love and support sent to me via text, calls, e-mails, messages, and posts. I could not catch my breath at times. I sobbed. I cried. I snuffled. I slobbered. I felt unworthy of the love that was being sent. I was overwhelmed. Those hot spots under my cheeks seem to have taken up permanent residence. I do not feel deserving of such love. I am humbled that somehow, I have touched so many people that they felt called to reach out to my family and me. You all have done for me what I asked that I could not do myself. You have prayed for me with words I cannot articulate. I do not know how to say "thank you" in any possible way but "thanks." I mean, with all the crap in the world, there are so many awesome, loving people that make it an amazing place. There is hope for the world with all the amazing children of God who have touched my family and me. The news shows can take their negative crap and shove it. Amazing, beautiful, and miraculous people live around us far more than the garbage that is highlighted on a daily basis. When I see people loving each other, supporting each other, and reaching out to each other, I have hope. I know the world is going to be a better place when I see awesomeness happen between people. You all are the hope of the world.

The most amazing thing happened from the messages I received. I saw a glimmer of hope. I was not feeling hopeful before. I could not see past the shock, the misery, the anger, or the despair. I was fueled yesterday. That is an irreplaceable gift. I heard stories of those that have been through the same thing as I and have conquered their cancer. I have heard positive statistics and I have heard God's love through the actions of my family and friends. I am still not happy with my lot. I would wish it away in a heartbeat and I still pray the doctors are wrong. However, I am wrapped in the loving care of my friends and family and for that, I am grateful.

Yesterday marked the first trip to the oncologist. The vampires descended on my veins. I was pumped with radioactive isotopes for a PET scan and learned that my cancer is further along than I had hoped. It has snuck into my neck, chest, and abdomen. Next week I head in for two surgical procedures: a bone marrow biopsy to see if it has invaded my bones, and another to remove my appendix (they fear there is a tumor on it and they want to make sure there are no tumors elsewhere in my abdomen). We are working out details and figuring out my treatment plan, and how I will get care immediately upon arrival in DC. I cannot believe we are moving to Washington, DC, and I have just found out I have cancer. I have no understanding of what is going on in my life. I feel completely out of control. I am so afraid. This is the twilight zone. I keep hoping to wake up from this awful dream.

I do know the prayers and love make a difference. Please do not stop. God hears you even when my own prayers are feeble. You are praying for me now when I cannot. I have not lost faith. I still believe fiercely in God. I am simply so angry at this that God is the only thing strong enough to withstand my anger and still tell me it will be ok. I know it will be okay because I've been taught that God's got this. I doubt because I am human. I just don't know what to do with these feelings. I don't know how to talk to God. Someone else praying for me makes the words that I cannot.

What I Learned . . .

Get people praying for you; prayer works. It will be really rather hard for you to pray for yourself at first, so let others do that. People want to help and support you. They want to love you through this difficult time. They will want to cook for you, clean for you, take care of kids (if you have them), run errands, do laundry, and shop for you. Let them do whatever they ask, and don't be afraid to tell them how you like it. If you simply cannot let them help you, at least let them pray for you. *Let them pray.* Tell them what you need prayers for: Get this cancer out of my body! Peace. Serenity. Strength. Faith. Trust. Fabulous doctors. Comfort. Healing. (These are all great things to pray about.) The power of prayer is amazing. Get people to pray for you. It makes a *huge* difference. Tap into social media and let the social media world spread the word that *prayer is needed for you right now for an indefinite period.* I've had cancer for three-plus years now, and people are still praying for my cancer and me—and it makes a difference.

Right now. Go and get people to pray for you right now.

Seriously, people praying for you will rock your world. I am convinced that prayer exerts powerful positive energies in the world around us and on us. Prayers are epic superpowers that your friends have. Your friends and family cannot take your cancer from you, but they can pray for you. Let them use their superpowers for you in prayer. Prayers will cover you in a defense shield that not even the Death Star can pierce.

As a side note to my story: my husband is an Army officer. Three days before I found out about my cancer, we had submitted a contract offer on a house we were buying in our new duty station in Washington, DC. We had orders to move about three months after my diagnosis. Experts would advise that moving in the middle of a crisis is generally *not* recommended. Heck, I do not recommend it myself. However, as you will see as my story unfolds, both my husband and I thought that God was pushing us to DC. The Army offered to keep us in Kansas to see my treatment through, but we both felt God was telling us we needed to go. Sometimes, you need to have faith in the middle of these things. God knows me far better than I know myself, and this move was as much a part of my cancer story as the disease itself. Don't be afraid to trust God in the middle of your journey; sometimes God is working in weird and mysterious ways. Prayer is communication with God; you will feel better when you engage in a regular prayer life as part of your disease journey.

Your Story . . .

Make a list of the people you can ask to pray for you:

_____

_____

_____

_____

_____

_____

_____

_____

_____

_____

Go call, e-mail, write, or text them right now. Get them to pray for you.

_____

_____

_____

_____

_____

_____

_____

_____

_____

_____

_____

DAY 4
A Litany of "God Bless"

Blessed be God, because he has not rejected my prayer or removed his steadfast love from me. (Ps. 66:20)

How I Felt . . .

I actually woke up in a good mood. I have been sleeping well since starting the anxiety medication. It is a blessing. I keep waking up expecting to feel sick. Although emotionally bruised and battered, I do not feel bad. I am strong (my exercise habits have paid off) and my energy level is pretty good. I do not feel sick. I will randomly crack jokes. I keep asking the doctors if they are sure they have diagnosed me correctly. Don't cancer patients usually look and feel sick? I do not really look or feel different—at least not yet. When they start pumping my body full of poison, I'll stop thinking this. For now, it still seems unreal.

I tried to have a normal day today. I got up early to go to work. I usually enjoy work and it can be cathartic. I do not mind the mundane. Normal is good. Normal feels like I have control in my life. Normal doesn't have drama, disease, blood draws, and doctor visits. Practicing whatever "normal" is right now seems to be restorative and makes me feel a little less like a patient, and a little bit more like myself.

Going back to work makes me find a sense of "normal" in my otherwise out-of-control life. I did have a moment when I totally went off on someone for bringing up "stupid" in the middle of what I was trying to create as a normal day. In my defense, I have been assured the person *was* being stupid, but I generally do not go off on people. My tolerance for stupid right now is low, I guess.

However, in the middle of trying to find this feeling of "normal," everything was working against me: time, my computer, my brain, technical upgrades to the software I use, people, and red tape.

I was a slow-burning fuse . . . and then I got a call to go back to the hospital.

It was not going to wait until next week as planned. I was called back to the hospital to fit my prep testing in today. Next Thursday I will get a CT-guided bone marrow biopsy under sedation and a full appendectomy with exploration of my abdomen for more abnormalities. I have just realized that running, weight lifting, and all the things I enjoy will be out for a while. I am annoyed. To hell with running and weight lifting, it seems those things I do to be healthy are tabled too. I guess my goal will simply be to put one foot in front of the other. It is a one-day-at-a-time sort of life I live these days.

They've called me back to the hospital. This is the third time in three days. I am a nurse and I hate hospitals. They bring back every memory of being a sickly kid. I want to apologize to every patient I have ever had over the sheer indignity of the medical experience. I like to think that I was a good nurse, but I still want to apologize. The medical environment is so hard. I mean seriously, as a staff member you know your way around a building; as a patient it is a maze just as foreign as Timbuktu.

I have had amazing doctors, nurses, and support staff, but I have also given my full medical history to about ten people. I have been poked, prodded, stripped down, examined, and looked on with pity as they read my age and diagnosis. "How did you think you had cancer?" they ask.

I never thought I had cancer. In fact, during the diagnosis period, I was on a walk with a friend. She asked me if I thought I had cancer and I replied, "No, I would know if I had cancer." So much for my intuition. Some days, I am convinced my doctors are wrong about my diagnosis; except I have this annoying lump on my left clavicle that reminds me the doctors are right. It has begun to hurt. I think it is my mind . . . my mind . . . it seems to play tricks. My mind is a huge part of this journey, as is my body.

I am thirty-eight. Thirty-eight-year-olds should not have cancer. (For that matter *no one* should have cancer—if I haven't said it before, I'll say it again: this cancer crap sucks. Let us not sugar-coat it—this stuff does not belong in *anyone's* body.) This is not just about me. This is for every single person that has it. We all have one heartfelt, longing thought: go away and leave my family and me the hell alone. Forever.

Every time I have been at the hospital I have had at least six people ask me if I have an advanced directive or living will. I fell apart on the first lady who asked me. Poor lady—I made her cry. Thirty-eight-year-olds should not need advanced directives and living wills. That sort of question is just plain wrong. I mean it is right, but just wrong in the place where I am in life. So, I bawled. Who wants to talk about how they want to die? Most people don't.

Then they ask me if I am an organ donor—which I am proudly. I am just not ready to give them up yet—and no one is going to want my organs after this. At least I don't think so. Who wants organs from a cancer girl? I might think I am a superhero, but my organs aren't acting like superheroes. Sigh.

The medical world we live in is so sterile. It is only made human by the kind people that work in this bureaucracy of healthcare . . . they are the only things that bring a humanistic sense of something warm and friendly to an environment that strips you of all that you are. God bless humans for being a part of that sterile world.

I do not miss working the clinical setting as a nurse, but I know if I ever go back, my patients will never be just patients to me *ever* again. They are people. People in the hospital are in a situation that strips them of any sense of normal, and any sense of dignity. Any sense of feeling they are in control. Between the decor, the questions, the garbage on TV, the waiting (waiting, waiting, and waiting), the smell, the fake lights, and the technology—everything screams that nothing natural goes on here. Except the people—the people give it some sense that I am not alone.

God bless my nurse today. Wendy let me put my head between my legs and breathe as she asked me questions while I almost hyperventilated. God bless Monique, the woman who joked with me about getting a tattoo, as she looked me up in the computer. God bless Theresa who cried all over me as I cried all over her when she asked me for an advanced directive. God bless Dr. Jax who promised he would not make any mistakes in my surgery. God bless Dr. Ludwig who called me in a prescription for Xanax without making me feel weak or stupid for needing help. God bless Sherri who has arranged all my appointments.

God bless Dr. Johnson who showed me how to be objective about my cancer in the middle of my meltdown. And y'all, pray for a good case manager for me who will help me seamlessly transition my care from Kansas to Virginia.

God bless my friends—I cannot say enough. And God bless Treb, my kids, and all my family. In the middle of this cancer garbage—I am blessed.

What I Learned . . .

I mentioned this above: *My mind is as much a part of this journey as my body.* I think this was an important learning point at this stage. I became aware that my mind could play into "having cancer" as much as my body. This is not to say that you should *not* listen to your mind. Rather, it is very important to be aware of your thoughts and feelings toward your body as well as your cancer; our emotional responses can trigger physical responses. You need to slow down and determine if what you are feeling is your body or your mind. Practicing mindfulness in the middle of these emotional responses can help you sort through the overwhelming thoughts, emotions, and physical responses you are having.

Your mind can be a huge asset in your journey forward. You are still allowed the time to grieve, be angry, or be frustrated. You should think and feel at every stage that this cancer journey is not fair; it is inconvenient, scary, anger-inducing, and on and on. I have always said, and probably will always feel, that no one has time for cancer. We all have better things to do. Because of your feelings, your tolerance for what you think is stupid may be low as well. You may find yourself impatient with others. Give yourself a pass. You have a disease. Your emotions may be high. Like me, you may go off on someone. You can always apologize, but don't beat yourself up if it happens. A lot of things may feel stupid when you have cancer.

However, even in the midst of high emotions, you can get your mind engaged with a heroic mindset that you are going to be a fighter and a winner. I am a believer that your vision of yourself can help you see yourself where you want to be. That may be as a warrior, or a survivor, or a hero(ine), or a tree withstanding a thunderstorm, or a clay pot that is transformed by the fire you have entered. See a positive image of yourself and hold on to this in your mind's eye. Do not give in to your cancer or whatever disease you fight. Your superpowers are greater than your disease. *You* are more than your cancer.

Recognize those who are fighting with you in your battle; you are not as alone as you may feel. As you develop this vision for yourself, let your mind also find reflections of God in your life, your doctors, nurses, case manager, friends, appointment technicians, and anyone else that touches you along the way. This is called counting your blessings. When you count your blessings, and focus on positive moments in your journey, it will help you focus your mind in a positive stance versus a negative one. Your mind and soul have power on your journey that you can use. I once wrote in *Christ Walk: A 40-Day Spiritual Fitness Program* (Morehouse, 2015) that your attitude and perception of events are directly related.

The Attitude/Perception Correlation

Your perception of this event in your life is directly related to your mental attitude about it. I strongly believe you can reprogram your thoughts and feelings about this cancer in your life and construct it into something purposeful.

After all, I believe you are more than your disease and there is purpose for you in God's world even with cancer. God loves you, I love you, and you are so much more than this.

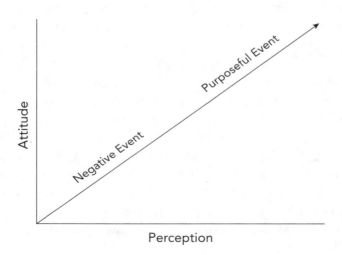

Your Story . . .

What are some things your mind is telling you right now?

_____

_____

_____

_____

_____

_____

_____

_____

_____

_____

What are some things your body is telling you right now?

_____

_____

_____

_____

_____

_____

_____

_____

_____

_____

_____

What are some blessings you have right now?

_____

_____

_____

_____

_____

_____

_____

_____

_____

In Sickness and in Health

For my thoughts are not your thoughts, nor are your ways my ways,
says the Lord. (Isa. 55:8)

How I Felt . . .

I am not sure what is going on in my life. I am hypersensitive to the passage of time and events right now. Important personal interactions are resonating in my heart on a deep level. I wonder in a very dark part of my brain if these are the last times I will have these experiences. I wonder secretly if things will go wrong, so each moment becomes extra special. I treasure my experiences deeply. I secretly fear this will be the last trip, the last adventure, the last time with friends, family, and loved ones. The fear is not reality, but it is there. I have never been an especially sentimental person, but now, when faced with this disease, events seem more important than ever.

On the one hand, I feel very alive; on the other, I feel incredibly broken. I feel as though time, events, health, life, and those things that really matter converged this weekend. It is the first time I have felt a glimmer of grace and hope in the middle of all the turbulence.

We flew to Seattle this weekend to celebrate the wedding of a dear friend to a wonderful woman. Ironically, at the time my lymph nodes were beginning to swell and grow with cancer, we were on our way through the Southwest and were stopping to see these friends at their new home. Unknown to us, the night before we had arrived, they became engaged to marry. We were some of the first people to get to celebrate with them on their new engagement. Over margaritas, red chili sauce, and *sopapillas*, we toasted the joy of two fantastic people finding each other. I remember how happy I was that Jason and Sarah had finally found each other. We were so excited for them. It reminds me how blessed I am to have found my husband. New love is a heady emotion. Love makes me smile.

As summer unfolded and I began to go through multiple tests to figure out what was wrong with me, we had continued to correspond with Jason and Sarah about their big day. We still had no clue there was cancer. No one really thought I had cancer, let alone me. Keep in mind, overall, I still feel fine. I have symptoms, but they don't seem dire.

I had told Treb long ago that when our friend Jason finally tied the knot, we would be there. We bought our tickets and got the kids excited about attending their first wedding. Jason and Sarah had asked us to do one of the readings during the service and we were honored to be included in their day. I love to read the Bible aloud at church. I can think of no better way to be a part of someone's wedding.

Three days before we were to fly out for this great event, I found out about my cancer. I looked at Treb and told him I could not get up in front of a group of people and read God's Word. There was no way the words would come out without me crying. At the end of the day, I did not want Jason's wedding to be about me. I wanted it to be about their love. We called Jason to tell them we would still be there, but that Treb would speak for both of us. My heart would be 100 percent there, if not my voice. Once again, I felt shame and guilt that I could not control myself, especially when I love God and the church, but I was still angry and hurt inside, and I knew this was the right decision. I did not want this day to be about me or about cancer.

As Treb stood up to read from Isaiah at the wedding, I cried because I could not do it myself. I cried because it was a wedding and because my heart is still so very raw. As Jason and Sarah pledged to love one another through sickness and health until death do them part, I could not stop the stream of tears. I turned to Treb and simply said, "Thank you." I am sure, when he married me eighteen years ago, he did not think he would *really* love me through *sickness*, but he is. As Jason and Sarah start their life together, I know Jason will love her through sickness and health as well.

What I Learned . . .

Not everyone is lucky enough to have a partner during their cancer or illness trial. I am beyond graced that my husband, Treb, was by my side. When you marry, you say the words "in sickness and in health" thinking that really, that will not be you or your spouse. When you are young, naïve, and filled with love, it is incredibly difficult to see the other parts of your love story unfolding with events beyond your control. When you get married, you do not envision a happily ever after stalked by disease.

If there is one thing I have learned (and would love to teach any young adult), it is that people are not the same people over time. I am not the same person I was when I was twenty. Young people have a tendency not to see the experiences of older adults, their own battle scars, their own tragedies, and how life has molded them. Young folks are insular, hyper-self-aware, and hyper-"in the moment." This is not a criticism, as I experienced it myself, and sometimes I still do, but there is a habit of looking at life through a microscope. Your life today is not the same as it will be tomorrow, in a year, in five years. Time changes.

There is an opportunity for love in the middle of all the cancer. If you have a spouse, partner, or other loved one(s), you can grow with them. You are not alone. They are a part of your story as well. They suffer too, as you suffer. They may not be ill, but their life changed when you got sick. They may not know how to respond, or how you will react to anything they say or do.

Remember, you are hypersensitive right now and sometimes our emotional reactions are fierce and strong, even to those we love. Try to be aware of that as you go through this process. Be together in your quest to beat cancer; try not to push people away. They want to help. Even if you just want to be left alone. Even if you are angry that they cannot understand what you are experiencing and feeling. Even if secretly you are angry that you got sick and not someone else. It is okay. However, be aware, as sometimes we say things to those we love that hurt them (often more than anything we say to anyone else), because we are so hurt ourselves.

I am fairly sure over the course of dealing with my diagnosis that I dropped many expletives and accusations, and hurled various profanities without thinking of what I was saying, what I was doing, or who I was aiming my words at. I remember sitting in the car trying to come up with the courage to tell my mom about my cancer and when I did, I screamed "@#!?ing cancer" at my mother. I do not think I have ever dropped the f-bomb in front of my mom. I owe her an apology. I generally do not like to cuss, but if there was ever a moment, I guess that was it. I don't recall a moment in my life I have ever been so angry.

Fortunately, my mom and all my other loved ones have forgiven me my words, my shortness, my anger, and my meanness. They will love you too through yours, but I think it is important for us, as patients, to also realize that they hurt too.

My mom, my husband, my best friends . . . they would have all taken my cancer from me if they could, but when they couldn't do that, they were at least there. These people are heroes too, because they stick with you through the good, the bad, and the ugly, and in the end, they still love you.

There will be times you will injure people with your words or actions. I know it won't be intentional, but at some juncture in your journey, you'll do something you regret. At some point, you should fix this. Apologize, if for no other reason than apologies release their own burdens on your soul. Most people I know accept apologies and move on. Those that don't, well, you cannot own their behavior. You can only own your own. If along the way, you did something that you think hurt someone, make the time to apologize. It's good for your soul.

There will be some friends that push away. I had friends that simply could not handle the force of my feelings and dejection and they stepped back. I don't blame them. I don't know what they have been through in life that may have triggered this response. Don't judge those that withdraw. They may not know that they withdraw or hurt you, or why they do it. You don't know where they've been on their journey. It doesn't mean that they don't care; not all of life is about you or your disease. It's hard to believe, but other people are struggling now too. Remember God asks us to love others as we would like to be loved. That's a call of action for you, not a judgment on others.

What I learned from this love story is that people care a lot. Their hearts are breaking for your situation. There is a part of your friends and family that have been attacked by this disease now even if it's not in their body. When you get to the right point, when you can step back and take a breath, be aware of those you love and how they feel too.

Your Story . . .

Who are your loved ones?

_____

_____

_____

_____

_____

_____

_____

_____

What are some things you've said that weigh on your mind?

_____

_____

_____

_____

_____

_____

_____

_____

What's your favorite cuss word or phrase?

_____

_____

_____

_____

_____

_____

_____

_____

Are there things you need to ask forgiveness for?

_____

_____

_____

_____

_____

_____

_____

_____

_____

Today I Felt Normal

He is the reflection of God's glory and the exact imprint of God's very being, and he sustains all things by his powerful word. (Heb. 1:3a)

How I Felt . . .

Today was a priceless, priceless gift. Today I felt normal.

A perk of attending a wedding in an old duty station was the opportunity to see dear military friends. We spent the rest of our weekend in the Pacific Northwest finding respite. Soon enough, hospitals and doctors will return, but for this little sliver of peace, we have been able to laugh, smile, love, hug, share, and be with friends away from the cancer. Sure, we have talked about it, but it didn't rule the weekend. For the first time in the last five days, I didn't feel defined by my diagnosis.

We spent our day hiking on one of God's most precious creations: Mount Rainier. Both Treb and I have a special love for this mountain from our time spent at Fort Lewis, Washington. I climbed to Camp Muir when we lived here, which was one of the most physically challenging feats I personally have accomplished in my life. I love that memory of climbing to Camp Muir. At 10,000-plus feet in the air, your perception of everything changes.

Going to Rainier for me was very healing. Hiking to Panorama Point showed me that my body was still strong. I could still do this. Each step affirmed me as a person. Each smell cleared my body—I felt as though I was breathing in the spirit of the world and the spirit of God. God smells like crisp snow. God feels like ice-cold air. God looks like the first buds of spring pushing through the passing of winter. God sounds like the birds that have returned to the mountain and the steps I took up the hill. I could hear each step I took in tune with the beating of my heart. The sounds resonate with my soul. I can experience

God with each of my senses when I am outdoors. These experiences of God nurture the joy I haven't felt in a while. I smiled without feeling as though it was forced or as if I needed to show everyone that I was okay. When I was outdoors, using my body, just being with nature, I was okay. *I was okay.*

I loved almost every moment of it, except the massive meltdown my little girl had halfway up the trail. (Her scream was so piercing you could hear it at the end of the trail. One old gentleman walked back down the hill to give me chocolate, she was screeching so loud.) This moment reminded me that my sickness doesn't affect just me. It affects my babies. This makes me resent my disease more than anything. Much like any other mom, I want to protect my children. I would shield them from every moment of it if I could. I hate knowing that they know their mom is different. I hate that they will always associate cancer and me. And I hate that every time they hear about someone dying from cancer, they wonder if the same will happen to their mom. Their world has been rocked as well.

But as we settled down and found our calm, both of us continued on to make it to our final destination at Panorama Point. The view was completely obscured by fog. We had made it, but couldn't see the view. Such are many things in life. You can set out on one journey with a specific goal, and you can reach that goal and be left empty. You can have all the plans you want in the world, but really, all you have are intentions. Things can change at a moment's notice and you will have no control over the outcome.

There is a lot to learn from climbing a mountain.

But as we descended again, the clouds parted and there she was. If you've been to Rainier, you know exactly what I am describing. If you have not, when the clouds part and Mount Rainier shows her magnificence, everything else seems smaller in comparison. People stop in midsentence. Breathtaking, speech-taking, thought-taking immenseness. Rainier is a magical place on earth. My husband prayed to see Mount Rainier because it is often hidden in the clouds. I told Treb to start praying as hard for me to get well as he prayed to see his mountain this weekend.

When Mount Rainier shows herself, you feel blessed.

When you see Mount Rainier, problems seem so much smaller.

My problems seemed smaller this weekend. I've been blessed by this trip. From being a part of a beautiful wedding, the hospitality of great friends, and a wonderful day hiking on Rainier, I found a sense of balance and peace I sorely needed. I'm sure it won't last, but it was a good reminder that there can still be great days even in the midst of darkness.

What I Learned . . .

If you have the means, the capability, and the time before your treatment, go do something fun. Do something that will remind you of what you love about life. This trip reminded me of friends, love, fun, hiking, and being active, as well as people and places that I care deeply about. For me, this trip was an invaluable reminder of why I want to live and why I really do not think it is my time to go. This cancer is a hiccup in the scope of my life. Your cancer, illness, or tragedy will hopefully also be a hiccup in the scope of your life. No matter what happens, or how you live and devote your life, even in the scope of disease it can be done from a place of being Christ-centered.

You can see your disease process as a participatory experience in the suffering of Christ. You can rise above this suffering as a dedicated moment to God. You can use your disease process as an opportunity for others to minister as Christ to you. Let go and allow others to love you deeply. It is an opportunity to love others deeply in return and share your journey with others. You are not the only person hurting, grieving, sick, or fighting during your disease. We are called to minister and be ministered to during all phases of life. Our disease should not be one of isolation.

I have said it before, and I will say it again: people want to be a part of your life with your diagnosis and you should let them. They will lift you up when you are down, and be there for you when you did not even know you needed someone. People will send you gifts. I have a collection of bracelets—one with guardian angels, one with an energy prayer, one with "brave" stamped in silver, another with "love," yet another with "faith, peace, and friendship" emblazoned as a prayer. I have a prayer shawl, books, food, caps and hats for if I lost my hair, gifts people made and knit, or long messages of uplifting prayer and love. One friend sent me a box of a whiskey and chocolate sampler that made me laugh and cry—sometimes you just have to face cancer with whiskey and chocolate. And I had friends who gave me their time with walks and ears and text fests, just listening to me whine through the year of coming to terms with my cancer.

And all this love made me uncomfortable. I had no idea how to say "thank you." It seemed woefully inadequate. Even as I write this, I am not sure that I will ever be able to repay the love and generosity of all the people who touched my life during this time. It makes me even more uncomfortable to know that there is no paying it all back. Just like Jesus died on the cross for me, and I am unable to pay back that gift, I am unable to repay the kindness of others. The only way I can hope to honor that love is to love as generously back to others in my shoes and to those that have loved me unconditionally so far.

When you are sick, it is difficult to let people in. When you hurt so fiercely, feeling that your body has violated you, love is something that hurts as much as it helps. It hurts because you are afraid of getting close. It hurts because you are afraid of losing people. It hurts because sometimes those we love are an emotional burden that we cannot deal with in the middle of our own emotional turmoil. It hurts because sometimes we don't know how to process all these feelings. It can be overwhelming.

Let others love you through this time. God tells us to love God and love our neighbor. You are letting others fulfill their call when they love you. And where there is love, there is God, and I think having God in the middle of your cancer is a really important thing. That love brings some fierce superpowers into the middle of the battle. Love is like Superman's kryptonite. The power it will have in this journey of your life may make you uncomfortable, but your life will be so much more uncomfortable without it.

Your Story . . .

Is there a "getaway" place you can visit either before your treatment or during a break? Is there a place that makes you feel alive again?

_____

_____

_____

_____

_____

_____

_____

_____

What are some ways you can let people love you?

_____

_____

_____

_____

_____

_____

_____

_____

What are some gifts you treasure so far?

_____

_____

_____

_____

_____

_____

_____

_____

_____

Answer This *One* Question

The Lord sustains them on their sickbed; in their illness you heal all their infirmities. (Ps. 41:3)

How I Felt . . .

One week into this journey and I need an answer. What do you tell your child when they ask you if the cancer is going to kill their mommy?

Where is the guidebook; the parenting book; the answer that won't scar them for life; the answer that isn't a lie; a response that will not make them hate God; or an answer that will not fill them with fear? I'm not equipped for this.

All the love in the world cannot promise my children that the cancer won't kill me. The probabilities are not in favor of the cancer winning. I have a treatable but noncurable cancer (it's a weird one; more like a chronic disease). I am young, healthy, and therapies get better and better each year. However, for all the probabilities and statistics, I cannot promise my children that this won't kill me. It might not kill me quickly, but it could kill me when I am old. Who knows? I could die crossing the street tomorrow. No one can promise my children that I won't die early. As my mom told me, we begin to die as soon as we are born.

However, it is cold comfort when you're faced with a serious illness. Everyone wonders what the disease will do to me. The worry of the unknown presses us down and I think too much. My kids think about it; we all think about it. I know I think about it way too much. No one likes to think about their death.

I know my kids are afraid and I know they hold it in. They are tough. My kids are the warriors. They look in my face and they know I am afraid and cannot give them the pat answer they want. Of course we laugh at it. Their mommy is too stubborn to let cancer kill her. We say, "Mommy is too sassy for cancer." However, I cannot promise them that nothing bad will happen. I do not have answers for this question right now and it eats at me.

I cannot say to them that if I die, it is God's will, because I do not believe that. This journey isn't just about me. It is about this disease and how it has infected all of us as a family. Of all the stupid stuff I've come to terms with over this week, this is the one question that stops me in my tracks. I bumble through my responses, I hem and I haw and I answer somewhere between "no" and "Mommy will fight this tooth and nail." And yet none of my responses feel right.

How would you answer it?

What I Learned . . .

What did I learn? There is no *right* way to handle this question and every parent in my shoes feels the crushing weight of this question. Every parent simply wants to raise their children, see them succeed, grow old, marry, have their own children, and find happiness. No parent wants to leave their child—at least not me. And I'd give anything not to have had that discussion or hear that question from my babies. No one wants to have this discussion of death.

Even healthy people do not really like talking about death even though it is inevitable for all of us. We all start to die the moment we are born. We just do not really think of the journey as having an ending when we have a life filled with work, family, kids, activities, prayer, mission, you name it.

Kids want to think their parents are invincible. A parent becoming suddenly ill rocks their world. They do not have the knowledge to process what is happening to the body. They often fear that what is going on with you will also happen to them. You may notice an increase in hypochondria in your kids once you are diagnosed. They may start searching for signs of cancer in their own body. They start to wonder what might happen to them if you die. This is incredibly scary for kids, let alone the parent(s) that need to have this discussion with their children. I loathed having to tell my kids about my disease. It did not even cross my mind that they would ask me if I would die.

It was a conversation I was not prepared to have. I'll say it again: no parent really wants to have this discussion with their kids.

In this situation, I am a real advocate that parents know their kids and will give them the information in a way they know their kids will process it best. I believe in being honest with our kids. We cannot protect them from the ills of the world, but we can love them and be honest. Kids are not stupid. They will know something is up if you try to keep your illness from them; this will create its own fear. Your hospital will have a psychologist or social worker on staff if you need help finding the right words to use for your kids' developmental level. There are tons of resources on the internet to assist you as well. I needed to have the conversation much more quickly than I had time to do research, so my husband and I just held hands and prayed fiercely that we would find the right words and hold our kids close throughout our sharing the information.

We answered their questions honestly. I showed them my surgical scars. I explained that many cancers are different. We told them that some of their questions could not be answered because we did not have that information yet. We talked about the potential hair loss (which *really* bothered my daughter). We shared how I would not feel well and could not lift things for a long time after my surgery. We made them a part of the process so that we were doing this together.

When it came to my son's question, "Are you going to die?" I still do not know if I answered it right. I did tell both my kids that we all die. It's important for all kids to understand that death is a part of life. It's a good opening for discussing the gift of eternal life that Jesus gives us through the crucifixion and resurrection. In this case, however, they knew that people died, but they wanted to know if their mother was going to die from this disease. I did what a lot of people do: I told them I did not plan on dying, I was going to fight, and we were going to combat it together, but we could not make any promises amidst so much uncertainty. I told my son I could die the next day from an accident. I would not promise I would be there forever. I told them that the most important thing we could do was to love one another fiercely. Then we coined a term: "Mommy is too sassy for cancer." To this day, my kids ask me if I am still too sassy for cancer and I reply that I am trying, every day, to be too sassy for cancer.

Come be sassy with me.

Your Story . . .

On a scale of 1–10 (or 100), how is your sassy meter?

_____

_____

_____

_____

_____

_____

_____

_____

On a scale of 0–100, how do you feel about dying?

_____

_____

_____

_____

_____

_____

_____

_____

_____

What's the one cancer (or other illness) conversation that you *really* don't want to ever have?

_____

_____

_____

_____

_____

_____

_____

_____

_____

_____

How are you feeling about your cancer (or illness) today?

_____

_____

_____

_____

_____

_____

_____

_____

_____

11
The Whispers of God at Midnight

"Let us be silent, that we may hear the whispers of God."
—Ralph Waldo Emerson

How I Felt . . .

It's three o'clock in the morning. I cannot sleep.

I'll say it again: I really cannot stand hospitals or doctors as a patient. I don't like depending on others. It's ironic because I love working in the healthcare field. Nevertheless, for all that I hate being in a hospital, my care has been fantastic.

Yesterday was a day I prefer not to repeat anytime soon. The bone marrow biopsy was a breeze thanks to sedation. I am assuming that my appendectomy was a piece of cake since my appendix is now gone. They told me that they found no tumors in my abdomen. Praise God.

However . . .

The recovery period bites. They told me I got sick between the procedures, although I have no memory of it. All I recall was awakening after it was all over in my hospital room in excruciating pain and getting sick over and over again. It took forever for them to get it under control. My body simply does not like anesthesia. I puke for hours on end. I have a three-inch incision in my gut. Puking and incisions just don't mix. They. Do. Not. Mix. Lord, have mercy, it hurts.

I have new respect for my friends that had C-sections. I cannot laugh, sneeze, or cough without excruciating pain. It's ridiculous that just two weeks ago I wrote on loving my body, scars and all, as the blueprint of my life on my skin. I now have five new ones to embrace with my lot. No bikinis this year.

Through it all, people I know and don't know have lifted me. I've felt the prayers from around the world. I am wrapped in a prayer shawl from the ladies in my church. I have Episcopalians, Catholics,

Methodists, Presbyterians, Lutherans, Baptists, a Buddhist, several Muslims, and my Jewish friends praying over me. Illness is the great ecumenical event. There are no denominations in cancer. I'm not picky where the prayers are coming from. I know God hears them all. I think God is a lot greater than any of us can understand.

I am wrapped in care. Now begins the road to recovery from step 1. Step 2 in this cancer process will bring a whole new set of experiences and prayers and trials that I hope to share. But for now, I feel like I've made it through a big one.

What I Learned . . .

I am a terrible patient. I am humbled by the experience. It can be the most degrading, humiliating, and dehumanizing event in one's life. Receiving medical care requires patience, which is the opposite of being in control. I hate it. I detested being dependent on all those people, no matter how necessary it was. I bet many people feel this way. It makes me want to go back to the years when I was a nurse and apologize to all my patients if I *ever* made them feel anything less than a precious human. The medical institution really is not designed to take care of the whole person. It fixes pieces of you at a time, unless you are really, really lucky to find a doctor that looks at all of you as a whole being.

I also learned that pain is degrading. Pain strips you of your strength. Pain can turn you into a blubbering idiot. Pain makes you irrational. Pain makes you short-tempered and irritable. Pain from abdominal surgery makes you constipated. Seriously, pooping hurts. Between the docs taking a spoon and stirring up my intestines, putting me on meds that send those intestines to sleep, and then trying to wake those intestines back up to do their job, it's excruciating. Pooping is the seventh ring of hell postsurgery, especially with an abdominal incision.

You will warrior your way through the pain. The pain is not forever; it is a phase of the journey. The pain may come and go. You may learn to tolerate the pain. You may not even have surgery as a part of your cancer treatment. That does not necessarily mean you won't have pain—it will just be different pain. Remember every approach to *your* cancer treatment is different. This was just mine. I like to think that when you have an idea of the experience, it helps you feel less alone, so I will continue to be frank about what I learned, because my goal is to help you—even if that includes a discourse on poop.

More than likely you *will* experience pain of some sort in your cancer journey. Be honest with your docs about your discomfort level, and be diligent about trying to stay on top of the pain cycle. This is one of those things that you need to address on a regular schedule. If you let it get out of hand, it makes it that much harder to control. Pain needs to be stayed on top of; don't let it sneak out of control. Take your painkillers on a regular schedule as decided by you and your doc and stick with it. If that schedule does not work, tell your doc. There are many options for pain control.

From my personal experience, drugs were not the most effective mechanism for dealing with my pain. I found acupuncture and a specific yoga regimen to be a better form of pain control, but that may require you to pay out of pocket for that expense if your insurance does not cover it. If it is a choice you have, try it. I like those kinds of choices; it makes you feel like you are more in control of your experience when you *do* have choices.

Pain is a serious matter during cancer treatment. Take it seriously and let the professionals take care of you and your pain. You are not being weak. You are being proactive. You will be a nicer person as a result of good pain control, more able to interact with others, and less irritable.

But take a stool softener, because you do not want painful constipation on top of it all—especially if you had abdominal surgery in conjunction with everything like me. Practice safe, pain-free pooping. Having cancer is bad enough—pooping should not hurt.

Your Story . . .

On a scale of 1–10 (or 100), how is your pain today?

_____

_____

_____

_____

_____

_____

_____

_____

_____

_____

Is your pain control method working?

_____

_____

_____

_____

_____

_____

_____

_____

_____

What do you need to tell your doctor about your pain?

_____

_____

_____

_____

_____

_____

_____

_____

_____

_____

How is your pooping?

_____

_____

_____

_____

_____

_____

_____

_____

_____

_____

DAY 12
Don't Play the Gambling Game

When you realize your guilt in any of these, you shall confess the sin that you have committed. (Lev. 5:5)

How I Felt . . .

I hate surgery. I hate coming out of the anesthetic. I get sick as the drugs wear off, and once it starts, it is really hard to stop. It's like once I've upchucked, my brain tells my stomach, "Don't stop!" And it keeps going and going and going. I hate puking about as much as I hate anything.

I've talked pooping. Let's talk puking. For hours. Just keeping this honest. My body does not like most chemicals. And so, I puke and puke and puke. I am going to suck at chemo. Zofran (an antivomiting medicine) is a Godsend. It takes the edge off. It did not keep me from getting sick, but it helped tremendously.

My whole body aches as though they dropped me off the operating room table. I actually asked my doc what else they did to me because while my abdomen hurts, my neck and shoulder are also on fire. My neck and back start to spasm from shielding my incision site. I cannot get comfortable. I cannot move unless I have help. I absolutely loathe not being able to do anything. I don't sit still well at all. It makes me a grumpy patient. I can't poop, I'm sick, and I hurt. Just stay away. I'm completely miserable.

However, it gives me lots of time to think and write. And it gives me the time to think through some of my private guilt over the cancer. I feel guilty. On top of all the other stuff, guilt eats at me.

I thought I had paid my health woe dues: asthma, hearing loss, and autoimmune disease are just a few to add to my history of chronic disease. I thought that the burden of illness on my body had been paid in full for a lifetime. My horrible preconceived notion that each of us has

41

our list of tragedies and they all balance out in the end is not working. In my mind, I play a statistics game of percentages; the likelihood that I would get cancer or some other additional disease was very small. In the statistics game, I'm an outlier, an aberration, someone where the numbers just don't add up. From the numbers game I play, I really shouldn't have cancer. Or so I think. I thought all my weird health problems covered the spread. I assumed I paid my dues by the time I was sixteen years old and lost all my hearing.

I guess this made me a little cocky about my health. Sure, I continue to balance the management of my chronic disease with a healthy lifestyle, but I figured I had already had my trial with my hearing loss. I had paid my dues, survived, and become stronger and more deeply involved in my faith as a result. God's will had worked through me and I was good.

I could look at a group of people and think that it would be someone else that would meet the statistic and not me. Now I feel shameful because it is a terrible way to think, but it was my weird, twisted way of dealing with an ongoing enduring illness. Someone else would have to pay the disease check because I had already paid my portion. I made a lot of assumptions about my health. Well, you know what happens when you assume. I made an ass out of myself. What an ignorant way to think on my part. And it's a shameful way to think. Hence the guilt.

The truth of the matter is the body is weird. It does weird things without reason. Different people react to different pathogens, viruses, and bacteria. Sometimes the body's response is illogical. Sometimes it just does not make sense or fit the statistics. Bad things sometimes happen to good people without reason. I'm trying to work through the realization that this did not happen to me because I am a bad person.

Sometimes crap just happens. There isn't a checklist of who gets what. We are all given talents and burdens commensurate with what we can handle with God's grace. In this time of my life, God is holding this together for me more than anything I've done for myself. I certainly could not walk this journey on my own. I feel ridiculously weak, broken, dejected, and rejected. I hold on to my faith like the security blanket of my youth. I curl into a pitiful ball of humanity that just wants mommy to take care of it all. I feel unworthy as a child of God.

Gambling with statistics is just a stupid way to approach the thoughts about my health, and it set me up for such great disappointment. Sometimes, things just happen. And in my case, I am young (relatively), healthy, and strong, and I have an amazing family worth living for. This isn't the end of the world for me. My story is not over. I really don't believe that God's work for me is done in this world. I am working very hard on trusting that God has a reason for all of this, even if I don't understand it myself.

What I Learned . . .

Superheroes are not invincible. There isn't equity in suffering or disease. I think we all go through something. And just so you know, almost every cancer patient has had this thought, even if fleeting, of "What did I do wrong to have this happen to me?" You didn't do anything wrong.

@#!? happens.

Good people suffer as much as bad people.

Suffering is a part of the human condition.

Disease and illness are a part of the human life cycle.

You are not the gambler. Know when to fold your cards to God.

But despite the shit storm that can happen, I also know:

God is faithful.

God keeps God's promises.

God is there even when we do not feel God.

God does not see shame in our thoughts and feelings. God sees the potential for growth.

God sees our purpose even in the middle of disease and infirmity. We are children of God at all stages of our life journey. God loves us in our valleys as much as God loves us on the mountaintop. God loves all of us. God is loving my cancer cells into oblivion.

God is not a statistic. God is not a gamble. God is a sure deal for the peace you seek in the middle of the firestorm that your life has become.

Don't give up. Hold on to God as your security blanket. Call out to God in the darkness of your nights blubbering like a baby.

Bad things happen to good people just like they happen to "bad" people.

But God happens to all. Don't shut God out. God is there.

Your Story . . .

Where is God in your story?

_____

_____

_____

_____

_____

_____

_____

_____

What are your secret thoughts about why you got cancer (or your illness)?

_____

_____

_____

_____

_____

_____

_____

_____

Do you feel like you are being punished?

_____

_____

_____

_____

_____

_____

_____

_____

Where do you see redemption in your story?

_____

_____

_____

_____

_____

_____

_____

_____

What Pain Will Do to You

He will wipe every tear from their eyes. Death will be no more; mourning and crying and pain will be no more, for the first things have passed away. (Rev. 21:4)

How I Felt . . .

I've lost track of the days. How many days has it been since my C-day? My cancer day; the day where my life changed. I don't know. My pain is worse. Things are not getting better; they are going downhill. The pain I feel has taken over my life. This isn't soul pain. My. Body. Hurts. Something happened in my surgery. They tell me I am wrong. They keep telling me it is cancer pain. I don't believe them. I don't think this is cancer pain. I think they messed up my surgery. Something isn't right in my body.

I feel terrible. This pain is such a discouraging sensation. When you don't feel well, it's hard to see greener grass. I can be trucking along with all the upbeat positive vibes in the world and my usual "can-do" attitude, and then the fear and pain takes my breath away.

It's a very physical sensation. My lungs don't feel as though they can fully expand. My breath hitches in the back of my throat. My heart squeezes tight and I am overwhelmed with the wrong type of thoughts. Dread engulfs me. My eyes bead with tears and negativity overwhelms me. I am a happy person. This is not me.

Every movement sends scorching pain along my nerves. I lose feeling from time to time in my hand and arm. I can't move right and every shift in my body as I try to adjust is agony. I think they stuck a hot poker in my shoulder and twirled it around like spaghetti on a fork. This is not normal. I do not know what is going on and I am not getting the help I need. They just keep upping my pain meds. I don't think that's what I need. This disagreement with my doctors makes me feel a little crazy. They are making me feel like this is in my head. They aren't listening to me. They are telling me this is the new normal. I am in denial. I am in rebellion. This is not the normal I accept.

The pain makes me think I cannot win. It saps my superpowers. It attacks God's grace in my life. I can see why people think of fear as the devil. Fear sinks into my mind . . . it makes me think that I cannot beat this unrelenting pain. My whole *self* feels covered in a black malaise. I am cloaked with a feeling that an intruder has entered my being. I am not in control of my body. I am a parasite in my own self. Terror snakes through my nerve endings. I feel it pulsing through my veins. Each breath pulses with the word: *fear*. I am crazy.

Fear. Fear. Fear. An ongoing echo takes over when the pain is out of control. This leads to worry.

Worry. Worry. Worry. I worry that I will kiss my children good-bye on my deathbed. I do not want this. I am in a constant battle with myself over placing all my trust in God and trying to control the outcome of this season. It is an impossible battle that rages in my heart. The battle is fierce, friends. It comes and goes. Sometimes I am better at it than others. Some days I need medication to help me. With pain, I am weakened.

Some nights my castle is strong.

Some nights the mortar crumbles.

I am scared. I am hurting. And I really think I am going crazy.

What I Learned . . .

I am not crazy. But pain sure as hell can make you feel like you are. Pain is a conduit to fear. Fear is a conduit to anxiety. Anxiety leads to worry. Worry brings doubt. Doubt makes you sad. And the sadness brings questions. It can turn into an endless cycle unless you are aware of it and harness it. The endless cycle makes you think you are losing your mind. Especially if your healthcare team isn't listening to you.

This is what I experienced. When I am hurting, it's far easier for the bleak thoughts to take over. At these times, I reread the notes that I have been sent to lift me up and remember that I am stronger than all this. I have angels watching over me. You do too. I know God knows the petitions of my heart (I have been a broken record about them). He hears yours too. I know I must be brave. You can be brave too. When fear clawed at me, I would practice a bit of a mantra with the experience (you can practice this too):

> With each breath of fear, strike back: "I trust in God." With each pulse of anxiety, parry: "My soul waits on the Lord." With every hitch of worry, throw up a shield: "God is my shield and strength."

Each time the fear came on, I would get up again and repeat my mantra: Trust. Shield. Wait. Lord. God. Over and over as though these words build a castle around me. I had to fight my fear. You may need to do this too.

I still believe my pain was not cancer pain. Some of my docs heard me, and others did not. To this day, we really are not 100 percent sure what happened. One doc thinks that my brachial plexus nerve was damaged during the surgery. But I have no proof. I didn't need proof then (or now), what I needed was a way forward for healing that didn't just involve increased levels of pain medication. There isn't anything wrong with pain medication—and I kid you not that nerve pain is *fiercely* painful—but in my situation, I felt that the pain medication was a lousy band-aid that really wasn't fixing the problem. In my own usual way, I did research and added specific yoga stretches, massage, chiropractic, and acupuncture to my treatment plan to get my nerve pain addressed. It took almost a year to feel normal again from whatever happened. It still burns from time to time almost three years later now, but it is more or less healed.

I was blessed that I had a couple of doctors that did not poo-poo the incorporation of alternative medicine into my treatment plan. There will be some docs that think the only way to fix a problem is through Western medicine, and I mean through *prescription* medicine. In my mind, this isn't the only approach to healing. I think healing comes in all shapes, sizes, and modes. You need to use what works for you. In my case, acupuncture was a Godsend. Don't be afraid to advocate for an approach that works for you. It doesn't have to be an either/or approach to your treatment plan; it can be an *integrated* approach. You do need to have all your providers on the same sheet of music so that it is a *coordinated* plan of care.

You really don't want to be trying Chinese medicines while getting chemotherapy, as there may be interactions between the medications. You don't want to turn your nose up at well-documented approaches to pain management because your doctor isn't informed on alternative approaches. Wellness comes from mind, body, and spiritual balances, even during things like chemo and cancer treatment. Get everyone involved in your care so that *your* care is made for *you*.

Finally, I wasn't crazy. You aren't either. Work at the situation until you get what you need to be whole. One of the scariest things in the world is feeling like you are losing your mind. Don't let your pain or fear overwhelm you.

Your Story . . .

On a scale of 1–10 (or 100), how crazy do you feel?

_____

_____

_____

_____

_____

_____

_____

_____

_____

On a scale of 1–10, how well do you feel your doctors are listening to you?

_____

_____

_____

_____

_____

_____

_____

_____

_____

Are there some alternative therapies you'd like to discuss with your doctor?

_____

_____

_____

_____

_____

_____

_____

_____

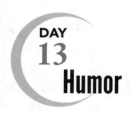

Humor

He will yet fill your mouth with laughter, and your lips with shouts of joy.
(Job 8:21)

How I Felt . . .

Every time I look at my husband, I want to apologize for this mess we are in together. When I start apologizing and falling into the "I am so sorry" and weeping mode, he gets sincerely annoyed with me.

First off, it's probably a little demeaning when I apologize for something I cannot control. It's also probably a little insulting since he takes his marriage vows very seriously. Sure, I bet he would like to take this from me, but he has vowed "in sickness and in health" and has not wavered. My husband is my rock. I know I am never alone with him by my side. In some ways, his journey is more difficult than mine. As my priest reminded me, Treb now has to pick up the pieces of what I physically cannot do and remain steadfast when I am too emotionally drained to deal with more. He has had to take on my household chores, the kids, telephone calls, answering multiple e-mails, and going to the grocery store. All of these are things he hates to do—especially talking on the phone and going to the grocery store. Not that we keep count, but the dude will have so many kitchen passes by the time this is through that he will be able to trade them in for a boat that he so desperately wants. *Grin.*

All of this leads to a litany of "I am so sorry" in my brain. The first time I said it, he swatted me with the kitchen towel as he was doing dishes. The second time I said it, he gave me the evil eye. And the third time I said it, he told me every time I said I was sorry he was going to go out and buy himself a new X-wing miniatures figure.

You see, my husband loves to play tactical board games. His newest favorite is the Star Wars X-wing miniatures game. He may be a little obsessed and before all this started, I was getting perturbed with the frequent packages from Amazon with a new ship for his collection.

So, I really need to be careful with my "sorry" comments. In one way or another, they may come back to bite me. The last thing I need is an entire room filled with Star Wars figures. If I am weak and start the apology nonsense again, at least he will be getting something he enjoys out of my moment of self-pity.

The Force is strong with that one.

What I Learned . . .

It is important to find humor even in the pitiful moments of this journey. I really was saying "I am sorry" every time I turned around. I felt so bad about all the pieces Treb was picking up as I was miserable. While you may want to apologize every time you turn around too, you may have a loved one who gets as equally annoyed at the apologies as my husband does. Instead, think about your blessings each time you want to apologize. I counted my blessings as a litany during this journey to remind myself of how much God has given me. Instead of all the things I wanted to be sorry about, I forced myself to start thinking of all the things I was blessed with on my journey. So many things could be so much worse.

I am blessed by my husband.

I am blessed by my children.

I am blessed by my family.

I am blessed by my friends.

I am blessed by my colleagues.

I am blessed by my writing.

I am blessed by my readers.

I am blessed by my doctors.

I am blessed by my nurses.

I am blessed by a strong body.

I am blessed by a strong mind.

I am blessed by God.

Your Story . . .

What are your blessings? Name them with purpose on your journey and they will help you through the moments of pity.

_____

_____

_____

_____

_____

_____

_____

_____

_____

What sort of things do you find yourself saying "I am sorry" about?

_____

_____

_____

_____

_____

_____

_____

_____

_____

_____

Goonies Never Say Die

Now when Job's three friends heard of all these troubles that had come upon him, each of them set out from his home . . . they met together to go and console and comfort him. (Job 2:11)

How I Felt . . .

It's three o'clock in the morning again and I cannot sleep. I'm beginning to hate three in the morning. Anyone who knows me well will know how irritating this is to me. I like my sleep and I rarely have issues with sleeping. Not so much lately. Insomnia bites. I don't know how people live with insomnia.

Yesterday was the two-week "anniversary" of my cancer diagnosis. It still seems a little unreal to me. It's not like we will be celebrating this "anniversary" with cake and champagne. Heck, most days I still ask myself, "Did they really call and tell me I had cancer?"

It's real all right, but it doesn't feel real. It doesn't feel like it could possibly be right. I still have far more questions than I have answers. I still don't understand why God has put me on this path—I'm still 100 percent sure I don't like having cancer or having to be on this journey. This is not the path I would have chosen. I'm still 100 percent sure that somewhere, someday, somehow, I will understand, but today is not that day. Yesterday wasn't either and I'm pretty sure tomorrow I will have many of the same questions. I still ask, "Why me?"

I am racked by guilt/anger/confusion/frustration/shame/shock. (I don't know—which one of those perplexing feelings should I pick today?) How I am supposed to lead people to a healthy life, as a nurse, as a wellness professional, as the author of *Christ Walk: A 40-Day Spiritual Fitness Program*, when I'm obviously broken in some way? I feel betrayed by my health practices. I have done what the experts recommend. I take care of myself. I eat right, I exercise, and I still got cancer.

I wax high and low between wanting to *go full on granola* with my approach to my cancer treatment and thinking, "Screw it, I got sick anyway." I'm pretty sure the balance is sort of somewhere in between, but I haven't quite gotten there yet. I look around my house and wonder if the plastic caused this. Is it because I use a cell phone? Is my Keurig dripping carcinogens into my coffee? Is my food really organic, or just another gimmick with more pesticides? Is my shampoo giving me cancer? Where did this crap come from? And *why*, when I've worked *so hard* for my health, would this happen? I want answers. *Who* is responsible for doing this to my body? *What* is causing this? *How* did this happen? *Where* was I negligent? I really want the answer to "*Why me?!*"

I have no answers. I may never have answers. That, right there, is what you call "embracing the suck." Soldiers, heroes, warriors, and people who make a difference, they all learn to embrace the suck. The suck is part of the achievement factor in tackling anything in life. I don't believe that good things come easy. You will have to fight for what you want.

Ugh.

And while I am fighting this reality internally, my body hurts. I'm sorry; maybe that's just too much information. Maybe I whine about it too much. I know I say it over and over. But I do. My body just hurts. It doesn't stop. It's probably one of the reasons I am up so early. In some ways, I'm bouncing back from the surgeries wonderfully. In other ways, I am so aware that my body is just not right. I can lay flat on a hard surface and everything feels out of whack. My left arm and shoulder constantly hurt since they took my tumors out.

I cannot get comfortable. And. I. Simply. Hate. Pain. Medicine. My guts feel rearranged. My mind feels fuzzy and my hands shake. My body, mind, and soul feel completely at odds with each other. I need a serious realignment. Where is God's chiropractor? Day after day, I've posted about the pain. Will it ever go away?

I know the things I can, and need, to do. I'm naming my thoughts and feelings. If I put my negative thoughts and feelings aside, maybe I can do it. I am an intelligent person; I know the healthcare field well. I know what I can do and things that will help. I'm just not thinking very clearly right now. I know that I can go to the chiropractor, massage therapist, or acupuncturist. I can try essential oils, yoga, relaxation breathing, and prayer (all of which I do some of the time and in some sort of way). But honestly, sometimes it is hard to find the time to do any of this when you are fielding phone calls from case managers, nurses, surgeons, movers, oncologists, and work, and then there is laundry to be done, naps to take, or sometimes just getting out of bed. My body needs many more hours to heal and I am impatient with that process. I don't feel like I have the time to take care of me. Clinically, I know what I need. I know this is a matter of time, but at my heart, in my inner core: I don't have time for this! And there lies my inner struggle.

I have yet to give in to, or embrace, my new reality. I am still fighting it tooth and nail. I want to wake up tomorrow (not at 3:00 a.m. hopefully) and have it be gone. And I mourn that it will not just go away. I feel like I have a big, fat label on my forehead.

In the psychological realm of things, I am somewhere between denial and grieving. It's a stage. A season. It will pass and there will be a new season. One of acceptance. The new season will be for the warrior. I know she is in me. She's just very tired right now. A little sore and a little beat-up. It will come. Just not today and maybe not tomorrow, but soon.

As 3:00 a.m. turns into 6:00 a.m. (it takes a while to write these days), and I pour my coffee into one of my favorite cups, I'm buoyed by its message, "Goonies never say die."

Not giving up yet . . .

What I Learned . . .

"I am still 100 percent sure I don't like having cancer. . . ."

That hasn't changed. I don't like my cancer. Even knowing where my story is now, I still wish it hadn't happened. It's changed my life in so many ways. I am fairly sure that you feel this way too. No one wants a cancer story. *But*, seasons change. The human body is adaptable. We find ways of dealing with pain, sorting out the grief, anger, and denial. We learn to dig deep for that warrior/superhero/fighting spirit and we come charging out, spitting fire at our cancer. You might not feel that spirit right now, but it's there—trust me.

Your inner warrior or superhero (or whatever you want to call it) will come charging out too. Embrace it. Your fighting spirit will help you weather the good, the bad, and the ugly that is to come. There will be days your fighter will be too tired to get out of bed. There will be days that your combatant hurts so badly from the surgery, the chemicals, the needles, the poking, the prodding, and the *invasion* of your body that you will just want to curl up in a ball. Those days are normal. Breathe through them. You will rally. On the days that you feel you are slipping in your fight, pray. If you cannot pray yourself, ask your friends and family to pray for you. There were many days that I could not pray myself and I swear the healing power of those that were praying for me carried me through the days of suck.

Three o'clock in the morning is a weird time. You will experience your bouts of insomnia. Worry and fear tend to prey in the middle of the night. I recommend you find an outlet. For me, it was writing. For others, they say books on e-devices that are backlit help soothe them back to sleep. This may be the perfect time for meditation and centering prayer practices. It may be the perfect time to cry and just let it go if you have been holding it together for others. You may knit. You may use a coloring book. Maybe you will listen to music, or feel like baking. I hated my insomnia and the worry that clutched my gut. But at the same time, it became "me" time. The house was quiet. I did not have to put on a face for anyone, and it gave me time to process much of my grief.

Through most of my writing and experiences, you'll see a theme of perception and attitude. When we perceive a situation in a positive light, or turn it on its side to see it from a different perspective, then we have the opportunity to improve our attitudes. Any improvement in our attitudes makes us far more likely to be successful in our goals and objectives.

Find your attitude and reprogram it to success. Define your perception of events so that your attitude contributes to your healing and wellness.

"Goonies never say die."

Never give up.

Your Story . . .

What is your cancer (or illness) motto?

_____
_____
_____
_____
_____
_____
_____
_____

What will you do at three o'clock in the morning, or when insomnia strikes?

_____
_____
_____
_____
_____
_____
_____
_____
_____
_____

On a scale of 0–100, how well do you like your cancer (or other illness)?

_____

_____

_____

_____

_____

_____

_____

_____

_____

DAY 18
We Are Groot

I lift up my eyes to the hills—from where will my help come?
My help comes from the Lord, who made heaven and earth. (Ps. 121:1–2)

How I Felt . . .

My son's godmother wrote me this week and said, "Girlfriend, it is time to stop feeling guilty."

She is right.

Guilt, when there is no transgression, is a wasted emotion. I may never know the why of my cancer. I may never understand this season and I may question God's plan for me during this time, but there is nothing to feel guilty about.

The guilt was weighing down my fighter spirit. And I am a fighter.

Even though I still cry, even though I have pain, even though I have my moments of distress and anxiety, this time has shown me that I have so many amazing people to fight for. My beautiful children, my amazing husband, my awesome family, and my phenomenal friends. I have been infused with the spirit of all these incredible people. I do not believe my time here is done—for whatever reason, I have been challenged *again* by my body and *again* I will make it healthy to do God's work in the world. I would not have this attitude if I did not have all these astonishing people in my life telling me I can.

My buddy Louie calls this, "We are Groot." Groot is the character from *Guardians of the Galaxy* who epically gives his life for his friends by binding them together in his roots. It is transformational symbolism of the power of deep friendships to save each other and lift each other up in times of trial. The splinter that remains of Groot is able to regrow into a new tree from the love of his friends. Where there is love, powerful things can grow. My friends are my Groots. Together, we are growing into a new tree. We will do this together. There is no "I" in this battle. I am not in this fight against cancer alone. This is not just about *me*. This is about *we* and what *we* will do *together*.

This togetherness is what I think God means by a community of believers. We have a bigger "church" going on than a brick building when *together* we are lifting each other up in love. We are called to be Groot to each other.

So, while the future will have its ups and downs, I will still question: Why? When? How? And I'm sure I will have days where I cry and gnash my teeth. Yet I have hope. I can't say that I don't feel guilty—it comes and goes—but I have hope, because of you all.

We are Groot.

What I Learned . . .

Reading back on this post makes me smile. What I continue to learn every day is that "Groots" are so important. We are *not* in this journey alone. I once wrote a blog post on how the greatest gift you could give someone with an illness like cancer is to tell them, "I believe you can conquer this. I believe in you." Having people (your Groots) believe in you is incredibly important.

But, it can also be a burden. Not all cancers can be beat. Not all illnesses are conquerable. Some cancers have to be lived with. Some cancers kill. Sometimes the disease isn't cancer, it's heart disease, mental illness, diabetes, a stroke, or any number of chronic illnesses that take over our bodies and upend whatever we call "normal" at that time. Sometimes trying to be a "cancer warrior" is a burden of its own, especially when we don't feel like warriors. Maybe you don't feel much like a superhero in the middle of your illness. Even if you don't feel like a warrior, or a hero, you still have friends. You have people that care about you, and it's this group of people that are going to help you through this journey/adventure/road to hell that you are on. They can believe in you, even when you don't believe in yourself.

It's true. We do far more together and are able to accomplish so much more as a community than we can ever do alone. Don't be a loner. When we believe in each other and in the power of the Holy Spirit to work through each of us, we are building something so much stronger than cancer or any other illness.

At the heart of the Christian tradition is the love for human life and our love for God. The love that knits us together makes us stronger. Even in non-Christian traditions, respect and care of the human life is essential. History shows us that when people are woven together in a common purpose, they are stronger together than alone.

This is completely true of the cancer experience, or any other illness, disease, death, loss, change, or challenge as well. Groots make us all stronger. Love makes us all stronger.

It is not an accident that the two most important commandments are to love God and love your neighbor (Luke 10:27). God taught us love through the gift of Christ's death and resurrection. The gift of love in Christ's resurrection is that things can be made whole again. God has a promise of "rightness" for us all. That doesn't necessarily mean rightness in the here and the now; it can take time. Jesus was made whole on the cross and through his resurrection a promise was fulfilled that all things wrong can be made new. The love that God teaches us is one we share with each other. If we love God, and we love each other fiercely, we can lift each other up through so many trials and tragedies. We are stronger together.

We are Groot.

Your Story . . .

Who are your Groots?

_____

_____

_____

_____

_____

_____

_____

Where do you want God to make you whole?

_____

_____

_____

_____

_____

_____

_____

_____

What do you think of God making Jesus whole again?

_____

_____

_____

_____

_____

_____

_____

_____

You've Got Your Good Days and Your Bad Days

Surely goodness and mercy shall follow me all the days of my life, and I shall dwell in the house of the Lord my whole life long. (Ps. 23:6)

How I Felt . . .

I just returned from a pavement-pounding, fierce walk.

Ten days post-op, some steps hurt more than others. However, I've yet to find any drug they've given me more effective in reducing pain, managing my mood, calming my anxiety, opening myself to prayer, and releasing tension than exercise. I am thankful that while I cannot run, today's "Christ Walk" was a good walk.

My mood has calmed. Not so much before I left. I was an irritable, anxious, pain-filled mess that was frustrated right, left, and center.

Cancer is killing one of my friends. Cancer killed a friend of a friend. Cancer is making people miserable. Cancer makes my hands shake and my body ache. The information on the internet is trying to leach my resolve to be a warrior. And I am still in pain. I never see things clearly when I am in pain and we are having a hard time managing my tumor pain. It's ironic, since two weeks ago I didn't feel much of anything. The surgeon thinks the surgery might have stirred things up. Yet another thing to discuss with my cancer doc. The list is getting long.

But, back to the research. All the information on the internet is overwhelming me and scaring me. It's hard to find resolve when you see so much negativity. There is so much scary information on the internet. It is difficult to process. I've been reading Kris Carr's *Crazy, Sexy Cancer* and decided to follow her advice and start a "cancer posse." These are the gals I can unload on and these are the gals that will do my research for me. I've told them I need to hear that I will survive and that I've got a much better chance than ten years. I need thirty or forty years. Fifty would be nice. I've got things to do and people to see. Books to write and kids to raise. That's not asking too much, is it?

Also weighing on my mind are the results from my bone marrow biopsy. Waiting has never been my forte. It seems God continues to try and teach me patience. I fear I am a hopeless cause. Waiting, wondering, and being unable to make plans drives me insane.

Hence my irritability. I'm not depressed—I'm pissed. But at least when you are pissed, you feel really alive. Being angry is a very tangible thing to deal with. Being mad helped me attack my walk and made me feel almost normal. In spite of the pain, frustration, and anxiety, I walked and walked.

It felt good. I might not be running any races anytime soon, but I've got a goal to try and do 10K steps per day. These steps will make me stronger and better ready to take on the chemo. And maybe next year, there will be a race to conquer. It will be nothing compared to cancer.

What I Learned . . .

The difference between this post and others to me is obvious. When you have cancer, your mood is all over the place. You've seen my highs and lows already. You will continue to see them in my story. I am, if nothing else, consistent in that my moods were all over the place from day to day. The cancer journey is a veritable roller coaster of emotions from one moment to the next. This doesn't change with remission. Your emotions and feelings still come and go with cancer. It might not be as drastic, but the hills and valleys are still present. I sometimes think we don't realize how long healing can take. The healing process is different for each of us. There is no "right way" to heal the hurt in your body, mind, and soul. It's a process of recovery.

From day-to-day your perspective of events will change. One day you may feel you can slay the world, and other days find you hiding in a hole. This is normal. I share this because I desperately needed someone to tell me that all of my feelings all over the place were a normal response to having cancer. I felt like I was going crazy. You will not *always* feel this way. Calm and equilibrium do come. But even when you find your happy resting place, your fear and anxiety can crop up . . . even when things are going well. This is also typical. When you are faced with a shocking disease, you'll always ask yourself, "What if?" What if things go wrong? What does this symptom mean? Have I relapsed? Is the treatment working? What if it doesn't? What if it makes me worse? These are all normal questions that will come and go, even when things are going well and even when you've entered remission. You see, curing your disease and healing from the process are two different things. And as I said before, healing takes time.

Having goals and friends throughout your journey is really important. It gives you something to see in the future other than the suckiness of doctors, treatments, blood draws, pills, and scans. It's called having your eye on the prize. It's an important part of success in your journey. When I was recovering from my surgery, my goal was to walk the block, then around the neighborhood, and then move enough to get ten thousand steps in a day. I built small, digestible goals that worked with where I was in my diagnosis. Think about something you would like to accomplish and make it your target. Break it down into smaller digestible pieces and keep your eye on that goal. You can set these goals in the middle of treatment, recovery, and remission. I'm a firm believer that physical activity aids in your healing process.

Finally, I've said it before and I can't emphasize it enough: having friends and family around you is important. Now it's time to learn to put them to work. Your friends and family *want* to help you. Give them roles in your cancer posse, but be clear about what you want. My research gals helped to filter out the scary nonsense and put it into perspective. They knew not to tell me I would cure my cancer with green drinks, coffee enemas (yes, this is a "cancer treatment"), and special supplements. That's just not my thing.

I wanted validated information to help me with my decision-making process and give another perspective to the information I obtained on my own. They ultimately acted as a filter between the internet and me. These are very special ladies in my life that know me better than I know myself. I trust them to tell me when I am really irrational, if I am just being silly, or if I am right on target in my thoughts and feelings. Since they knew me well, they knew how to frame the information in a way that wouldn't completely freak me out. To this day, I've been known to call up my cancer posse, tell them I am having a can-anxious (anxious cancer) moment, and they put things back into perspective for me. There is value in a group of friends that you trust to do this for you. It helps break things down.

If you don't like the research methods of your cancer posse, put them to work doing other things: writing thank-you notes, making meals, *praying*, making calls or e-mails or Facebook posts, driving you or being with you at appointments. Have them send you funny daily jokes, or go on a trip with you when you have time or a break in your treatment. Let them be involved in your journey so you won't be alone.

Your Story . . .

You've identified your Groots. Which of your Groots do you want to be in your cancer posse?

_____

_____

_____

_____

_____

_____

_____

_____

_____

_____

_____

What do you want your cancer posse to do for you?

_____

_____

_____

_____

_____

_____

_____

_____

What is a goal you would like to have in the middle of this insane journey?

_____

_____

_____

_____

_____

_____

_____

_____

Three Weeks. I Want My Mama

Honor your father and your mother, so that your days may be long in the land that the Lord your God is giving you. (Exod. 20:12)

How I Felt . . .

I do not care how big you get in life, there are days when all you want is your mama. Yesterday was that day for me. My blog is full of comments about all the pain I've been having since my surgeries. I really try not to talk about it much because I know all the talk is just plain wearing on both my friends and me. I repeat myself a lot. Who likes the doom and gloomy friend? So, I keep it in check, or I blog about it. Misery loves company, especially on the internet.

Regardless, I have been in pain for about two weeks now and I have not been able to get it under control with just Tylenol and Ibuprofen. It's been a vicious cycle. So, I finally gave in on Monday night and upped the ante to Percocet. Percocet is a hardcore pain med. I *hate* drugs (which I'm very aware I need to get over in the coming months, but hey—this is an honest post; I'll never lie here about what I think and feel). I took the Percocet as prescribed every four hours by my doc. And yep, the pain went away. *But*, it brought with it dizziness, vertigo, and hours and hours of being violently ill. For the life of me, I cannot figure out how people get addicted to Percocet (I know we all have our vices, but . . .). This crap makes me feel *vile*.

Like "curl up in a little ball and whimper for your mommy" kind of vile.

Which I did.

I called her and told her I just wanted to hear her voice. I think I made her feel bad because she's a mom just like me, and she doesn't like her baby hurting any more than I like having my kids hurt. We were pitiful together. She told me how people were amazed at how strong I was. And I laughed. I told her, I don't think people would think I'm all that strong if they saw me now. A pale, shaking, barfing, stooped shadow of myself. There was no strong in this picture . . . a lot of pitiful. A good bit of whining and a lot of feeling like a little kid that just wants mama to take it all away.

My mama is one of the greatest formative forces—not only in my faith but in me as a person. I love my mama and I am not afraid to say it. So when I am pitiful and not remotely strong, she is the person I call to get a good dose of sympathy or a swift kick in the rear.

I worry a little bit (*ok, a lot*) about how I will tolerate the chemo. I am a puker. It is the one side effect that I would choose to avoid at all costs. I was on chemotherapeutic drugs back when I lost my hearing. I have lost chunks of my hair (just not all of it), puked, have scars on my skin from the medications, suffered infections, and the rest of the nine yards. The meds I was on when I lost my hearing have a lot to do with why I hate drugs. On top of that, it takes three antinausea meds to keep me from puking from surgery and that does not always work. I hate to throw up. Because once it starts . . . it does not stop for at least twenty-four hours or longer for me. I worry that if the Percocet would do this to me, it will be infinitely worse when my system is hit up with something far stronger.

It is what it is and I won't know till I know . . . but I'm pretty sure that if it is bad, the first thing I'll want is my mama.

What I Learned . . .

Pain is often a part of the cancer journey. Not always, but more often than not, you will experience pain at some point. There is *no shame* in having pain and needing medication to help it. I had a really hard time with this. I felt that I was less than strong when I broke down and took the pain medication. It did not help that narcotics and I really do not get along. It works for many people, but not for me. But let me repeat this: *there is no shame in needing pain management.*

You are not weak. You are not seeking to be propped up by drugs. You are seeking pain relief. I have had doctors tell me that cancer pain is part of the journey and I should get used to it. I have had doctors tell me that I should not be experiencing pain. Regardless of what a doctor, or nurse, or other professional tells you, your pain experience is *your* pain experience. As I've mentioned, I also recommend that you seek out alternative forms of pain management if you are like me and do not like the drugs, or are seeking other ways to wean yourself off the drugs.

In my case, I sought out chiropractic, acupuncture, and a special yogi that came to me and showed me healing poses to relieve the agony. My body was in pain from the surgical wounds, but the constant guarding of the surgical sites, poor positioning, my anxiety, and poor sleep contributed to muscular pain as well. My body was a knotted mess of misery. I found more relief from these alternative methods than from the pharmacological approach. It took a lot of time and patience to get things fixed. We found that either the tumors themselves or their removal damaged the nerves in my shoulder, causing me constant pain and loss of function. Almost nine months passed until we got my arm working again, and although I still have some residual pain and discomfort, it works like normal once again. It was a process to get there though. It took me being proactive, diligent, and determined to find something that worked for me.

I have learned that everyone is different. My experience with medication throughout my life may not be yours. There are people who fly through chemotherapy without issues. There are those that cry for their mommy like me. There are those that have countless side effects and there are those that have peaks and valleys in their experience. *You* are *you*. Be an advocate for yourself. Tell your doctor how you are feeling. Tell your doctor if you want to explore alternative medicine. Many hospitals have access to these integrated therapies now, and if not, seek other avenues. It is not money wasted to try and get you back to the best you.

Since we are talking side effects, another side effect of treatment is going to be nausea and quite possibly vomiting. Either the medications and chemo will destroy your appetite or, as it was in my case, anxiety and pain made it incredibly difficult for me to eat. Unfortunately, good nutrition is very important to your cancer health and battle. A balance of protein, carbohydrates, and fats is essential to your energy levels throughout treatment, and it is essential for when your body needs to build healthy cells to replace the cancer cells. Think of your nutrition as something else you *can* do to help your body fight the cancer and build new cells that are strong and healthy. There are also a plethora of medications, essential oils, and acupuncture/pressure points that can help with your nausea and appetite. Coordinate these methods to ensure you have a period of time when you can attempt to eat.

However, when you are sick, nauseated, anxious, or in pain, eating blows. The last thing I want to think about is food when I am feeling any of these things, but here is my list of go-to foods in a situation where I need to eat, but have no appetite. These are also easily digestible:

- applesauce (no sugar added—sometimes sugar additives can give you the runs. You don't need runs on top of the runs.)
- saltine crackers
- ginger ale
- baked potatoes
- mashed potatoes
- scrambled eggs (I like to add shredded cheese for additional nutrients and protein, but dairy may be hard for your gut.)
- yogurt without excessive sugar
- chicken broth or chicken noodle soup
- bananas
- oatmeal
- smoothies (see my recipe for Anna's Smoothies on page 75)
- Mom's Baked Egg Custard (see the recipe on page 75)

These are my go-to "I'm sick and I need comfort food that works" food items. You might have your own. It may take some trial and error to find those things that give you the energy and nutrients you need. As always, if you have special allergies or nutritional needs, work with the oncology or other disease nutrition specialist and your doctor to make sure you have options that work for you. As gross as food may be right now, you do need the nutrition. Good nutrition is important for healing.

Finally, I learned it is okay to still want my mom. There is no shame in a forty-year-old woman who desperately wants mom to fix the mess she is in. Or maybe a sixty-year-old man, or wherever you are on the spectrum of gender or age, wanting comfort or the memory of a loving parent, friend, or companion to help you through the hard times. There is no shame in your pain, tears, fear, crying, whimpering, or moments of weakness when you do not feel strong.

These times will pass.

Your Story . . .

What side effect worries you most, or causes you the most discomfort?

_____

_____

_____

_____

_____

_____

_____

_____

_____

Have you told your doctors about your side effects?

_____

_____

_____

_____

_____

_____

_____

_____

_____

_____

What sorts of alternative therapies are you interested in exploring?

_____

_____

_____

_____

_____

_____

_____

_____

_____

What's keeping you from trying them out?

_____

_____

_____

_____

_____

_____

_____

_____

_____

_____

ANNA'S SMOOTHIE

INGREDIENTS:

- 1 banana
- 1 cup mixed berries
- 2 scoops organic, plant-based protein powder
- ½ cup plain Greek yogurt
- ½ cup to 1 cup unsweetened almond milk (now, you can use any liquid you want, but cow's milk may upset your stomach. Try soy or coconut milk—use whatever works for you.)

DIRECTIONS:

1. Throw everything into the blender—buzz it.
2. Drink.

Variations: Add peanut butter powder for more protein; freeze the bananas and berries for a colder version; add avocado for more fat; add mixed greens (spinach, kale, collards) if you want more roughage (I cannot do this—too many of these greens will tear up my stomach, so keep that in mind when thinking about what your stomach can handle). Add honey for more sweetness. Switch the berries for peaches, nectarines, or whatever is in season. Add cocoa powder for fiber and flavor.

MOM'S BAKED EGG CUSTARD

This egg custard recipe is one both my mom and I have eaten through our cancer experiences. It's comforting, super easy to digest, filling, and is a great way to get protein. She will make the recipe with Ensure, or Breakfast smoothie packets, to increase the nutrients and protein. It's a great win, when you really don't feel like eating, but you need to put something in your body.

Continued

INGREDIENTS:

- 4 eggs
- ¼ cup sugar (you can use raw organic cane sugar if you want to make this a cleaner version of the existing recipe; in fact you can use all organic versions of the eggs, milk, and sugar if you want it to be super clean eating.)
- ¼ teaspoon salt
- 2½ cups milk
- 1 teaspoon vanilla
- Sprinkled nutmeg

DIRECTIONS:

1. Preheat oven to 300 degrees F. Grease a 1-quart casserole or six 6-ounce baking cups with butter or organic oil spray.
2. In a mixing bowl, beat eggs until thickened and lemon colored.
3. Add milk (with the instant breakfast packet or protein powder mixed into the milk beforehand) and vanilla.
4. Beat the egg/milk mixture until smooth.
5. Pour into casserole or baking cups; sprinkle with nutmeg.
6. Place casserole or baking cups in pan containing 1 inch of hot water.
7. Bake in preheated oven for 1¼ hours for casserole, 45 minutes for baking cups, or until a knife comes out clean when stuck in the middle.

You could call this stuff comfort custard. It's the bomb.

David and Goliath

But David said to the Philistine, "You come to me with sword and spear and javelin; but I come to you in the name of the Lord of hosts, the God of the armies of Israel, whom you have defied." (1 Sam. 17:45)

How I Felt . . .

I received great news today. My bone marrow biopsy shows no signs of malignancy. Take that, cancer! It was a total "fist pump" moment. My thoughts and prayers are with my brothers and sisters who also have received news that buoys them and also with those that received news that did not pump them up.

News can go either way.

My thoughts these days have been a lot about the mind-body-spirit connection of my disease. I have been engrossed with the injustice that my body would do this to me when I have spent the last five years altering my family's environment, food, and lifestyle so that we are all healthier and cleaner eaters. We are all inundated with information on how we can live healthier lives and raise healthier kids. Since I've been diagnosed, I am flooded with information on how to be healthier with cancer. It's overwhelming. All the directions on what I should and should not do are anxiety producing. But, as a health professional, I take these kinds of recommendations to heart. As someone with a bad immune system, the sort of healthy changes I made in our life as a family have been critical to living a healthy life for the last thirty-eight years.

And yet, I still got cancer. I have been so wrapped up in the negativity and injustice of it all. I've done everything right, taken care of myself, and cancer still happened. And I have been secretly fearful that the diagnosis would discredit my approach to a healthy, Christ-centered lifestyle. Who takes health tips from a cancer patient?

What I have come to learn—a light-bulb moment—about this diagnosis is to turn my thinking around about it and my health practices. Instead of thinking that I got cancer even though I practice all these healthy behaviors, how about thinking how strong my body is to defeat this disease? My blood work is amazing. I show no signs of the disease except in my tumors and scans. I have my fitness and my mental strength, great vitals, and an amazing can-do attitude (when I haven't buried it under self-pity). Yes, my history of autoimmune disease makes me more susceptible to lymphoma, but I can control what I do. It's insanely frustrating to read all these books about getting away from the "standard American diet" and eliminating processed food, eating clean and organic, and avoiding chemicals and pesticides, and on and on. Well, I do all this, and this disease still happened. It can still happen to me or to anyone else in this same position. I know many, many, many people who follow a healthy lifestyle and still get disease. It happens.

I am learning to think of my health practices in terms of how healthy I have made my body to defeat this disease. Instead of beating myself up about what I've done wrong, I need to think about what I do right. Over and over again if need be. I am starting from the top of the mountain in facing this disease, not the bottom of this hill.

If I change the mindset about the situation I am in, I can move from feeling defeated to feeling like a warrior. Attitude completely determines perception of events. My attitude is bigger than my cancer. Sometimes a positive attitude makes you David over Goliath.

What I Learned . . .

Attitude is everything. You will be hit from all sides with the feelings, information, attitudes, and emotions of yourself and others. You will be hit with opinions and recommendations from many people who mean well, but haven't got a clue about your situation. Your attitude is going to reflect 100 percent your perception of the events of your cancer or illness journey.

A crappy attitude makes everything worse. Remember when I said that fear and anxiety feed a vicious cycle? It is true. If you stay in that vicious cycle long enough, your perception of events starts to be colored by anxiety and fear. Anxiety, fear, sadness, guilt, anger, and regret: these are all normal parts of the process.

But.

But.

But.

But.

Do not let them last forever. The more often you tell yourself "You can do this" and pump yourself up with good news, good thoughts, and a good attitude, the better your perception of the events will be.

Your Story . . .

Say this (out loud): I am more than my disease.

_____

_____

_____

_____

_____

_____

_____

_____

_____

_____

Say this (out loud): I can do this.

_____

_____

_____

_____

_____

_____

_____

_____

_____

_____

_____

_____

Ok, so now that you've talked to yourself, how did those things make you feel when you said them?

_____

_____

_____

_____

_____

_____

_____

_____

_____

_____

_____

What triggers your anxiety moments?

_____

_____

_____

_____

_____

_____

_____

_____

_____

_____

One Month In

I am weary with my crying; my throat is parched. My eyes grow dim with waiting for my God. (Ps. 69:3)

How I Felt . . .

It's day thirty on this *Journey with Cancer*. My life has turned into an ongoing roller coaster ride. It's one high after a low after a high after a low kind of ride. It's exhausting. There are good days and there are bad days. I have to remind people that even when I have a bad day, it doesn't mean that I am not fighting, or that I don't believe I can't beat this, it's just that some days you have a bad day and it sucks the life out of you.

We are in waiting mode. I hate waiting. As Dr. Seuss said in *Oh, the Places You'll Go*, "a most useless place . . . the waiting place." Waiting for an answer. Waiting for a treatment day. Waiting for a treatment plan. Waiting for information. Waiting for a doctor. Waiting for results. Waiting for news. Waiting to heal. Waiting for a moving date. Waiting. Waiting. Waiting.

Right now, we have to wait for our move. My doctor here won't start me on treatment in the middle of the move, and my doctor in the new place won't make a decision until I get there on what that treatment will be. We have gone from "You must get there by the beginning of December to start treatment—you can't wait!" to "We'll make a decision about your treatment when you get here. Just let us know." To say this is conflicting messaging is an understatement.

I have two very different doctors with two different opinions on what to do and neither of them gives me any sort of peace. So, I am calling on God for patience, because God knows I have none of my own. And I sit in this waiting place, where one doctor seems very comfortable with waiting and watching for me to become symptomatic and all I want to do is kick this parasite out of my body as fast as I can. If I could claw it out of my chest, I would. Watching and waiting doesn't resonate with me for a number of reasons. And I disagree with them completely when they say I am asymptomatic.

The first doctor would start treatment in two to four weeks. She would treat me if I was not moving and if I wasn't recovering from open abdominal surgery. But moving gets me closer to family and help, good schools for my kids, and a good job for my husband. And since my cancer is so slow-growing and indolent, the move doesn't seem impossible. But then I wait some more. And wait and hear things like "This cancer isn't curable." "We'll get you into remission, but you'll relapse." And my mind gets spun up on "This is my life now" and "This is not how it's supposed to be."

And then there is the other doctor. The one I haven't met yet. I am putting my faith and life in hands that I have not seen. I am putting my trust in a woman from two thousand miles away, hoping she will see me as a person and not a patient. I am clinging to this belief that she will fight for me as hard as I am—fighting to live a life with my family without cancer. I have to hope and pray that I am not just another clinical trial to her. I have to wish and contemplate that she will have my best interests at heart and that she will become one with my cancer posse. I have to pray that God has this all under control because I have *none* of it under control.

I'm in a roller coaster in my mind, my heart, my spirit, my soul, and my body. I am either high or low and I struggle to find the equilibrium. And each day I walk. I walk to get myself off of that high or out of that low. I walk to pray, and I pray to continue to be able to walk. And I wonder, wonder, and wonder some more what my life will be like. This waiting place makes you feel like you are in a stuck place.

And I still just want it to go away. People, I have made plans, and cancer wasn't part of any of them. And it still isn't. I want this crap out of my body now. And this makes waiting a tortuous place.

So the questions I ask: "What's the plan?" "What's next?" "What are you going to do?" I don't have answers. No one can seem to tell me what the plan will be. We will move and then we will hopefully find out what is next. And so, I wait, and I pray. Maybe in this interim of waiting, God will make my cancer go away. I desperately want the imaginary Santa Claus God to wave his magic wand and make it disappear—you know, the God who is sometimes like a magician, a wizard, a Santa Claus. But that's not God. God is something else. Maybe God has bigger plans for me than I can understand. I still pray for the cancer to go away. I know God hears me. I am learning to wait and see what those answers will be.

What I Learned . . .

As I write this, it has been three years now. I still hate waiting. The waiting place sucks.

However, sometimes waiting is a good thing. Taking time with your diagnosis allows you to get second opinions and look at many alternatives available to you. The Cancer Treatment Centers of America[1] recommend second opinions. Second opinions can improve your prognosis and expose you to alternative treatment plans, clinical trials, and other insight on your courses of action. Second opinions give you the opportunity to have choices in your care. When things feel like they are spiraling outside of your control, sometimes having that second opinion and choices make you feel in control of your situation. Second opinions can give you hope.

I also learned very clearly that God is not a magician. I have always known this, but in a situation like cancer, or any other difficult illness, you desperately want someone or something to wave a magic wand and take it all away. You want a magic elixir. You want a charm. I diminish God in my life when I make God only a part of the good in my life. God is no more than Santa or a fairy godmother when I beg God to fix my life. We are called to honor God no matter what. We worship God. God does not worship at our own altars. God calls us to love one another and live the life we have, with whatever body we have (no matter how broken). We are far more than a person with disease to God.

My faith and my understanding have grown exponentially over the last years of dealing with my cancer. God has been faithful, even

---

1. *www.cancercenter.com*

when I have not been faithful. God has constantly whispered to me to "Trust in God." And each day with my diagnosis is a day where I can honor God with my trust, and use my broken body to still love others.

Your Story . . .

Have you pursued a second opinion?

_____

_____

_____

_____

_____

_____

_____

_____

What are some options for a second opinion?

_____

_____

_____

_____

_____

_____

_____

_____

What do you think about God right now?

_____

_____

_____

_____

_____

_____

_____

_____

_____

The Number One "No-No"

The Lord is my shepherd, I shall not want. He makes me lie down in green pastures; he leads me beside still waters; he restores my soul. He leads me in right paths for his name's sake. (Ps. 23:1–3)

How I Felt . . .

Information can be hugely helpful in any disease process. Information can also make you crazy. There is soooooo much information out there. It's ridiculous. I have a *very* hard time with doing research on my cancer on the internet. The data and information available makes me anxious, fills me with fear, and leaves me feeling defeated. With the glut of information available, I have to figure out what is good information and what is not good information. I really need to turn to my cancer posse to do this for me. I know I cannot do it on my own without ending up in a very bad place in my mind and heart.

Getting on the internet and "googling" lymphoma scares the hell out of me. I can take only short bursts of information before panic takes over. It's the surefire way to beat down my warrior attitude.

But every so often, I start to think I am strong enough to handle the information and I go searching. And invariably, something comes up that jolts me and makes me fall apart. And as a former oncology nurse—my knowledge as a *former* oncology nurse does more harm than good. This specialty has come so far from when I worked in an oncology practice. But my memories and knowledge are far more of sick people that were fighting for their life than those we helped. Selfishly, I recall wondering why anyone would put themselves through this treatment. Before my children were born, I remember telling my husband I would rather die than go through any of the cancer treatments I saw during those years of practice. How little I knew.

I want to apologize to every one of my patients for that thought. I have kids now. I have more experience, friends, and goals to accomplish now. I understand you will do *anything* to have more years with those you love. It's a fierce desire. I will fight unfailingly for time with my family. It's not that I am afraid to die, or afraid of God—it's just that I love my kids and husband that much. We have so much more we want to do together.

My disease is considered incurable. Yes, I will get remission, but this is my life now. And scientists quote numbers of five to ten to twenty years. But this isn't good enough for me. My children will be twenty-nine and twenty-seven in twenty years . . . I want more. More, more, more. And I pray about this insanely. I want to see my kids grow up, my grandkids too, and enjoy retirement with my husband. I hold on to this want fiercely because it is based in love. I cannot think that God will not understand this because I love my family so intensely that I cannot and will not let them go yet. God commanded us to love one another. It is this ferocious love that calls me to fight. This cannot be wrong.

But this love is also the center of my fear. I am not ready to go. I am not ready to consider my mortality, but being diagnosed with cancer and reading the various websites—*that fear creeps in because all you love is threatened.*

Research on the internet feeds this fear. When you feed a fear, it becomes larger than it really is. You build a monster in your mind that feeds the cancer and gives you one more thing to fight in this battle.

When my fear gets too great, I cry. I'm not the strong warrior people see. I'm a mess. I curl up on the couch. Sometimes I kick the couch while I rage at my situation. Fear is of the devil. It's not pretty. It's red noses, boogers, slobber, many tears, hot flashes, and cold streaks. Panic takes your breath and freezes your mind. Your voice is raw from crying and screaming, and your body aches from the grief. Fear seems so much bigger than it really is. I *must* remind myself that *my God* is bigger than *my fear*.

My mantra: give my fear to God. God is asking me to trust my Lord through these times. I am being called to put my faith in something I cannot see or feel. The internet can't feel or talk or know *me*. I am a person. The internet is not a person. God and God's grace is experienced through my interactions with people. More often than not, people will help assuage your fears. More often than not, the Bible will also help assuage your fears. I am reading over and over in the Bible how God assures us that we will be delivered. God will be my strong rock and a castle to keep me safe; God will lift me up in his time and deliver me from my fear; God will comfort me when I am down and heal me if I put my trust in The Lord.

Gotta love the psalms.

I just need to stay off the internet in the interim. Don't feed the fears.

What I Learned . . .

To this day, I believe that the internet is both a curse and a blessing. As much as I've learned over the last several years, as much data that unfolds on my cancer each day, it still scares the crap out of me to search the internet. I can be doing oh-so-awesome with dealing with my cancer, and decide I have the mental *cojones* to handle anything they throw at me. I'll find some article on what happens when my lymphoma mutates, and I turn into a cower-in-the-closet-scaredy-cat.

I do believe knowledge is power. The internet is awesome, because there is so much information at your fingertips. It is a gift from the devil as well, because there is so much information at your fingertips. You need to remember that you are *you*. *You* have your own story, your own cancer, your own disease, and no two people are the same. Statistics can cover a wide variety of people and situations. Large correlations can provide you with some degree of probability, but you are still you within the scope of that probability. You could be an outlier on either end of the spectrum, so take care of you. If the internet feeds your fear—get off of it.

This is where your cancer posse can come into play. My cancer posse rocks. To this day, I'll sometimes have them look up stuff for me to provide reassurance when I'm having one of those "I'm gonna be one of those awful statistics on the bad end of the spectrum and my children will be motherless" moments. These people are awesome. They have *mucho* cancer posse qualities.

Cancer posse qualities: these peeps will take your moments in stride. They know how *not* to enter into your drama. They will listen, do research, and then reassure you that while your superhero cape is a bit tattered today, they've got some awesome thread to sew up the holes and send you on your way. They will know exactly how much info you can handle, what info would help, and what info will hinder. They will send you wine (or whiskey) and chocolate. Did I mention they have excellent capabilities for listening? They also know that *you* are *not* your disease. These people will still see you. Find your cancer (or other chronic disease) posse and keep them close.

In those moments I do decide to delve into information on the internet, it's usually through high-quality, well-documented sites. Look for evidence-based organizations that share the most recent research and results. But overall, I belong to very few cancer pages, blogs, and/or information sites. I like the Lymphoma Club[1] because nine times out of ten, it includes positive stories of superheroes and success stories. It is an uplifting page of courage, perseverance, and "can-do" attitude. After years of being an oncology nurse, this is the sort of information I need to keep me strong in my battle.

I, personally, *don't need* the statistics that draw me down. These statistics might not bother you at all. You need to decide that for you. But whatever you do, no matter the information you need, make sure you identify the information sources that *feed the fears*. Do not, *do not,* feed the fears. Bad juju, my friends. Let your cancer posse read the information that can feed the fears and digest it for you. It is not putting on blinders; it is breaking the information up in digestible pieces that keep you in fighting form. I have always said the most useful information you need at any given time is, "You can do this." Regardless of any disease or cancer, you need to hear, "You can do this."

You can do this. Trust me. I can do this. You can do this. We can do this together.

---

1. *www.facebook.com/lymphomaclub/*

Your Story . . .

So how does the "You can do this" statement roll over for you?

_____

_____

_____

_____

_____

_____

_____

_____

Good? Bad? Ugly?

_____

_____

_____

_____

_____

_____

_____

_____

_____

_____

What information scares the crap out of you? For me, the words "incurable" give me an ache in my stomach. I don't want to hear that.

_____

_____

_____

_____

_____

_____

_____

_____

What information pumps you up?

_____

_____

_____

_____

_____

_____

_____

_____

Making Bad Good

A generous person will be enriched, and one who gives water will get water.
(Prov. 11:25)

How I Felt . . .

Today I was able to go back and serve at an outreach opportunity that I have been involved in at my church. Once a month, we host a free community meal. I have been understandably absent the last two months and I have missed my kitchen peeps. Cooking in the kitchen for this meal is truly one of the highlights of my service to God. It is a physical expression of everything I believe. It was so good to be back in the kitchen.

And my kitchen peeps told me they missed me—my salty humor and all. And I missed them. It was a bittersweet day because a) I didn't have the energy to stay there all day and b) it was my last time serving before we move.

I've found that in the midst of the chaos of my life, including the grief, the anger, and the pain, two things make me feel real and normal again:

1. Serving others. Everyone has sorrow going on in their lives. Yeah—I've got a load of crap on my shoulders right now, but looking outside of myself keeps me from wallowing in self-pity. I am human—I can make this *all about me* with the best of them. Serving others reminds me that I am not the only person in pain, with tragedy, or with frustrations. We are all in this human condition together.

2. Exercise. Physically—after cooking all morning—I had to come home and take a nap. I have found my cancer makes me tired. I either take a nap or go to bed really early. It is what it is. Today I

got a nap and a second wind and headed out for a walk. I miss running and weight lifting, but this is my "Christ Walk" now. I walk as I am able, and still use my body for God's work in the world.

I know when I have not been able to walk. My mood is down. I feel physically drained and I don't cope as well with my anxiety and fear. My walk keeps me off my personal roller coaster. And it makes me feel normal and alive. My cancer may be my personal parasite, but it's not going to own me. I own it. And when I walk, I am able to pray. I am able to pray in some really deep ways that I am unable to do alone in my room or as I lay down for bed at night. I am able to cry behind my sunglasses and tell God how much I would really like to just put my head on God's shoulder and rest. I am able to say that I really just don't want to die. I know I'll have my place in heaven, but I have so much more to do here. I am comforted on my walks that God is with me and I am free to be me. Tears, anger, frustrations, fears, and all. And I always come back feeling better.

So, I think the two things I've learned to cope with this, no matter how things progress, is that to continue to serve others and to walk with God (and pray and cry) will get me through my bad days.

Everyone asks, "How are you?" My honest answer is there are bad days and good days and I think that will continue no matter what.

But for now, I give thanks because today was a good day.

What I Learned . . .

I think it is fairly clear what I learned from the above. Making time to do something for someone else outside of you is a sure way to feel better. We are called to serve others even when we aren't well ourselves. Was I able to volunteer for as long or as hard as I have done in the past? No, not at all. But I got out there for a bit, did something, and it felt better than any drug.

When we go out there and volunteer, even in small, seemingly meaningless ways, we recognize that we aren't the only people suffering. Walking a step in someone else's shoes really gives us an opportunity to get out of the funk that is our lot in life at the moment. There are many, many people who are hurting right now.

You are not alone. Volunteering and giving of your time, even in the middle of treatment or posttreatment, can make you feel a little bit like your old self. Feeling like your old self is a sure way to feel like you are giving cancer the bird.

Make the commitment to give cancer the bird.

Just like volunteering and giving of your time when you feel you are able, you should take every opportunity to get some sort of exercise. Walking is the most perfect exercise. When my mom was getting her bone marrow transplant (my mom is also a cancer survivor), she did not have a whole lot of energy to exercise, but she put a stack of five pennies in the corner of her room window. Her goal each day was to walk five laps of the hospital wing she was in. When she walked one lap, she would move one of those pennies to the opposite window. It was a strong visual representation of what she was able to accomplish in a day. Some days, she was able to move more than five pennies, but moving those five pennies was her goal. Even small things like this give you purpose in the middle of treatment and contribute to your overall wholeness and wellness.

Every step you take that is active helps to keep your body strong. As long as your doctor does not prohibit exercise, I encourage you strongly to stay as active as you are able. The fresh air will help with nausea; the activity can help with pain control. Simply moving makes us feel more alive. And exercise sometimes keeps our bodies busy so that our minds and hearts can pray. I wasn't able to pray well sitting still, but somehow the activity broke down my walls and opened my heart to the words I was afraid to say to God.

I wasn't flipping tires, lifting weights, or running marathons. I wasn't winning any races, but every step I took was a small step of victory in my journey back to me. Cancer and disease have a way of making you feel like you've lost yourself along the way. All these types of activities that you can continue to maintain in some shape or form will help you feel more and more like yourself.

Your Story . . .

What sorts of things would you like to try and volunteer to do during this journey of yours? What takes you outside of yourself?

_____

_____

_____

_____

_____

_____

_____

_____

What sort of exercise would you like to try on your journey?

_____

_____

_____

_____

_____

_____

_____

_____

_____

Identify a daily goal you can set for the next ten days:

_____

_____

_____

_____

_____

_____

_____

_____

_____

The next thirty days:

_____

_____

_____

_____

_____

_____

_____

_____

_____

_____

The next sixty days:

_____

_____

_____

_____

_____

_____

_____

_____

_____

_____

The next ninety days:

_____

_____

_____

_____

_____

_____

_____

_____

_____

_____

"So, How Are You?"

Will it be well with you when he searches you out? Or can you deceive him, as one person deceives another? (Job 13:9)

How I Felt . . .

If there were three words more loaded with conflicting answers, I am not sure what they would be:

"How are you?"

There should be a guidebook on how to answer this one: *The Dummies Guidebook to Answering Questions in a Socially Appropriate Way.* They need a special chapter for those of us with something going on. I feel like a deer in headlights when approached with it. Is it someone that really wants to know? Is it someone that can handle full kahuna? Is it someone that will understand "how I am" changes from moment to moment? Or is it someone that *I* need to reassure that everything is going to be ok? I often wonder if it's socially acceptable to really answer the "how I am" question in an honest manner—do people *really* want to know? Some days I am not really sure how I am because I'm still in the dreaded waiting place. How I am and how I *want* to be are two different questions.

"I'm okay" covers a lot of ground with anyone going through something. It's also the lottery ticket out of a conversation if you don't want to answer the question straight up. There are some people you just don't want to get into detail with about how you are, and then there are other people whom you need to buy a new shirt because you've just blubbered everything out on their shoulder.

So, how am I?

I am beyond blessed. God sent me a freaking neon signage saying, "It's going to be okay" that I will blog about at a later date, but it has put me in a calm waiting place rather than an anxious one. For any of you doubters out there . . . there is a God, God does care, and I am confident in God's plan . . . even when I don't get it.

I am tired. Frequently just tired. Mentally and physically tired. I love going out and being social, but it makes me tired. I am much more selective about what I do and whom I do it with because I am tired. I often take a nap in the middle of the afternoon before my kids get home so I have energy for them. They remain my priority. If I don't take a nap, I don't make it past nine o'clock most days. I'm learning to manage my energy levels so I can do what *I* want to do. My body controls my life right now. I'm learning to surrender to its needs.

I still hurt. It's manageable, but it is still there. My tumors sit on top of a damaged nerve, we think. After a day of working at the computer, my shoulder is a tortured mess of tangled fibers. I swear by acupuncture, massage, and yoga stretches. And Advil. We cannot forget the Advil. But I am rarely unaware of the parasite that sits on top of my clavicle. It reminds me daily that yes, it's still there, and yes, I have to wait to get rid of it.

I still get anxious, but each day it's better. I am not going off the deep end, even when I have a bad day and let it all out for everyone to see. If you want to know how I am, don't freak out if I tell you the truth. It can be a loaded question.

I still swear by my walks and talks with God. The best advice by far I've been given is to pray for others during this time when my anxiety is overwhelming. It works. I practice this vigilantly. Life is more than just about me. Praying for others takes me outside myself.

I am weak. While I am coming out of the toxicity of anesthesia, and my body heals from all the surgeries, I'm working on my fitness level, or rather what remains of my fitness level. I ran about five hundred feet for the first time. My first push-up was an utter failure, but I am learning to modify and listen to what my body can do. This is especially hard for me as a health and fitness professional. What I define as healthy now is very different from how I've perceived it in the past. I just ran a half marathon four months before my diagnosis and spent the entire summer doing a hundred-day burpee[1] challenge. I'm used

---

1. A burpee is a squat thrust exercise.

to being strong, not weak. It's humbling. I wrote a chapter on this in *Christ Walk*—about exercise for where you are now. And that's what I am trying to do. No, my fitness level is *not* where I would want it to be, but I am plugging away with it daily. It's a journey, not a sprint. I need to exercise with the body I have right now, not the one I wish I had, or the one I had before cancer.

I am still waiting. Waiting, waiting, waiting. I don't wait well. And because our life is not complicated enough, we are moving in three weeks to a new home; we are in the throes of managing movers, cleaning, and getting rid of things. We are registering kids for new schools, closing on a house, and still waiting to find out what they will do with me. I still have far more questions than answers, which makes "How are you?" very difficult to answer. There are so many moving parts in the waiting place right now.

I evidently look good because people tell me this all the time. Like, "Wow, you don't look like you have cancer." I'm not really sure how to answer that one . . . how are cancer people supposed to look? I jokingly tell my doc that I don't look bad because a) makeup is amazing and b) I still (*still*) question that I have cancer. If I hadn't read the pathology reports, I'm not sure that I would believe it because I felt fine until they started messing with me. But yeah, I look good. They haven't done anything to me yet, so when I look like a cancer patient, I guess I'll let you know. But this is a great lesson: we have no idea what people are going through solely by the way they look. Makeup and clothes make for great armor around whatever you are carrying in your heart.

I have a sick sense of humor. Gallows humor puts cancer in its place. I won't apologize for cracking jokes about my cancer even if it makes someone uncomfortable. When I can make jokes about death, dying, and cancer, it allows me to face the cancer and tame the beast. It's a "take that" response. So, if I drop my cancer into a conversation like a bomb, don't cringe. Let's beat that beast back together. I've learned my friends are scared just as much as I am. We aren't going to tiptoe around this crap. We are going to slap it down and own it.

I have amazing friends and family. I'm certainly hoping I haven't hurt any of their feelings about the "How are you?" question because *everyone* asks this out of a sense of concern and love. I don't get upset when questions come from a place of love, even when I'm really not sure how to answer them. People mean the best when they ask you how you are even if it makes you a little crazy to answer it. Some days you want to answer it with a four-letter word or two, even when it's not polite to answer that way. It is what it is. When you have no control over your life, it's a roller coaster of responses.

"How am I?" is a complicated question. I am a lot of things. And it depends. It depends how I am at any given moment. It depends on what is going on around me and it really depends on how much you really want to know.

That's how I am today. How are you?

What I Learned . . .

Three years into this journey, I still don't really like this question of "How are you?" I am still not sure what the right answer is. My situation is complicated. It's less dire, but still complicated. I have moved from needing to rapidly treat my lymphoma, to learning to live with it. My tumors still sit on my clavicles. They still remind me of their presence at odd moments. I have learned that my cancer will always be a part of me. I have learned that people don't always want the truthful answer to "How are you?"

I have realized it's okay for people to feel that way too. Sometimes people do not really want to know out of a desire for self-preservation. Your feelings may be a lot for them to bear. You will learn, if you haven't already, that there are certain people you can let it all out with and there will be other people who would prefer that you stick with "I'm okay." The people who have no clue what your journey is like will never really understand. Don't hold that against them. This is your journey, not theirs. You will also become increasingly comfortable with your cancer. As I've said, it is a part of me now. It is a part of my story. It just *is*. It will become less important to you to answer that question of "How are you?" You will save the answer for those people who are your Groots.

When I have difficult moments going into checkups, or I worry that my cancer is growing, I can answer my Groots truthfully when

I am not doing well. But it isn't the sort of thing I share all the time with everyone.

My mom found her own catchall phrase when asked, "How are you?" She says each time, "I am enjoying each day." For me, it's along the lines of "I am still watching and waiting, and every day learning to trust God more." It really doesn't cover all of it, but it's a socially appropriate response. When I am able to say those words, it puts the cancer in its place. Trusting in God is far more important to me than worrying what my cancer is or is not doing at any given time.

Your Story . . .

Really, *how* are you?

_____

_____

_____

_____

_____

_____

_____

_____

_____

_____

_____

On a scale of 1–10, how stinky are you feeling about your situation?

_____

_____

_____

_____

_____

_____

_____

_____

_____

_____

_____

On a scale of 1–10, how annoyed are you when people ask you
how you are?

_____

_____

_____

_____

_____

_____

_____

_____

_____

_____

_____

_____

What's a phrase you can use that answers people's questions, but doesn't get into the details if you aren't interested in sharing? (Remember to be nice—most people are asking from a place of love.)

_____

_____

_____

_____

_____

_____

_____

_____

_____

_____

Crazy Things That Happen When You Have Cancer (or Other Diagnosis)

First of all, then, I urge that supplications, prayers, intercessions, and thanksgivings be made for everyone, for kings and all who are in high positions, so that we may lead a quiet and peaceable life in all godliness and dignity. (1 Tim. 2:1–2)

How I Felt . . .

I have started drinking green tea. This is what I call my "kick cancer's a$$ tea." It is not bad, but I do not really like it. I am a coffee drinker at heart. But just about everything you read about green tea talks about its butt-kicking, anticancer properties. Each afternoon I sit down with a cup of my tea and imagine it destroying cancer cells like the Death Star blowing up. This is only one of the many crazy things I have started to do in this journey of healing and faith. I have discovered that when you feel out of control with your life, controlling the small things is quite empowering. Drinking my tea, whether or not it works, makes me feel like I am doing something other than sitting here waiting.

I also decided one day that my Keurig coffee maker was a culprit in my cancer diagnosis. (Disclaimer: Keurig coffee makers do not cause cancer. These are my feelings I am describing.) It up and got itself sold. No more coffee dripped through cancer-causing plastic for me. When I told the lady I sold it to that I was worried it was causing my cancer, I thought she would throw the thing back at me. She was very gracious with my crazy cancer thoughts, but I learned that some of your crazy, you keep to yourself.

Along with the Keurig, all the plastic in my house turned evil overnight. The plastic storage containers went into the garbage; I tossed my plastic water bottle and opted for a glass one. I have begun looking at my water faucet through squinty eyes—there might be cancer chemicals in my water. We might just need a water filter in the future.

I have started taking an organic whole foods multivitamin and digestive enzymes. Those suckers are supposed to eat up all the junk in your gut that might cause cancer. Bring on the probiotics.

The next to go was any deodorant in the house. No more aluminum deposits for me. No sir—I promptly purchased an all-organic deodorant that leaves me smelling great but does not do a whole lot for sweating. Of course, since my cancer has been growing, I sweat 24/7, so it is part of the cancer thing, more than my antiperspirant, but hey, a girl can hope.

In a true fit of crazy, I tossed my mascara too. I have a nice tube of organic mascara now as well. Organic brown. It even looks organic. It works great and now I won't get eye cancer. I will neither confirm, nor deny, whether my other beauty products will take a hit in the future. I am eyeing all products the same way I look at my water: with suspicion.

I have determined I will embrace my grey and forego any chemical treatment of my hair. It is just one more of those things I can control.

We already eat very organic and I am not huge on processed foods to begin with, so our journey down the *real foods* approach to living started long ago. We really have an overall healthy house. I avoid chemicals when I clean, I believe in organic produce and locally sourced products as often as I can get them, and I am very conscientious about what I buy and what is in what I purchase. In fact, my son recently said to me, "Mommy, there's something I don't understand. You are the healthiest of all of us—why did *you* get the cancer?"

Indeed, why did I get this cancer? It is a question I ask myself a lot. Why did I get this cancer, even after all the things I do right? Things just happen. A lot of things in life happen that we cannot control. A lot of things happen that we will never understand. A lot of things we have to just have faith in God that a greater purpose is in store for us than we can ever fathom.

In the meantime, with those things I do not understand, nor can control, I will continue with the sort of things I can control. They may not work and they may look like crazy cancer girl thoughts, actions, craziness to everyone else, but to me they are things that make me feel like I am doing something to beat the beast.

What I Learned . . .

There is no way to control every cancer-causing thing in your environment. There is no 100 percent way to prevent cancer. It sometimes just happens. In my case, I have a medical history that predisposed me to my cancer. In my case, my healthy living has probably kept my cancer at bay for a long time. I still ask myself, "Why?" I will probably always ask myself why, because I will never be content that I have cancer. I may live with it, I may be at peace with it, but I will never be okay that I have cancer. I will never be okay that anyone has cancer.

I can tell you with 100 percent assurance that incorporating habits of good exercise, healthy eating, prayer, stress modification, and tobacco cessation are distinct actions you *can* take to either reduce your risk or improve your response to the cancer or illness experience. There are a lot of things we do as humans that are bad for our health. There are actions *we* take and choices *we* make that can both help or hinder our journey. However, there are a lot of things people have no control over in their lives that you will never, ever be able to fix. There will be no green juice, no magic pill, no change I can make, or something that I should have done that will fix the flaw in my genetics. There is no perfect way to prevent cancer (at least not right now).

Sometimes, crap just happens.

I still drink green tea, although not every day. I still prefer glass to plastic, although you will find random Tupperware in my cabinets. I still aim for mostly chemical-free living. My hair is greying. I have not dyed it in three and a half years. I still have organic mascara, and most products I use are purchased with an eye for cancer-causing chemicals. But I am a little more relaxed about it all. I do not blame myself for causing my cancer with anything I use or do not use. I no longer think there is a special juice or miracle pill that is going to fix what happened. It just did. I believe that we should do what we are able to do. Make changes in your life that are reasonable, attainable, sustainable, and contribute to your overall well-being while on this journey.

The changes I made in my life made me feel like I was *doing* something to my cancer while I waited. The changes you make in your life may empower you as well. If a green smoothie every day floats your cancer boat, then do it. If not, there are plenty of other healthy things you can do to support your wellness. And let me stress this: you *can* support, improve, and focus on your wellness and well-being, even with disease.

With confidence, I can share that stressing about any of it makes things worse. I did the green juice thing. I loaded my body up with kale, collards, and all sorts of green stuff that was supposed to kill my cancer cells—it made me sick. I tore up my stomach in this over-enthusiastic pursuit of a natural approach to cancer care. With all my focus on trying to be extra healthy, all it did was stress me out. This is not good and was definitely not good for me. Sometimes you can go over the top trying to be healthy and lose focus on the important things in life: joy, love, relationships, and just feeling well. Try to focus on those things that bring you joy and reduce your stress load. This will contribute more to how well you respond to your treatment and the outlook you have on your journey. Do those things that work for *you*.

All sorts of people are going to e-mail you with articles on magical, all-natural approaches to cancer care. Some of this advice will entail supplements, diets, coffee colonics (yes, you read that right, squeezing coffee in your you-know to cleanse your intestines out along with the cancer cells . . . I like coffee, just not that much), and much more. People will tell you all sorts of crazy things to try. People do this because they desperately want to help you, but many people do not realize that this kind of advice can often make you feel like you did something wrong. At least that is how I interpreted it. While people were trying to help me, all I heard was, "You weren't leading a healthy enough life and look what happened to you." I saw big fat fingers pointing at me everywhere.

Some of the advice was just crazy. My organic mascara might be crazy, but the coffee colonic was *really* crazy. Many things made me roll my eyes. Some things seemed promising. Other things did not make sense for me. What I did learn was talking through options with my doctor made a huge difference. She was completely supportive of yoga, acupuncture, my vitamin therapy, and continuing my healthy choices. She did not think I was going to be able to "cleanse" myself of my cancer, but she did listen to me, because when people offer you those "magic" cures, they sound really exciting and hopeful (well, maybe not the coffee colonic). When things are exciting and hopeful, it is easy to get your hopes up because all we want at the end of the day is for our disease to magically disappear.

Your friends and colleagues reach out to you with their own level of crazy out of a place of love. I try very hard not to get upset with anyone's advice, because I realize they just want the best for me. That is not really very different from what I want for myself as well.

Remember, the key to health, with or without disease, is reasonable, attainable, sustainable, achievable choices, focused on your overall well-being. Your decisions need to be things that you can live with for the rest of your life in order to promote health inside and outside your home, body, and mind. I believe those choices are different for everyone, but it does require you to think about your life and what needs changing in order to be successful.

Your Story . . .

What are some crazy cancer (or other illness) changes you are thinking about making, or have made in your life?

_____

_____

_____

_____

_____

_____

_____

_____

_____

_____

Are these changes reasonable, attainable, achievable, and sustainable?

_____

_____

_____

_____

_____

_____

_____

_____

_____

_____

What are some suggestions friends made for you to change that made you mad or anxious or upset?

_____

_____

_____

_____

_____

_____

_____

_____

_____

_____

What was it about their advice that struck you as wrong?

_____

_____

_____

_____

_____

_____

_____

_____

_____

God Advertises in Neon Signs

And he said to me, "These words are trustworthy and true, for the Lord, the God of the spirits of the prophets, has sent his angel to show his servants what must soon take place." (Rev. 22:6)

How I Felt . . .

Let me just put this out there if you have not realized it yet: I believe in God. I believe that God is all around us, and I believe that God walks with us every step we take.

I have been going through a lot lately. Digesting a cancer diagnosis is not quite as palatable as digesting a piece of chocolate cake. But we still need to swallow it and work through whatever has been thrown at us to conquer. I have known theologically (or rationally or clinically) through all of this—God is with me. My heart has been another story. At times my heart was so hurt, so angry, and so disillusioned that all that negativity was keeping me from feeling the love of God during this time.

I think this is normal. I think God understands that. I think God knows that we are so fragile, so sensitive to our emotions that we need time to process and digest before we can realize that there is more to this moment than what we are living right now. I am reminded of the time my mother-in-law and I made a cake. It was going to be this beautiful chocolate roll (see the recipe on page 121) that is a family tradition. Well, I ruined the cake. I saw failure in the crumbled pieces of my expectations. There was not going to be a chocolate roll with the cake in crumbles. In that moment, I could not see possibility. I saw failure. When time passes, however, things unfold. The chocolate roll became a chocolate roll bowl (à la trifle-style) and was just as delicious, if not as beautiful as the original plan.

"Life is what happens to us while we are making other plans."[1]

---

1. Allen Saunders, 1957, *Reader's Digest*.

It is difficult to see my illness as a possibility. I am fragile. What I am experiencing does *not fit right* with my senses. Everything feels out of balance. When I am overwrought with emotion, I need to feel, touch, hear, smell, taste, and see God to believe that God is with me on my journey. I need that tangible evidence because when I am fragile, I doubt. Sometimes, I need some sort of neon sign to see that God is there.

Sometimes it takes a long time for me to see those neon signs in front of my face, but they are there. Sometimes the hardest thing about my faith is to believe in God and know God is with me without those experiential senses tied to it. There are times when my senses are overwhelmed with God right here, right with me, and in the moments I need it most. These are moments of grace. God comes to us through grace.

I have said it once, I will say it again: I am far too flawed to understand the *why things happen* in the world, but I believe in grace. Grace is God's action in the world. Grace is how I experience God through my senses. Grace happens through people. God is grace in action in people.

Grace happened to me last week. Grace showed up in my life like a big neon sign for a cupcake bakery. Grace came to me frosted, with pink roses and sunshine and smiles and promises *that everything was going to be ok.*

Grace rocks, people.

Grace came to me in the form of a letter. My husband and I are moving from Kansas to Virginia with the Army. We have been holding off on my treatment (with the approval of my doctors) until we get to our new duty station. My husband's leadership had offered to advocate for us to try and keep us in Kansas. However, in my gut, I knew (remember grace . . . listen to your gut) that we should move anyway and we would figure out how to do that around the cancer. The move was something I had mixed feelings about. It was an added complication to an already complicated mess and it did not help with the struggles with anxiety I continue to have.

Then this letter came . . . this beautiful letter that had grace coming from it out of every sentence. The executors of the estate that we were buying the house in Virginia from had found my blog. And they had reached out to me via my blog e-mail to send me a message.[2] The previous owners of the house were a lot like Treb and me. The previous owner was a retired military man—a WWII decorated veteran—and his wife was a nurse. They were a strong Christian family with deep ties to the area where we are moving. This lovely lady wrote me a letter that this house was meant to be ours. *She said my cancer would be healed by the love in that house.* (Ok, so that was not what she wrote, but it was the message I received. God's grace sends messages.) *Grace happens.* Grace comes like an advertisement in neon when you need it, and I desperately needed this message from God that everything was going to be ok:

Hi Anna

I understand you are the new owner of my late uncle's home, as our family fondly refers to the house on P Lane. My cousin, the executor of my Uncle's estate, shared your Facebook page with me. Wanting to know more, I went to your blog page. I am touched deeply.

Since I have not met you, I was not comfortable posting on the blog, but I feel compelled to reach out to you. I want you to know about the tremendous love and blessings and celebrations that were shared in your new home. The home where you will rest your head, where you will return after your treatments for the cancer which has invaded your body, where you will recuperate and, God willing, beat this beast, where you will raise your children, where you will nurture and strengthen your marriage, where you will seek and find the peace of Christ.

My dear Uncle and Aunt, my mom's only sister, showed me the true essence of sacramental marriage. Never have I witnessed a couple more devoted to one another or more in love. Nothing was more important to either of them than their love for the Lord, their love for each other, and the love they had for their children. Their doors were always open to our large extended family as well as the hundreds of friends my cousins had. Not only was their door open, but their hearts as well. Their love was so great that it could not be contained within their home but spilled over into the community

---

2. The e-mail is shared here with her permission.

and beyond, in service to the poor and the homeless, in the establishment of prayer groups to bring others closer to the heart of Jesus Christ, in ministry to the sick and homebound. The list is long.

I believe with all my heart and soul that God has a plan for each of us and that His plan is perfect. Many times we can't comprehend this or see His light because of the darkness that we allow to overwhelm us. But I am certain that it is no coincidence that my beloved Uncle was called home a few months ago and that his family home was available just when you needed it.

So, Anna, know of my prayers for you and for your family. May you find comfort knowing you now reside in a home that has been blessed in so many ways. May you continue the legacy of love for the Lord, for your spouse, for your children and for the Kingdom, which began so many years ago by my Aunt and Uncle. May God bless you and give you strength.

Lord, I heard a man say, "I give you my heart." But this morning I feel I cannot give only my heart. I offer my whole self.

What I Learned . . .

Even as I reread my post, I am brought to tears. God sent me a sign through another person that I desperately needed in the middle of this chaos and I and my husband were touched beyond measure. God does send signs. Yes, some are bigger and bolder than others, but I know if we open our hearts to these signs, we will see them, be comforted, and brought peace. God never promised me a rose garden in my life, but God did say the Lord would be there with me through it all. When we love one another, we are sending God-signs to each other. And when I got this God-sign from Gail, my anxiety and fear abated.

Look for God-signs on your journey. There will be many times that grace is in action in your life so that you can touch, see, hear, feel, and taste God along your journey. You may be struggling to feel God during this season. You may be like I was: very angry, confused, frightened, and anxious. This does not mean that God is not there. When we can count the grace in action in our lives, the love from other people, and the actions of others on behalf of us, we sense God's presence. I can feel God in the hug from my friend. I can taste God in the food brought by a neighbor after my surgery. I can hear God in the words of my children as they whisper, "I love you, Mommy." I can see God in the words that people have written from afar. I can smell God in the prayer shawl knit by my church. I know God through these acts of grace. You will know God, just as we love one another as God loves us.

Your Story . . .

Name some acts of grace:

_____

_____

_____

_____

_____

_____

_____

_____

_____

How do you see God?

_____

_____

_____

_____

_____

_____

_____

_____

_____

_____

How do you feel God?

_____

_____

_____

_____

_____

_____

_____

_____

How do you taste God?

_____

_____

_____

_____

_____

_____

_____

_____

_____

_____

How do you hear God?

_____

_____

_____

_____

_____

_____

_____

_____

How do you smell God?

_____

_____

_____

_____

_____

_____

_____

_____

_____

_____

How do you know God?

_____

_____

_____

_____

_____

_____

_____

_____

_____

THE COURIE FAMILY CHOCOLATE ROLL RECIPE

This is the recipe for the chocolate roll I described above, unless you have to turn it into a trifle because the cake falls apart. It's a celebration cake. It's a cake made with love, one you should absolutely make when celebrating each of your victories.

INGREDIENTS:

- 6 eggs at room temperature, separated
- ⅔ cup sugar and ⅔ cup sugar
- ⅔ cup self-rising flour
- 7 tablespoons cocoa
- 3 tablespoons hot water
- 1½ pints whipping cream

DIRECTIONS:

1. Beat yolks and add ⅔ cup of sugar.
2. Add 3 tablespoons of hot water.
3. Mix flour with cocoa and add yolk mixture.
4. Beat eggs whites in a separate container and add the other ⅔ cup of sugar and a pinch of salt; fold whites into the chocolate mixture.
5. Grease and flour a 17 x 11 (cookie sheet) pan lined with waxed paper.
6. Bake at 375 degrees for 10 minutes.
7. When the roll comes out of the oven, turn onto a wet (damp) kitchen towel and remove waxed paper. Then roll into the towel and set aside until it cools, but don't wait too long before you unroll it and fill with the whipped cream. Otherwise, it falls apart (see exhibit A described above). Beat the whipping cream to thick consistency and add sugar. Pour into the roll and roll back up. Frost with chocolate frosting.
8. *Whipped cream:* Beat 1 to 1½ pints whipping cream until stiff; add sugar until sweet. Add ½ teaspoon vanilla. Put into cooled chocolate cake and roll over.

Continued

CHOCOLATE MOCHA FROSTING FOR CHOCOLATE ROLL

INGREDIENTS:

- 1½ teaspoons instant coffee granules
- ⅓ cup boiling water
- 3 squares unsweetened chocolate
- ¼ cup butter
- Dash of salt
- 2½ cups sifted powdered sugar
- Chopped pecans

DIRECTIONS:

1. Mix together and set aside the instant coffee and boiling water.
2. Melt together the chocolate, butter, and salt until creamy and set aside to cool.
3. When cooled slightly, stir in coffee and sifted powdered sugar.
4. Beat until smooth.
5. Spread over the chocolate roll.
6. Sprinkle chopped pecans over it.
7. For Christmas, add green and red cherries for a Yule Log.

Enjoy! And make sure you celebrate things on your journey.

Happy Thanksgiving!

Enter his gates with thanksgiving, and his courts with praise. Give thanks to him, bless his name. (Ps. 100:4)

How I Felt . . .

On this day of Thanksgiving, I remind myself I am blessed. In the midst of everything going on, we are still blessed by God, our families, our friends, and the love we have. We remember the sick, the hungry, the lonely, the oppressed, those who are afar, and those who continue to work on this day. We remember our soldiers, our sailors, our marines, our airmen, our nurses, doctors, police officers, and firemen; we remember the young, the old, and those we may have forgotten. God bless us all.

Happy Thanksgiving to you all! And don't forget your Christ Walk today. You need to burn off that slice of pie.

What I Learned . . .

Holidays are going to come and go during your diagnosis and treatment. The rest of the world does not stop. Holidays, birthdays, and anniversaries do not get put on hold just because you are sick. People will be celebrating, when all you want to do is mourn.

Some of you will dread the holidays. You may not be able to be happy. Some people will not know how to find joy in the middle of celebrations, holidays, and parties. There is a weight to the joy and excitement of people around you that is soul crushing when you feel horrible and when you are scared and full of anxiety. It's hard to respond to people's joy when you just do not feel the same way. Sometimes you will just feel like crap and be unable to physically participate. But the holidays still happen.

My advice for holidays: celebrate them however you feel you are able. But do not pretend they do not happen. You will feel worse trying hard not to acknowledge a birthday, holiday, or anniversary. You want to stop time and pretend you are not losing parts of time to your disease, but unfortunately, time keeps moving on.

Sometimes we want time to stop. Sometimes, we want to freeze this part of our life so that we can compartmentalize it as "the disease time." That way, when the "disease time" passes, we pretend we can forget about it and restart life where we left off. This isn't anywhere close to the truth. You never forget that you have your disease. Even when you are cured of it, it has become a part of you. Your experience right now is shaping you as an individual. Don't wish time away just because you are sick right now. Remember that where you are right now is not where you will be forever.

With these special occasions, I really did not want to participate in them. I did not have a lot of energy. I was frustrated by this lack of the enthusiasm and zeal that I usually have. It was a constant reminder that something was not quite right. Yet, I never regretted when I did rally and participate to the best of my ability. Was it the same? No, not at all. I scaled back with preparations, plans, presents, and expectations, but I still celebrated. The important part of these occasions is that they are a reminder of life. And those reminders can beef up your superpowers to keep fighting.

Holidays are a reminder that we are more than our cancer or disease, and yes, that is an important thing to be reminded of frequently. *You* are worth celebrating.

You are worth celebrating. And your friends, family, and the life you have right now are worth celebrating. Each breath you take, the steps you make, every moment of this journey is worth celebrating because your life is precious to God. Even when things go south, we have this opportunity to fully live our lives in a godly manner. We can proclaim the gospel from hospital beds, couches, and chemo rooms. Every day is an opportunity and a gift to celebrate because our life is here, complete with God's will to do great things, even with the crappiness that might be going on inside the body.

You are worth celebrating. Use each holiday as an opportunity to celebrate and share love. Celebrate yourself.

Your Story . . .

What did you do for your birthday during treatment?

_____

_____

_____

_____

_____

_____

_____

_____

What did you do to celebrate your anniversary?

_____

_____

_____

_____

_____

_____

_____

_____

_____

_____

_____

What did you do to celebrate a holiday?

_____

_____

_____

_____

_____

_____

_____

_____

_____

How did you feel about those celebrations?

_____

_____

_____

_____

_____

_____

_____

_____

_____

_____

Wearing Yourself Thin: What Not to Do

Now, even if I boast a little too much of our authority, which the Lord gave for building you up and not for tearing you down, I will not be ashamed of it. (2 Cor. 10:8)

How I Felt . . .

Life was not complicated enough, so we decided to fly home to South Carolina for Thanksgiving to see family. In our defense, we bought the tickets long before we knew about my cancer or our move schedule. We will fly back to Kansas today; tomorrow the movers come. We have been packing for two trips, taking pictures off the walls, cleaning basements and garages, and ensuring the house is ready for inspection. To say there are a lot of moving parts is a bit of an understatement. Moving is hell.

But with going home for Thanksgiving, I got to hug my mama. Even though I am thirty-nine years old, I still want, need, and love my mama. Her hugs make it worth it.

And we got to go back to my alma mater, Clemson University, to attend our rival college's football game. It has been over two years since I have been back and I was astounded by the changes and additions to campus. Even so, Clemson still feels like home. Or maybe I am just sensitive to the need for a home in the middle of a move. Or maybe I am just more sensitive to the need for home in the middle of this diagnosis. When the Army is done with us, Clemson is one of those places I could call my forever home . . . there is something in the hills. My happy factor was bursting.

I got to see some surprise friends I did not expect to see; I got to cry all over my old roommate and get hugs from so many wonderful people. We got to visit with many who have supported me from afar the last several weeks. And I guess I still do not look like I have cancer because everyone still says I look good.

I got to see my Tigers win their football game. It was great to see those around us whom we have sat with over the last sixteen years (on and off), and now their kids are grown and in high school or college. Since I still look twenty-one—or so I think—I am confused that everyone else is looking older. Ha!

Things were going so well, and then I had to fall asleep during halftime. I am sure everyone thought I was a terrible fan, but that is what my body does now. By evening my back and arm were a knotted mass of pain. There were times I had to walk off the tears. I dislike (yes, still do) the interference of my disease on my plans. I have managed to get a cold, I am pooped, and my back and arm will take at least a week to get back to being manageable. But to hug my friends, shed tears with those I love, and see "where the blue ridge yawns its greatness" was a weekend of thanksgiving for me.

The real world returns tomorrow, but my heart is full (even if my body aches).

What I Learned . . .

Sometimes you overdo it and push your body to its limits for a chance you might not have for a long time. I do not think there is anything wrong with this. Your doctor may have other thoughts when you share your plans, but I do think it is very important to live. Life does not stop just because you have cancer or disease and require treatment. In fact, the most important part is doing things you like, to the best of your ability, during this time. So what if you have to take a nap in the middle of it? Do it anyway. You want to go see your favorite singer, actor, or sports hero and you fall asleep? Do it anyway. These moments are about enjoying life. Do not lament the fact that you are not where you were before. Just enjoy doing what you can, the best you can. This time is not forever.

Now, having said that, you may have repercussions from the choice you made. In my case, my whole body rebelled against the added stress. I got a cold, the problems with my shoulder postsurgery flared up, and my entire body hurt—but I cannot say it was not worth it. Every hug was worth every ache. I needed to see my family and friends. You may have that same need for something in your life too. Go get it.

Your Story . . .

What is something you feel like you want or need to do?

_____

_____

_____

_____

_____

_____

_____

_____

_____

What is something that your situation makes you feel like you cannot do?

_____

_____

_____

_____

_____

_____

_____

_____

_____

_____

What are some ways to do that in your current situation, and maybe change your expectations so you can enjoy it?

_____

_____

_____

_____

_____

_____

_____

Where Is My Breaking Point?

How long will you torment me, and break me in pieces with words? (Job 19:2)

How I Felt . . .

Where do my breaking points lie? I have been flirting with them on and off lately. I am in a rough patch. I am old enough to know that eventually it will pass, but young enough that it still entangles me; consumes me; grabs me by the throat and tries to rule me. The devil and I are dancing the tango.

The last two weeks of my life fit this hashtag: #youcannotmake thisstuffup. I am living my own personal soap opera and even I am left stunned by the crap that stalks me.

There are various reasons why. Number one: *I don't like to relinquish control*. Number two: I think I walked under too many ladders, crossed too many black cats, broke too many mirrors, or something. I do not really believe in jinxes, omens, or anything, but really, lately stuff is just stupid.

When you have cancer (or any other kind of tragedy, disease, problem), you instantly lose control over your life. Consequently, you try to retain tighter control over those things in life that you can. For a control freak such as myself, this presents problems.

I am sorry, but the whole "Let go and let God" approach is like Mount Everest to me. It is my sin; I know it and I try to tackle it daily, but when I lack control, I find myself slipping closer to my personal breaking point. Plus, stupid things can make me a little crazier than normal as well.

This week has been our move. I am used to moving. My son and I counted up fifteen moves in my thirty-nine years this week as we talked about our newest adventure. I am an old salt. A vagabond at heart. This life suits me, so do not think I am complaining about my lot. But it does not make it easy. The process of moving is inherently exhausting: mind, body, and spirit.

And my body is tired. It feels old and fails to respond with the vigor I know. In my heart, I know my cancer slows me down. I resent it immensely. I have no place in which to focus my fury. No outlet for my angst. I am stuck in this short period of time that is called my move. I am trying to focus my energy on my children, who are also struggling with yet another move. This will be the fifth in six and a half years. During all this, my husband is wrapping up school—all so we can leave earlier than planned in order for me to try and get the right treatment. It is the perfect storm.

And the storm began brewing when we decided to stick with our plans to go to South Carolina for Thanksgiving. I overdid it as usual and then to cap the cake with more frosting, we missed our connection by five minutes; the plane was still on the tarmac waiting when we arrived, but they would not let us on the plane. This led to a six-hour layover and arriving home about one o'clock in the morning of the day our move started. On top of that, I came down with some nasty virus.

At the prodding (well, really demanding, forcing, cajoling) of friends and family, I did what I truly *hate* to do—I have asked for help this week. I could not do it on my own. It was more than I could handle. I set up friends for dinner, coffee runs, companionship, and childcare. And I asked our transportation/moving coordinator for *one* thing:

I played the cancer card—not in jest. We simply said, "I have lymphoma. We need a smooth move to DC with as quick of a delivery of our household goods as can be so I can see my doctors and get treatment." (Treatment is the only thing on my mind these days—I want this crap out of my body fiercely.) The only thing I asked of them was to send me a good team, make it as stress-free as possible, do a good job, and get my stuff to DC.

Well, this is how it played out:

Day 1: "Ma'am: we will be there between 9 and 10 a.m." Ok. Good. This will work. Hour after hour passes. Finally, at 1:45, they show up with three people and work for three and a half hours. Maybe a fourth of my house is complete. No worries: they tell me that they will come back the next day between 9 and 10.

Day 2: 10 a.m. passes by . . . and then another hour and then another. Finally, they show up at 12:30. With two guys. Evidently, the third has been banned from entering a military installation. All day the lead packer is calling around looking for help. He wants this job done today. There is no way with two guys. Around 2:30 p.m., four more guys show up. Things pick up, but still not enough to finish packing. At one point, they are telling me how they are not getting paid enough to come help "me" out on this extra job. It is everything I can do not to tell them that I have had to take two days of leave without pay to wait for them to come do the job they were contracted to do. They want to stay until 10 p.m. to try and finish the job. I am exhausted. My body hurts. My kid is falling apart. We tell them to come back the next day. You do not get to stay all night when you cannot show up at the time agreed upon.

Day 3: They actually show up at 9:40. I am elated. But there are only two guys and the second guy has the flu. I give him medicine. Fluids. He goes to work. I keep being told that they will be done by 1:00. This from the same guy who told me they would be done by 6 the previous day. No time management skills. When you show up for work four hours late two days in a row, there is no getting done early. I think we all hated each other at this point. It is really difficult to love someone when you are not feeling well, and expectations are not being met. Hours roll by. They finally finish packing around 6:15. A lot of things were left undone.

Day 4: Loading van day—"Ma'am, we will be there before 9 a.m." Time passes. At 10:40, the van shows up. It's two-thirds full of other people's stuff. There is no room for all of my household goods. Plus, they spent a good hour taking things off and rearranging other people's belongings that were just thrown in the truck. At 11:00, I officially lose it. I spent half the morning yelling at people on the phone that said they would take care of this and make this an easy move because of my cancer. It has been the worst move ever (and remember, I have done this seven times as an adult). They fill the first van. My stuff is scattered across my lawn in boxes and pieces. It is like looking at your life as a broken puzzle strewn across the ground. I already feel broken. Now my house feels broken too. At 4:30, a second van finally shows up to load the rest of my house. So instead of one move with one delivery date, I will now have two delivery dates and two unpack dates all around three huge doc appointments that wait for me at our destination. The sad thing was that our loading team was great. If they had a van that had fit our stuff, then they actually would have been done on time. Both our loading team and my family got screwed today.

To the man that said he would "take care of this and make sure I had nothing to worry about." Thanks. You did a bang-up job.

From there, our driving adventure ensued. Because the moving fiasco was not enough, I am driving one car and my husband is driving the truck pulling the boat we cannot get rid of.

I loathe, *loathe* driving. Three days, twenty hours were ahead of us. It was totally a bear-down-and-get-through-it deal for me. My stomach still hurts from the incisions. I still cannot move my arm without pain. I am embracing the suck with the attitude of "Let's get this done."

So, I'm trucking along on my end of the trip with the plan to meet my hubby at our first destination. I thought he was about thirty minutes behind me . . .

He is four hours late . . . WTHeck???? The boat trailer broke. I kid you not. The wheel fell off the dang thing! YGTBKM!!! Thankfully, my husband had the great wisdom not to inform me of this until we were reunited. I do not handle that sort of thing well. (Control freak, remember?) The boat got left behind to get fixed. It was going to take several days to get the parts needed in the middle of nowhere Missouri. We will figure out the boat later, I guess. Two more days of driving commence . . .

Then upon our arrival to DC, we are greeted with a traffic jam. The number one reason I have resisted DC to date is the traffic. I loathe traffic. #countrygirl

This lengthened our eight-hour trip to ten. And I am already pooped. Grumpy has nothing on me at this point.

I hate these moments. They bring out the worst in me. I cannot find my Christian charity. I cannot find my patience. I cannot find my kindness or my understanding. I am tired. I am sad. My family is sad. We both love and hate to move. On the one hand, a great adventure awaits: a new home and new friends are around the corner. On the other, we leave dear people behind who have been a lifeline, not only during these last weeks of finding out about my cancer, but also during this move. I simply cannot thank them enough.

As we arrived at our new home, it was ready for us. Finally, something has gone right. Friends had left gifts, welcome notes, and beer. The house itself is everything we were promised.

(I'd like to end the post here, but I'm still irritated at my moving coordination so I will close with the below and say several prayers of forgiveness tonight.)

For the dude that promised to help, and then turned this into hell—well, the sinful side of me hopes you have a move just like this one in your future, and I will hope and pray you have people by your side because these last few days were awful, and the only thing that kept my toe from crossing the breaking point were the peeps I had by my side. I am not a Christian on my own. It is the people around me that call me to be something better.

What I Learned . . .

I have a breaking point. I did not exactly break, but I certainly flirted with the line those days of that move. It still ranks as one of our worst military moves, and I have no desire to ever repeat the experience. There is no part of me that recommends doing what I did in the middle of battling a disease. It ended up being the absolute right thing for our family as you will see, but it was still highly stressful and not something I recommend without serious thought about your health, your mental stamina, strength, and what you feel like you can handle in your life.

I also learned that being a Christian, and following the Christian way of living, is really difficult when you are tired, mad, hurting, sad, scared, and anxious. Regardless of moving, you will probably feel these things at any given time during your journey—and maybe all at once. I sometimes wished some of these people could feel how truly horrible I felt so that they were able to understand that all I wanted was some compassion and help during this really complicated transition. I think one guy had a really hard time believing I had cancer because like many of you, I do not *look* like I have cancer. Appearances on the outside can be truly deceiving for the battle that rages underneath. Whether it is cancer, diabetes, heart disease, depression, or some other horrible disease, we really have no idea the war that lies under the surface of our human brothers and sisters.

As a result, even when we do not feel like being Christian to someone else, we really need to focus on God's guidance. Even when we are sick and struggling, we *do* have control over the choices we make as individuals and how we react. It does not mean it isn't hard. It does not mean we will be able to do it, and we may fail to respond in a Christian manner (I certainly failed), but we are called to try. In *Christ Walk* I write that I believe God smiles every time we try. I still believe this. Try to not break. Try to use kind words. Try to understand. Try not to judge others by how they look on the outside. Try to be compassionate, even when people make you angry. Try to find joy, even when you feel like crap. We do not stop being Christians because we have an illness. We are still Christians in spite of it. That illness is just along for the ride. Let being a Christian define who you are, not the illness.

Your Story . . .

Do you let your illness define you, or do you define yourself in different words or context?

_____

_____

_____

_____

_____

_____

_____

_____

_____

Who are some people that you need to work hard on finding compassion and understanding for, even though you do not feel you have the patience for their drama in your life?

_____

_____

_____

_____

_____

_____

_____

_____

_____

How do you define being a Christian?

_____

_____

_____

_____

_____

_____

_____

_____

_____

Ten Bits of Advice to the Healthcare Industry

So let us not grow weary in doing what is right, for we will reap at harvest-time, if we do not give up. (Gal. 6:9)

How I Felt . . .

Between my personal health and my professional resume, I have been around the healthcare field for a long time. I have noticed things come and go over the years, but I have a running list of thoughts that would improve anyone's experience. Here are some of these suggestions:

1. Be a patient for a day. You have no clue what the other side is like until you have traversed it yourself. Try getting lost in corridors. Or have a technician get mad at you for a doctor putting in orders wrong. Being a patient can be one of the most dehumanizing experiences you can imagine. It is not always, but it is something we should remember when working in the healthcare field. The people who are traversing the corridors of the hospital have scary things going on in their lives. Be kind. Experience the healthcare process for the day as a patient. Finally, do not presume to know my body better than me after five minutes with me. This is a partnership, not a dictatorship.

2. Do not put flavor in contrast fluid. It does nothing to help the experience of sucking down bottles of that crap for over two hours. A straw would be nice too. Never underestimate the power of a straw. Especially a pink one with an umbrella on top.

3. *Always. Always. Always* serve good coffee. Life is too short for the patients, doctors, nurses, or other staff to be served terrible coffee.

Everyone will be happier. Happier people equals a happier organization. This will always start with good coffee.

4. If you have to make a patient wait in a clinic for two hours for a procedure, consider offering recliners instead of hard chairs. I can squeeze a nap in while I wait or put my feet up when I am hurting. Your patients will appreciate the comfort when they are stuck in the dreaded waiting place.

5. For God's sake—I know healthcare is expensive, but do not try to save a few pennies by turning off the heat. Or at least tell us to bring gloves and a blanket. These places are like waiting in an icebox. Turn on the heat in winter and the AC in summer. Add it to my bill.

6. Serve good food. People go to hospitals to get well. If you are serving terrible, fake food, that is never going to happen. You can make yummy food that does not look like cardboard. Then people will spend more of their money on your food instead of on fast-food that they bring in, thereby reducing waste at the cafeteria. It will also be better for their health as a whole.

7. Make everyone in the hospital take a customer service class. And I mean everyone. *Your* attitude makes a huge difference in how I am handling my health. Your attitude makes a huge difference in whether or not I send a nastygram following an event. People are far more likely to tell you what you did wrong than what you did right. A lot of miscommunication can be smoothed over with good customer service.

8. Provide integrative medicine. Teach your providers that things like acupuncture, massage, and chiropractic are not all "woo-woo" techniques. (Yes, I've had a doc ask me how my "woo-woo" techniques were working for me.) They work. And they can make me a better patient if they are included as a part of my care plan.

9. I am all for patients that are proactive and engaged and informed in their treatment—but that is not a pass for patients to do a provider's job. It is *your* job to make a patient's healthcare experience a good one. And it is your job to make it run smoothly from referral to diagnostics to treatment. Do not tell me I am responsible for doing your job.

10. Finally, it's okay if patients cry. You do not have to send them off to mental health or chalk up every symptom to their emotional state. Sure, if a patient needs serious counseling, they should get it, but sometimes patients need to cry with the doctor and see that they care about them as a person, and not just as a disease. Dealing with your health is scary. Think how you would feel in their shoes and act accordingly. Compassion goes a long way in this business and we will remember you far longer for your smile and understanding than we will for your credentials or education.

What I Learned . . .

I penned this list while sitting in radiology waiting on a two-hour CT scan process with multiple levels of contrast that turned into a four-hour ordeal because my orders were put into the system incorrectly. None of it was my fault—a lot of it had to do with poor communication between providers across departments—but I got the brunt of a really bad attitude. I was cold, in pain, nauseous from the contrast material, and alone. I had just moved to a new area, and the facility was a maze of the unknown. I had not yet bonded with my doctor, and I was scared.

The receptionist yelling at me really did not help.

Everyone has bad days. Everyone. While I still think a lot of this "top ten list" would be really important for every hospital to digest, I also recognize that hospitals are big organizations with many people going through their own stuff in life. People do not always know you are going through a rough patch, especially when they may be living through their own difficulty. I think sometimes when we are dealing with cancer, we expect a bit of a free pass, or things to be made a little easier for us. I know I felt that way from time to time.

Have you ever heard of the cancer card? The cancer card seems like an immediate pass to being treated well. (In my own experience the cancer card has been pretty useless. With having cancer, or some other horrible disease, it is easy to get used to the world revolving around you (or me in this instance). I have said it before, and I will say it again: it is very easy for you to think that everything in life is about you and your illness. It is not. I say that with all the love in the world.

There is a whole boatload of crap going on while you have cancer. That is why I think it is so important for us to reach outside of ourselves while we go through this and see the experiences of others that may be suffering as well. You may find that your well of compassion grows beyond understanding as you go through this journey. You may really start to see that there are many people hurting, crying, dying, and struggling—which is a good thing (for you). The compassion that our healthcare industry needs is the same compassion we need to grow and share as individuals. Sprinkle compassion with abandon. You just may be the only person who says to another, "I understand when things are bad—you aren't alone."

Just because we got this sucky deck of cards called cancer doesn't mean that our purpose for God ends. Indeed, God will continually tell us to "go" and minister even in the middle of our messes. God is good with mess. The Bible tells us that pretty consistently. When we are dealing with the mess of our healthcare, it is good to trust in God to help with the chaos, and good for us to continue to minister to others as well as we are able.

Your Story . . .

Did you play the cancer card yet? How did it go? How did it feel?

_____

_____

_____

_____

_____

_____

_____

_____

_____

What are some things you'd like to tell the healthcare field about taking care of people who are sick?

_____

_____

_____

_____

_____

_____

_____

_____

What's been your biggest pet peeve so far?

_____

_____

_____

_____

_____

_____

_____

_____

You Will *Never* Believe What I Have Chosen

I am the Lord your God who brought you out of the land of Egypt, to be their slaves no more; I have broken the bars of your yoke and made you walk erect. (Lev. 26:13)

How I Felt . . .

God works in mysterious ways. Without a doubt, both my husband and I believe that God wanted us to be back on the East Coast and in the DC area (despite all the freakishness that happened—and continues to happen—with this move). We are here for a reason. And part of that reason was to create a waiting place between Kansas and DC.

God placed me in the waiting place for a good reason. And I have chosen (believe it or not) to stay in the waiting place. I dread the waiting place. I loathe the waiting place. There is not enough action and activity in the waiting place. There isn't enough "doing." I am a doer.

However, the waiting place has become my friend. Upon arrival in DC, we immediately set upon meeting my new oncologist. (She is a rock star that looks just like a blond version of my sister-in-law. It was comforting to see a new, but somewhat familiar-looking face.) My doctor and I both had questions regarding some of my test results, so we decided to rescan my body and take a closer look at my tumors. While we waited for the results, she had also set up an appointment with the National Cancer Institute at the National Institutes of Health (NIH) in Bethesda, Maryland. Let me tell you, that place is amazing. While it is an *all-day* event to go into the clinics, it was worth *every* minute of my time to spend the day with incredible researchers, doctors, nurses, and other staff that walked me through the entire cancer protocol process. Remember last week where I wrote about the top ten things every hospital should do? Well, NIH knocked these out of the park (and yes, they had Starbucks coffee too).

Following additional testing, exams, and a review of my history, my doctor at NIH looked me in the eye and said, "Anna, I'm thirty-nine years old too. I have a wife, kids, and a job. If I were you, I would not seek treatment for your cancer. Your cancer is not extensive enough. The staging you were told is not correct. I believe you are stage I, not stage III. Your 'good cells' in your tumor far outnumber the 'bad cells' in the tumor and you are young. This needs to be your decision, and if you feel you cannot wait for treatment, then we have treatment for you. But if you can watch and wait, you slow down entering the treatment cycle."

Wow.

With my kind of cancer, once you enter the treatment cycle, you begin a cycle of remission, relapse, treatment, and then start over again. I do not have a cancer that is considered curable. So, when I start treatment, it is very likely that for the rest of my life I will be in and out of remission and treatment cycles. This is very hard on the body and exposes the body to a lot of toxicities. I am young (despite what my joints tell me). My tumors are not causing me to be severely symptomatic at this time; it behooves me to watch and wait. Watching and waiting also allows my body to fight the cancer if I take care of my body.

My NIH doctor shared hope with me. He wants me to be a part of a natural history study to explore *why* I have this cancer. He explained that when the time is right, there *will* be a treatment for me. It could be a multitude of different things, but when you have the opportunity to wait, you also have the opportunity for new research to be released for public protocols each year, with better and better treatment becoming available. One day, there will be a *cure* for my kind of cancer. The waiting place gives me a chance to be a part of that "one day."

My local oncologist concurred with my NIH doctor that the repeat scan found only a small, 2.3 cm tumor cluster in my neck. Nothing was seen in my chest or abdomen, contrary to previous scans. My blood work is beautiful and both doctors concurred that my shoulder pain was a physical ailment versus a tumor ailment: a result of my surgery and not my cancer. My scans *did* show arthritis of my C7–C9 vertebrae, so we *do* have conclusive evidence I am getting older—ha! It is not all in my head.

All of which leads me to the dreaded waiting place. I have never liked the dreaded waiting place. As a doer, the waiting place blows. But I am amazingly at peace about this decision to watch and wait.

The waiting place allows me to grow closer to God. I am putting my trust in God that the waiting place is right for me. The waiting place allows me to physically hand over my cancer and my care to God and trust in the Lord God with *all my heart* and *all my body*. This gives me joy (at least most days, when I do not let my anxiety take over). I still have worry and fretfulness. I still wonder if I am doing the right thing, but in this waiting place, it allows me to *practice trust* that God has a greater plan in store for me than anything I can possibly understand. God has led me to this place, to these doctors, and to this plan. The waiting place will allow my tumors to either get smaller or disappear, or they may get bigger and we'll look at whatever might happen after that. Without the waiting place, I would be starting treatments that I might not be ready for. In this waiting place, we have the chance (albeit small, 8 percent) of spontaneous remission. In the waiting place, there is hope, there is peace, and there is a chair with God by my side (or me by God's side). In the waiting place, I can hang up my coat of worry and busyness and rest a little. In the waiting place, there are all sorts of levels of healing.

Some might say my story is one of misdiagnosis. One can say that. I would rather think of this part of my story as a testimony to prayer. I have simply *thousands* of people praying for me all over the world: of all types of faith and belief, and all sorts of denominations. God has heard every one of those prayers. A friend described it as "storming heaven" with prayers. Y'all keep storming heaven for me. This isn't over. This isn't a sprint. This is a long haul, for the rest of my life, and prayer makes a *huge* difference.

This has also been a wonderful example of the power of social media. We have a prayer chain without end when we share our lives over the internet and ask us to pray for each other. *Your* prayers matter. They have made an amazing difference in my life and I cannot express my gratitude enough.

Does this mean I will be in the waiting place forever? No. I am okay with this. I will probably have treatment at some point in my life. But today is not that day. Does this mean my cancer will grow? Possibly. But today is not that day. Could things still go terribly wrong? Possibly. But today is not that day. Could things possibly get even better? Maybe, but today is not that day.

Today is a waiting day. Today, I am okay with the waiting place. God is there.

What I Learned . . .

This moment in my story is so very pivotal. I learned so very much.

1. God is faithful.

2. Prayer matters.

3. Second opinions are lifesaving. In fact, some research indicates that second opinions can improve outcomes from treatment plans. Second opinions often give you options, when sometimes you think you have no options in the world.

For patients dealing with a serious and life-threatening disease, second opinions can often help you feel like you have a say in your treatment plan. This opportunity to take action with your treatment plan is critical. The more engaged you are, the better things will turn out. And you will feel more confident about what you are going through as well.

The other thing I learned was every cancer is different. My approach to my lymphoma would be very different for someone with breast cancer. Brain cancer is not the same as leukemia and ovarian cancer is not the same as testicular cancer. The approach to treating all these different cancers is very different. And it differs within that type of cancer depending on the stage, location, whether it has metastasized (spread), and the underlying health and age of the patient. There are so many things that are important to take into consideration when deciding on the best thing to do with a cancer treatment plan. What is best for you may not be best for me, and vice versa. You can say this of many chronic and stage-serious diseases. This is why I think it is so very important that you become an advocate for your own care and your own self. No one knows you better than you, so please make sure you have a voice in your treatment. Do not be afraid to ask for a second opinion; do not be afraid to ask your care team to propose your treatment plan to an oncology board to seek a consensus among the experts on what is best. You need to know what your goal is from your treatment and communicate that to your team.

In my case, I distinctly remember saying to all three of my oncologists that what I wanted most of all was to raise my kids, kiss my husband, and grow old to see my grandbabies. I told them five years wasn't good enough, ten years wasn't good enough, and twenty years wasn't good enough. I wanted many more years. (Why ask for cake when you can ask for chocolate triple chocolate cake? I wanted the best of the best outcome from my treatment plan.) I think they got the message loud and clear, and God opened up this door to watching, waiting, and continuing to take care of my body to reach that goal.

I am three years in to watching and waiting now. It isn't as easy as it sounds. Learning to live with cancer versus trying to defeat cancer is its own battle. The battle is more in my brain than in my body, although my body has its own symptoms. A large part of my disease right now is my attitude. I needed to learn to look at my cancer not as an acute event, but as a chronic event that I manage on a day-to-day basis rather than eradicating it from my body. Each year, I go in for scans to monitor the progress of the disease. Every four to six months I go in for blood work to make sure my tests aren't spiking, which indicates the cancer cells have sprung out of control. This new rhythm is the rhythm of my life. My cancer is a part of how I am every day. I have to figure out how to live with it because otherwise, I am always in a holding pattern of stasis, and I don't think that's what God wants for me. God gave me my hero cape, and I think God expects me to use it with or without my cancer.

You may be in a similar boat where you live with a disease that just doesn't go away. A large part of your success with your disease is learning to live with it, ensuring your attitude is more or less positive, and continuing to strive to do those things you feel called to do by God. Don't let your disease stop you.

I have not had the miraculous remission that I hope for, but so far, I continue to pray fiercely for that trust in God, trust in my doctors, and trust that the waiting place will get me to that goal of raising my kids, kissing my husband, and seeing grandbabies somewhere in the future.

Your Story . . .

Do you have concerns about your treatment plan?

_____

_____

_____

_____

_____

_____

_____

What options do you wish you had?

_____

_____

_____

_____

_____

_____

_____

_____

_____

What are some resources for a second opinion?

_____

_____

_____

_____

_____

_____

_____

_____

Do you have a waiting place? Is God there? What is God trying to show you in the waiting place?

_____

_____

_____

_____

_____

_____

_____

_____

_____

_____

COURIE FAMILY RECIPE: CHOCOLATE SOUR CREAM POUND CAKE

As you can tell, I have a love affair with good chocolate cake. A little bit goes a long way with me, but a little bit is all you need. When I refer above to asking for the cake of cakes, I am talking about my mother-in-law's chocolate cake recipe that I am sharing with you here. While you are hanging out in the waiting place, a piece of this cake might make waiting just a tad sweeter.

INGREDIENTS:

- 3 sticks butter, softened
- 5 eggs
- 3 cups sugar
- 3 cups all-purpose flour
- 1 teaspoon soda
- ¼ teaspoon salt
- ½ cup cocoa
- 1 cup boiling water
- 2 teaspoons vanilla
- 8 ounces sour cream

DIRECTIONS:

1. Cream butter and sugar together.
2. Add eggs, one at a time, mixing thoroughly after each addition.
3. In separate bowl, mix flour, soda, salt, and cocoa.
4. Add to creamed mixture alternately with sour cream.

Continued

5. After this has been mixed thoroughly, add the cup of boiling water. (Be sure your mixer is on *low* when you do this!! You will feel as though you have made a monumental mistake at this step. You have not. Keep going, as the boiling water will ensure you have the moistest, most delicious cake in your life.)

6. Stir in the vanilla.

7. Bake in a 10-inch greased and floured tube pan at 325 degrees for 1 hour and 20 minutes, or until cake tests done.

8. Frost with the chocolate fudge icing recipe that follows.

CHOCOLATE FUDGE ICING FOR THE CHOCOLATE SOUR CREAM POUND CAKE

INGREDIENTS:

- ½ stick butter
- ⅓ cup white cane syrup
- Pinch of salt
- ½ cup cocoa
- 1 pound powdered sugar
- 2–3 tablespoons milk or brewed coffee

DIRECTIONS:

1. Blend butter and syrup together; add the next ingredients and blend well.

2. A little more milk may be added if needed, but add sparingly.

3. There is usually frosting left over and I just dump it into the hole in the middle of the cake!

Remember that disease loves sugar, so enjoy your sweets, but do so sparingly. Celebrate your life, but follow good nutrition too. It's all about balance. There are periods of feasting in the Bible and there are periods of fasting too.

On the First Day of Christmas . . .

Therefore, since we are surrounded by so great a cloud of witnesses, let us also lay aside every weight and the sin that clings so closely, and let us run with perseverance the race that is set before us. (Heb. 12:1)

How I Felt . . .

. . . It was time to get in shape. What? Are we really going to talk about fitness and health on the Lord's birthday?

Yep.

If there is one thing I know about, it is getting back into shape after a hiatus for health reasons. Sometimes fitness and health are where you are in your life at that moment.[1] It may not always be in the fighting shape you want, or some perfect body you imagine, but I can still work on being healthy, even with disease. For me, this Christmas, I have decided to take a very literal view of Jesus's birth and look at my own body and life that needs to be transformed as I head into this season of waiting.

I could wait on my butt and feel sorry for myself as we hang on to see what the cancer does. Or I can look at Christmas as the beginning of a new chapter of my life. Now that we are settled (mostly), my body has healed from the surgeries (mostly), and life is returning to some form of normal (sort of), I am ready to focus on getting back into shape and making this body a lean, mean, cancer-fighting machine.

In cancerville, they call this the "wait and watch" treatment. Well, "wait and watch" and see what I can do with my body and me over the next couple of months. It is "watch and see" *me* transform over time.

---

1. I write a lot about this in *Christ Walk: A 40-Day Spiritual Fitness Program* (New York: Morehouse, 2015).

That means daily walks with God, goals of ten thousand steps or more, healing fruits and vegetables from God's earth, building back my push-up strength one push-up at a time. It is learning to run again. It is learning to do burpees again and it is learning to find some "om" from yoga again. It is a time of rebuilding and this does not happen overnight.

It is a slow and often frustrating journey to look at what I need to do in my life to be healthy again, but it is worth it. It is often frustrating to look back and see where I was versus where I am now. I need to find a way to live on this path that I am not wishing for something from the past, or dreaming of a future that's unattainable. Being stuck wishing I were the old, precancer me really keeps me from moving forward in my journey.

I am physically going to turn myself around and look to a new direction of where I want to be, and take that step toward it. I'm giving myself the gift of health, one step at a time. I'm hoping this goal will help me learn to deal with the waiting place. Because God knows, I'm terrible at waiting.

What I Learned . . .

Your Christmas will come. There will be a point when the treatment is over and you will need to begin the rebuilding phase of your life. Perhaps you were at a certain level of fitness before your illness and it has been destroyed by the chemotherapy. Maybe you were like me, where surgery was debilitating and crippling for a period of time. If your heart and soul still ache so much, you may be struggling with finding the motivation to learn to live again. Possibly fear chokes your throat and you do not want to invest too much in a body that may soon betray you yet again. When you are ready, you can set goals to gain your fitness level back to where you want it. It will take time. Fitness is not a static moment in time. Fitness is not a status quo moment. Fitness comes in all sorts of shapes, sizes, and skills at varying points in your life.

You will come to an end in the road of this portion of your cancer journey. I wish I could say that "beating cancer" equals leaving cancer behind forever. However, I do not believe that, and I do not believe (from what I have discussed with others that have cancer) that you ever really stop having cancer. You may be cured, but something about it will always be with you. Your diagnosis has changed you irrevocably. Perhaps like me, you've found that your faith was broken and then built up again. Maybe like me, you have softened as a person. Perhaps you've slowed down, begun to smell the roses or the bread baking. Conceivably, you have new meaning in life, or renewed purpose, or perhaps you have no idea what to do with yourself now that you are at a crossroads. Possibly you are like Rey in *The Force Awakens* where you deeply want to follow the Jedi path, but are afraid to do so. The fear you have for your family and the unknown ahead may be holding on to you.

I understand the "stuck" spot deeply. I vacillate between feeling trapped and moving forward *all the time*. I can be a veritable yo-yo in my emotions. I only hope that even though I get stuck, I have moved ahead enough steps that the progress is always forward and not back. Going forward means taking that first step toward the life you want.

For me, that means physically taking that step toward building my body. Staying strong, finding the balance between peace and action, trusting in God, eating right, and focusing on my family is essential to my way forward. If you also take that physical step forward, you are one step closer to obtaining a level of peace that you seek in your remission, the waiting place, or wherever you may be on your journey. Physical steps to wellness make a huge difference in getting you back to where you want to be. Taking care of your nutrition and your stress levels is essential to living with cancer and the threat of cancer long-term.

Even though you choose to take those steps, you need to *not* beat yourself up if you are "never the way you were before." You might not be the same as the precancer you, but that does not mean you cannot find a level of fitness for where you are now. It also doesn't mean you are any less of a person. You are just a new version of you, battle-tested and finding yourself. You will get there by setting goals for yourself. Only you can know what you are capable of doing, but if you work with your doctor and physical therapist, you can rebuild yourself: one step at a time.

Your Story . . .

What frustrates you most about your body right now?

_____

_____

_____

_____

_____

_____

_____

_____

What would you like to try and accomplish to find your new normal?

_____

_____

_____

_____

_____

_____

_____

_____

_____

_____

How long do you think it will take you?

_____

_____

_____

_____

_____

_____

_____

_____

In all honesty, it will probably take you a lot more time than you expect depending on the side effects from your treatment. Be patient with yourself. Set a goal to build up to walking thirty minutes on most days of the week. Then see where you can go from there.

Saying
Good-Bye

Trust in the Lord with all your heart, and do not rely on your own insight.
In all your ways acknowledge him, and he will make straight your paths.
(Prov. 3:5–6)

How I Felt . . .

There's nothing quite like facing your own mortality with cancer as
you watch a friend succumb to hers. One of the greatest fighters of
cancer that I know will die soon. She is the one who taught me that
half of the battle was a fighting spirit and believing you can knock this
sucker out.

Unfortunately, while she's going out her way, with her head held
high, my friend will soon die. She is dying on her own terms with her
husband and children by her side at her home. But she is still dying.
This isn't the result we all prayed for.

I have no answers for this. A beautiful, young, courageous mom of
three, devoted wife and army spouse, will lose her life shortly to her
cancer and I have no answers.

I have grief, fear, and sadness in my heart. My soul screams at the
unfairness of it all. My faith has little spider veins of doubt because we
have prayed so hard and so long for my friend to beat the beast. And
the very weakest part of me nurses fear. This could be me. I have drum
mallets in my psyche trying to beat the fear away. I pray in God's name
and pray out my fear, but it crawls and claws at me trying to reach
all of me.

I don't want my friend to die. I'm certainly nowhere near, nor
even ready, to accept any thoughts of my own mortality, but this is
what cancer does.

Cancer forces the "what if" question front and center. Cancer
forces you to really look at yourself and answer honestly: what do you

believe? It's like Indiana Jones with the Cup of Christ and the Grail Knight . . . what do we believe? Are we ready to drink of the Holy Grail and see what's on the other side? Are we ready for the kingdom of heaven? Do I have a place reserved for me with the company of angels?

While I cannot begin to understand why this world will be bereft of a beautiful spirit from such disease, nor why other spirits are wrest from us when we so desperately need their contributions to make this world a better place, I believe all are surely going to the arms of a loving God. There will be no pain, no fear, where my friend goes. There will be peace. Eventually there will be peace for her family as well and for us. We just aren't there yet.

Part of the Great Thanksgiving Eucharistic prayer in the Episcopal Church includes these lines: "Therefore we praise you, joining our voices with Angels and Archangels and with all the company of heaven, who for ever sing this hymn to proclaim the glory of your Name."[1] In my heart, I believe that my friend will be a part of this company in heaven. And there will be a song on her lips and probably a wine glass in her hand. My friend's smile will light up heaven, along with so many other smiles.

I, too, hope that one day I will be a part of that company. Just not today. Nor any day soon. I'm just not ready. But my friend's death and dying has made me think of this a lot today. I'm sure others share or have shared in this grief and fear. Yes, I am well. Yes, things seem to be in a good place. However, I still live with this beast in me and when a friend dies from that beast, well, fear has this nasty habit of finding a foothold.

Just like many people in this world, my friend was a shining beacon. Her light touched many and for this we are very blessed.

What I Learned . . .

When you have cancer, suddenly you seem to know a lot of people with cancer. Or who have had cancer. I find this weird. I am not sure why, but there are a lot of sick people in this world struggling.

---

1. The Book of Common Prayer (New York: Church Publishing, 1979), 362.

It reminds me that I am not alone in this journey. The cancer experience opens you up to a lot of people living with this disease. I had one friend lose part of her tongue, another lose a leg, another lose her thyroid, several who have lost their lives. Cancer is all around us.

Some of these people you meet will die. It is incredibly scary to be on this journey and have a fellow cancer warrior die. It will shake your bones a bit. It may shake your bones a lot.

But everyone's story is different. Their death does not make them any less of a superhero. They have fought the warrior's fight, and in those times when cancer claims a friend, we need to remind ourselves that God has promised us that there is something more than this life—there is something better. If we trust in God, God will be there for us. I believe that our family on earth will hurt, but hurt is not forever. Even if you die, there is an opportunity for God's grace to work in the middle of that grief. We need to fiercely hold on to God's promise to us that there is much, much more to our story than this earthly one. God will be in the midst of our families when we are gone and provide grace and healing to them. Let us all believe that God can work in the ugly happenstances of life (and death).

If there is one thing God consistently tells us, it is that we need to trust God. It is not always easy to trust God, but God repeatedly tells us to do so. God handles this messy stuff really, really well. My friend's death hit me hard. I felt horrible that on the one hand, it wasn't me. On the other hand, I was frightened it could be me, and on another hand (or finger, or foot, or whatever body part you want to count), I was so deeply saddened and shaken that despite the intense prayers in Ivey's name, she still died. What if the ferocious prayers that were being prayed for me right now weren't enough too? And yet, God says, "Trust me."

My problem with trusting God was that it was in direct conflict of the storyline I wanted. This storyline of death for my friend became a real storyline for me. When we get these storylines, our immediate, gut response is, "Where is God?" Indeed, the psalmist reflects our cries. In Psalm 42:3, the person cries out: "My tears have been my food day and night, while people say to me continually, 'Where is your God?'"

Where is your God? Have you wondered? Have you thought this? Is it somewhat familiar? Psalm 42:10: "As with a deadly wound in my body, my adversaries taunt me, while they say to me continually, 'Where is your God?'" Indeed, where is God in health and human suffering? I've muttered, "Where is God?" in this story I have shared with you many times. You'd be amazed at the times where my initial response was, "But God, this isn't the story I want." I have cried, "Where is my God?" "Hellllloooo God! It's me, Anna! Where are you?" When Ivey died, I questioned a lot. During this entire journey, I have questioned and questioned.

The psalmist speaks to me.

You see, I want *my* story. Not God's story.

In *my* story, I can hear without hearing aids. I can eat cake, cookies, and ice cream and not have to run. In my story, my parents don't get sick, and there are no mental illnesses. There are no wars, no conflict, no political discord. In my story, there isn't adultery, death, terrorism, or abuse. In my story, I don't have cancer. In my story, Ivey doesn't die from her cancer, nor do any of my other friends. In fact, no one has cancer in my story. In my story, God and I are in sync over everything that goes on.

In my story, I'm rather large and in charge and God's along for the ride. Does this sound familiar?

This is how God's story goes: trust me.

God doesn't say there won't be war, illness, death, poverty, pain, or suffering. In fact, the Bible tells us pretty clearly these things will never go away here on earth. The Hebrew scriptures and New Testament tell us how people have learned to trust God in the middle of these storylines. God can work in the middle of all stories and make them better. You see, when you really look at scripture and think about the stories, you hear the accounts of people struggling to find God in the middle of a mess.

The Bible is filled with mess. And it consistently tells us a story of grace in the chaos.

The prophet Isaiah tells us, "Do not fear, I am with you, do not be afraid, for I am your God; I will strengthen you, I will help you. I will uphold you with my victorious hand. . . . For I, the Lord your God, hold your right hand; it is I who say to you, 'Do not fear, I will help you'" (Isa. 41:10, 13).

Where is God? God is holding our hands. God is weaving grace through these stories of pain and fear, anxiety and loneliness. God is telling a consistent story: trust me.

I would be lying if I didn't say I want to hear without my hearing aids. I would not be telling the truth if I didn't say that I wish I didn't have cancer. I am not okay with Ivey dying. However, I am 100 percent convinced God is engaged in all of it, and God's grace is working through it all. You see, I've learned my story is incomplete without God.

If I trust in God, I have to recognize that I trust God in all aspects of my life—and death. Should my cancer take me, I have to trust in God that my family will be taken care of. God will take care of my storyline. I have learned to be at peace with the unknown in my future, to come to terms with those that have been lost along the way, and honestly to be okay with my cancer by looking at the story of Jesus.

Jesus was made whole. The resurrection of Christ is a promise that all storylines will be made whole. God's grace and salvation will make us whole. The resurrection of Jesus promises to restore us to wholeness. What we are living now is not the end of the story; there is much, much more to come. I believe that Ivey is there now and has been made whole, along with Linda, Josh, Sheila, and Heidi (all friends who have been taken by cancer along this journey). Their deaths are not the end of the story. "For mortals it is impossible, but not for God; for God, all things are possible" (Mark 10:27).

God can do your messy, your change, your transitions, your illness, your anxiety, your fear. At every stage of life, God is weaving through our stories. "Trust in the Lord with all your heart, and do not rely on your own insight. In all your ways acknowledge him, and he will make straight your paths" (Prov. 3:5–6).

Hold your peeps tight, my friends. While there is a grand place waiting for us in heaven, life is very precious here on earth—hold it close. Friends will die from cancer. I might die one day too. We might not understand why, but God will always be whispering, "Trust me."

Your Story . . .

We've touched on a really uncomfortable part of the cancer or serious illness journey: death. How does that make you feel?

_____

_____

_____

_____

_____

_____

_____

_____

Have you lost a friend to cancer? How did that make you feel?

_____

_____

_____

_____

_____

_____

_____

_____

_____

_____

How does it make you feel to give it all over to God, and listen to the whisper, "Trust me"?

_____

_____

_____

_____

_____

_____

_____

_____

Another Day with Cancer, or Just Another Day?

O give thanks to the Lord, for he is good, for his steadfast love endures forever. O give thanks to the God of gods, for his steadfast love endures forever. (Ps. 136:1–2)

How I Felt . . .

I had every intention of writing a blog post marking the four-month passing of my diagnosis with lymphoma. That day passed without me realizing it (January 7) until several days later when I realized my friend Ivey died from her cancer on that "anniversary." I will not wander through that coincidence. Ivey's death hit me far harder than I was prepared for. Her memorial service was beautiful and just the thing to say good-bye to my friend. Although her death roused my own suppressed fears, it was necessary to look at them and remind myself that I am trusting in God. No matter how little I understand, nor how little I can comprehend of God's intentions, I am learning contentment in trust. *Everything* I cannot control or handle goes into God's hands.

With that said, thinking back on my "four-month diagnosis anniversary," I have realized that although my cancer still lies in my body (a sleeping giant?), life goes on. The move came and went. Life goes on. Christmas came and went. Life goes on. Families came and went. Life goes on. Births, deaths, work, and school have come and continued the cycle of life. Life goes on.

The fact that my 120 days passed without my awareness is a good thing. It means I, too, am moving on. My cancer is still *very* much a part of me. There are days it rears its ever-loving head and says, "Hey, you, you've got cancer, pay attention to me!" And I pull out my metaphorical baseball bat and beat it back into submission. It is nice that more days go by when it is just a passing thought than something that stalks my brain every day.

It means life has gone on for me. That is good. I'll continue to wait, watch, and mark the passing of each month of my diagnosis anniversary, because each month means I am closer to passing a year of staying healthy with my tumors. This is my kind of goal for the New Year: health with illness. I do not exercise and get fit to have a better body; I exercise and get fit to tame the illness that rests within me. The exercise and fitness ensures that illness does not take a toe-hold in my body that it won't let go of. The exercise helps me deal with the anxiety and stress of living with this thing so I don't go crazy. I don't find myself driven by hypothetical Personal Records (PRs) anymore. Exercise isn't about being a beast or a stud in the gym anymore; exercise is about whatever I can do to stay fit and sane. Every day that I am active and another diagnosis anniversary passes is a win for me.

I've actually turned into a calmer, more contented version of myself as each day passes. God has answered those prayers of mine for peace and acceptance. I asked to be able to live my life, even with this beast in me. And God has granted me those prayers. Even with cancer, another day is another day.

What I Learned . . .

Writing this book as a reflection on what I experienced after the fact has afforded me the opportunity to really look back on each of the things I was feeling and realize what I learned. This is important because sometimes you do not realize what you are learning in the middle of the experience. Looking back and reading this specific post, knowing what comes next, makes me realize that the experience itself is a roller coaster.

Here, I am completely upbeat. I am determined to live with my cancer and not let it get me down. It presents the picture that I am always this fierce, determined hero of the cancer story. It isn't remotely true. I believe we all have ups and downs on the cancer/illness journey. Sometimes there is no stopping us; sometimes it just becomes a part of who we are and sometimes it overwhelms all of our being with fear and despair.

This is one reason it is important to write down how you feel throughout your journey. It is important to be able to go back and remember the high points, your fighting-stance, aggressively empowered, can-do attitude that makes you feel like *you* are in charge of your journey and not the cancer or disease. I have to remind myself when I get overwhelmed with worry that I don't *always* feel this way. I am not *always* living in the low points of my journey—there are high points. Reading back on my thoughts reminds me that I have a life outside of my illness.

So don't be discouraged if one day you feel like Superwoman/Superman, the next day you feel like the Joker or Loki, and the next day you feel like you experienced the death of an Ewok. The ups and downs are normal patterns in your experience and they do even out over time. When you've ridden the roller coaster sufficiently, you start to learn strategies for when the emotions try to take over. I personally do a couple of things: I go for a long walk, pray the rosary, and focus on my breath. With each breath I say, "Here, God, take this." Getting my body back under control isn't an immediate response to my tricks, but they help. They help me put things in perspective so that I do realize that each day is just another day, even with cancer.

Three years later, I still practice these strategies. I still have my highs and lows. I have noticed that those lows coincide with my checkups as I begin to worry what the scans will find this time, but I get better and better equipped to deal with the lows when I use my strategies effectively.

Your Story . . .

What are some of your high points on your journey?

_____

_____

_____

_____

_____

_____

_____

_____

_____

_____

What are some of the low points?

_____

_____

_____

_____

_____

_____

_____

_____

_____

What are some strategies that work for dealing with the low points so that they don't take over?

_____

_____

_____

_____

_____

_____

_____

_____

_____

It's World Cancer Day

When I came to you, brothers and sisters, I did not come proclaiming the mystery of God to you in lofty words or wisdom. (1 Cor. 2:1)

How I Felt . . .

It is World Cancer Day today and I have no clue what to do with it.

You would think that since I have cancer, I would have something profound to say.

You would think that since I have a mother who is in remission from cancer, I would know what to say.

You would think that since I have a friend who just died from cancer, I would have something eloquent to say.

You would think that since I worked as an oncology nurse, I would know the right thing to say.

You would think that since I have friends, family, and colleagues who have supported me through my illness, I would have a clue what needs to be said.

I really do not. Cancer still sucks. I wish it would go the heck away, but it seems that with one in two people getting cancer, in this day and age we will all be dealing with cancer in our lives. I really think this is the new chronic illness of the decade.

It is weird to me to have a day devoted to cancer awareness because for me, I am aware of it every single day. I never have a day that it doesn't cross my mind and there isn't a day that goes by where I'm not still trying to figure out the new norm. And with my kind of cancer right now, I wonder if the precancer me is really all that different from the postcancer me. I don't fit in a survivor category. I don't fit in the treatment category. I fall in the waiting category. I wait just as terribly without cancer as I do with it.

169

But God has given me some sort of strength to deal with it. I follow my cycle of prayer, exercise, and connections that helps me when I feel especially "cancerous" some days. I don't feel especially strong. I don't really know if I'm managing it the right way. It's more like I don't know any other way to deal with it.

For me, every day is cancer awareness day and that's about all I have to say about that.

What I Learned . . .

I am not a huge fan of awareness days. I am not sure why. I probably am a little bit of a cynic in that I believe every day is an awareness day when you realize that everyone is going through something in life. On the other hand, these days do bring much needed awareness to the research being conducted with various diseases and causes. When there is something near and dear to your heart, you will be more likely to raise money to support the efforts toward a cure.

The research being conducted on cancer is amazing. One of the greatest fears in learning my diagnosis grew out of my experience as a bone marrow transplant nurse seventeen years prior. I experienced many patients going through some truly horrible treatment experiences, and many dying along the way. There were also those who beat the odds of their cancers and got many more years with their loved ones. This is another example of the roller coaster of cancer. Some people thrive and make it; others do not. Some people stay on the treatment cycle forever, others do not; some people have horrific side effects and others do not.

I recall at that time thinking there was no way I could ever put myself through the treatment my patients did—how naïve, young, and foolish I was at the time. Now I understand why many sought experimental therapies when traditional therapies failed. It was the love of their families that called them to try things no matter what, for the elusive hope that something would give them just a few more years with their loved ones. When you love fiercely, you are willing to do just about anything for more time with those loved ones.

I was very aware with my diagnosis of what I was willing to do to see my kids grow up. I wanted time. At the same time, I was very afraid, because I had seen firsthand what the research therapies could do to someone. I had a very unusual view and experience of cancer treatment, a vantage point that was usually reserved for those where the traditional therapies failed. This was a problem for me because I had no experience with those where therapies were successful: I just had a vision of chemo and bone marrow transplants as a last-ditch effort that often failed.

I could not have been more wrong. Thanks to things like Cancer Awareness Days, research funding has brought cancer treatment and side effect therapies light-years away from where I was working seventeen years ago. The treatments are tailored. The options really seek to understand the patient, their disease, the stage of their cancer, and their preexisting risk factors, and create almost a boutique approach to the treatment of that individual's disease process. It is simply amazing where we are today in the treatment of cancer.

There is so much more hope with every kind of cancer than there was twenty years ago, and even just last year. Science takes Goliath steps toward the cancer cure each year. Maybe I am a Pollyanna, but hopefully I will live to see those cures come to fruition in my lifetime.

If you are like me, and you see this Cancer Awareness Day and you mutter, "Well, duh, I am aware of cancer every day," know that these days do make a difference. They empower people to support the very thing you care so much about so that one day there will be a cure, and books like these won't need to be written.

Your Story . . .

What would you like for people to be aware of on Cancer Awareness Day?

_____

_____

_____

_____

_____

_____

_____

_____

What sort of cure do you hope they find for your cancer/disease?

_____

_____

_____

_____

_____

_____

_____

_____

_____

What part of your treatment do you wish they had better research regarding? Maybe there is a side effect you wish they could have prevented or diminished? (For me, it's the puking—the advent of Zofran as an antiemetic has changed the life of so many cancer patients. It isn't a cure-all for vomiting, but by God, it is a life changer for those of us who have stomachs that revolt.)

_____

_____

_____

_____

_____

_____

_____

_____

_____

_____

My Six-Month Cancerversary

But the day of the Lord will come like a thief, and then the heavens will pass away with a loud noise, and the elements will be dissolved with fire, and the earth and everything that is done on it will be disclosed. Since all these things are to be dissolved in this way, what sort of persons ought you to be in leading lives of holiness and godliness. (2 Pet. 3:10–11)

How I Felt . . .

My six-month cancerversary has come and gone this past week. It was marked by illness for me and my son, a blood transfusion for my dog (she may have cancer too—cancer just sucks), and a torn calf muscle for my husband. It has been a week that I would like to forget.

But a six-month cancerversary is worth writing about. Every time I think of that phrase, or see it in writing, I long to insert "cancer-free" into the statement. If I am honest, I want to bang my keyboard that I am unable to put those words in writing. It is like standing at the end of a long race and being unable to cross the finish line. It taunts and teases me. I am not cancer-free. I'm not sure what to celebrate.

I fall into that nebulous category of individuals who are not survivors. We haven't beaten our cancer (yet). It is still with us.

I call it my pesky parasite. There is no fist-pumping moment of definitive success in my cancer story because there isn't anything I can do to fight it at this time. I have to wait and watch. Waiting and watching is its own treatment option. It's a viable one in my case that points to a greater quality of life and a better long-term prognosis. Don't get me wrong, I'm thrilled to be in the treatment shoes I wear . . . but in the secret, dark places of my heart, I yearn to yell the words, "I'm cancer-free!"

No such luck.

Instead, the six-month point in my journey is marked by a tight-rope-balancing act of moving on. I still find myself searching for the new norm. Routine and structure keep me focused on positive activities, and not those things I cannot do anything about. So, my routine and structure is now defined by a training plan for a local ten-miler. I have secretly been going out each week checking off long runs on a racing plan, praying that I do not fail. Each step is a powerful thought of squishing cancer cells under the sole of my shoe. Success is marked with each step and each mile. When I run, my cancer cannot stop me. My cancer posse cheers me along the way, telling me, "You go girl." But each step is marked by at least being able to do something. There is no sitting on my butt doing nothing in my world. Running the race fills me with a sense of accomplishment and purpose. I will not sit back and take this diagnosis lying down.

Let us run with perseverance the race that is set before us. (Heb. 12:1b)

And yet, even with every step toward a fight for normalcy, I find that it intrudes itself on my awareness more than I like. I'm a lot weaker physically since my diagnosis. My pace is a lot slower and it takes me far longer to build up my endurance. I am also finding (to my grief) that I'm a bit more susceptible to pesky germs. A bronchial infection laid me up the last week, derailing my running plans that kept me sane. Yet again, I felt like I was looking at a finish line, unable to cross. And let me tell you about night sweats—waking up two to three times a night in a pool of sweat because my body no longer understands how to regulate temperature is just gross. And annoying. Did I mention annoying? I like my sleep.

But here I am six months later, still in the weird waiting place. I hope to tick off the "cancerversaries" in an annual fashion from here on out. I'm hoping that with each passing year, I'll decorate the weird waiting place with race medals, tiger paws, sunshine, beaches, friends, family, and memories with my husband and kids. Hopefully in time, this weird waiting place will look no different than the walls of my house, or the love in my heart. Hopefully in time, the weird waiting place feels comfortable.

Will I ever be a "cancer survivor"? I don't know. But I sure hope, for as many years as God gives me, I'll *thrive* with cancer. It's the best revenge to thumb my nose at it and say, "You aren't going to stop me."

So at my six-month cancerversary, not crossing the race finish, not crossing the treatment finish, not really doing anything, but learning to go on in life, let me take a moment to fist pump and yell:

"I'm *thriving* with cancer."

Take that. Cancer still sucks.

What I Learned . . .

The hardest race you run is one where you don't cross the finish line, but you still figure out a way to go on. That's what I've learned. I still have my ups and downs, both a love and hate relationship with my cancer. Three years in, I continue to learn to live with it. I still think cancer sucks. I still long to yell, "I'm cancer-free!" It is an ongoing process. I wish I could tell you that at some point it all will be some sort of normal living, but I am not sure it will be. It's just living with cancer. Going on and living life. This is the new norm. For me, cancer will always be there and always be a part of me, no matter if I get to pump my fist in the air and say, "Yes, I am cancer-free."

That is not what I get to type now, nor have I been able to say that for the last three years. It confuses people to hear that I have cancer and I live with it along with its set of symptoms, watching closely to make sure that it doesn't get out of control. People often tell me, "But you don't look like you have cancer." But I do, and much like you, one of the things you will need to get used to is a sense of being hypervigilant about your health and symptoms. If you've had the opportunity to beat cancer, you will still be sensitive to your body and fearful of the symptoms you exhibit. One of the things I talk to my doctor about frequently is, "When will I know when things go south?"

You see, leading up to my diagnosis, I had symptoms that were truly vague: fatigue (I have two kids, three part-time jobs, and am a military spouse—who isn't tired?), weird sweats (not the usual night sweats, but all-day sweats—basically my body cannot control temperature well), and nosebleeds. All three, for several months, were chalked up to premenopausal symptoms (let me tell you, as a thirty-something, to hear "premenopausal" is the kiss of death to the female ego). Now, I am hypervigilant about these symptoms because I think they will clue me in on when things go south. My doc keeps telling me I will know. I keep telling her I am a little crazy and my mind may think things are going south when my body is still trucking along.

You see, since my body has already let me down, I am not sure how to trust it; you become a little suspicious of its every tweak when it has already given you grief once. I remember telling a friend when I got my biopsy, "Oh, I'd know if I had cancer." Well, I was wrong. My reluctance to believe my doctor when she tells me I will know when things start to grow out of control still leaves me skeptical.

You, too, are sensitive to your body and its messages to you. The hypervigilance of what is going on and the things you are experiencing is normal. You will dissect everything you experience within the context of having cancer. You will have to determine if what you are experiencing is your cancer or disease, or if it's just the common cold or virus that everyone catches. You will wonder, wonder, wonder if the cancer is coming back, or if your disease is trying to take over your life. This is normal. It is part of the phase of learning to live with cancer (or whatever disease you have) or learning to be a cancer survivor. The fear that it will come back and change your life again is normal. You've blown up the Death Star; it is completely normal to fear the evil Republic will begin building cancer cells in your system again. It is okay to be vigilant. It's okay to be super watchful. It's *not* okay for you to stop living your life.

You've probably figured out that I believe strongly in being active as a means for coping. Whether that's walking, running, swimming, praying, doing yoga, volunteering, or meditating, it's vitally important that you release your fear and vigilance in an active way. You need to put your anxiety and the crazy thoughts in their place so you really can *thrive* with cancer.

Your Story . . .

What are your fears?

_____

_____

_____

_____

_____

_____

_____

_____

What are symptoms you feel you need to keep an eye on as you either "watch and wait" or live in remission?

_____

_____

_____

_____

_____

_____

_____

_____

_____

What are some strategies for dealing with your fear?

_____

_____

_____

_____

_____

_____

_____

_____

Somewhere around Nine Months

The king said to his servants, "Take me away from the battle, for I am very weak." And immediately his servants took him out of the line of battle. (1 Esdras 1:30)

How I Felt . . .

This post is private. As much as I have talked about my anxiety, I don't know how to post about it now. Partly, I am at a point where I feel like people are tired of hearing about my cancer. Sometimes, I get tired of talking about my cancer. Sometimes I just want it all to go away.

But around the nine-month period, I have to be honest. This anxiety is coming and going. I am sad; I'm not coping. My exercise is focused on punishing my body for betraying me and not about taking care of myself. I am extremely frustrated because I feel like I am doing everything "right" and this anxiety stills creeps up and knocks the wind out of me. Something is going on.

I've never been afraid to go talk to someone about my emotions. I am a big believer that therapy is a good thing. I have decided to get help. Regretfully, for a huge, long list of reasons, the therapist that I was referred to was a crackpot. The sessions were a disaster and I was essentially told I needed to suck my lot up, that my cancer wasn't that bad, and that I should be thankful it wasn't worse. I've been around the medical profession a long time. That's not how those sessions are supposed to go. *It's supposed to be a safe haven to talk.* I wasn't safe, and I walked away from it. That leaves me with a whole lot of emotion to try and deal with. If I'm honest, I'm depressed.

I pray and pray and pray. I talked to my oncologist a bit about the failed therapy and she agreed that person wasn't what I needed. She offered me a referral to someone else, but honestly, I was burned. I walked out and internalized it. I am a tough sister. I am a "pick up the pieces and move on" kind of girl. I wish I could say I have the magic bullet. I don't. I still have anxiety. I worry. I get mad. I think too much and "what if" too much about the future. It isn't an everyday thing, but it happens. I don't think I'll ever get past getting cancer. I am not sure I'll ever stop worrying, even when (if) I go into remission. There is always the looming darkness of the future that includes a storm cloud of "what-ifs." I find God missing in those moments. I go searching. I seek the echo of God's beacon in the fog of my anxiety. Sometimes I feel God strongly; other times, I have a real hard time finding God, because I get caught up in a major hurdle: this is not the story I wanted for my life.

Sure, I have grown. I have a deep faith that provides me with comfort, peace, and a trust in God that was immature before. My story helps others. This is important. My story is a story of God's grace in my life. I am a living testament of God's grace at work in an individual.

But I am also human. This really isn't the story I want. I'm selfish, and petulant, and irritated. This wasn't the way I wanted to testify to my faith. My sin is fear and worry. I fear where this story will take me. This sin of mine is where God is working the hardest. I fear greatly the future of my life and what it holds because I really don't want this cancer story.

When we are growing up as children and envisioning the white bridal dress, the wedding of our dreams, the cute kids, a career trajectory in our chosen profession, maybe a dream of being a missionary, of fighting battles, making a difference in the world, or being our own version of a superhero—we aren't dreaming of being cancer heroes. People don't dream of a cancer story in which to make a difference in the world.

This isn't the superhero story I want. And so I struggle. I struggle to find where to share my angst. I struggle with depression. The highs and lows are killing me. I struggle between being honest with my feelings and focusing on the hope and grace of God. It is a roller coaster that goes at different speeds and different directions, and I am not always sure when it will show up in my life.

The fear of cancer never goes away. It comes and goes, but it never really goes away.

What I Learned . . .

The nine-month moment still comes and goes in my life. I still find the need to talk about my worries and fears. I don't know that it will ever go completely away, although I am told by those who are further on this journey than I that the periods of time between the worry and anxiety get further apart (this is true!). Coping does come, but it comes in different ways for different people.

I think it is very important for me to address the nine-month mark in my journey because it isn't really something I want to share. I like the story to be all rose-colored glasses, sunshine, and hope. We need hope on this journey of disease we have been given. Don't get me wrong, the hope is there, the joy and grace of God is there. But we are all human, and our humanness has a tendency to want to overwhelm what we know to be true about God and God's promises to us.

I don't want to dive into this month and be honest, because it means being honest with some of my not-so-healthy coping mechanisms. I don't really want to talk about it because I perceived myself to be weak during this time. It's not a trait I like to recognize in myself because it means my superhero self has some things she needs to work on. But I am human, just like you, and I get depressed and anxious, and I had to learn how to deal with it, because it wasn't going away. If you let your depression and anxiety spin out of control, it can become a gateway to addictive behaviors. These behaviors include misuse of your medications, alcohol, self-mutilation, illegal substances, or other behaviors that are *not* healthy coping mechanisms.

There was a really dark point at this nine-month mark where alcohol was a really attractive mechanism for dealing with my anxiety rather than addressing it. It scared me because I have never thought of drugs and alcohol as an option for dealing with my life. All of a sudden, alcohol was an easy way to blunt the feelings that were out of control in my body. Alcohol wasn't judgmental. Alcohol took the edge off. It crept into my life rather insidiously. At first, I wasn't even aware of it, but then, for some reason, I was joking about having a drink following a rough day, and I realized it wasn't a joke, and I really didn't like that I was thinking of drinking to deal with my day. I am not a teetotaler—I enjoy a glass of wine, beer, or a nightcap—but it is different to enjoy drinking responsibly than to drink to deal with issues you aren't addressing. And this is what I was doing, and this is when I came to realize my thoughts were not healthy thoughts, and my behaviors with alcohol were not healthy behaviors.

Cancer patients have access to a lot of drugs. It is very easy to slip into letting the drugs numb everything. It is easy to up those doses. I've read countless stories of individuals that came out of their cancer journey with a substance abuse problem they didn't really know was happening, because they were so focused on getting through their journey.

I knew that if I didn't address the anxiety and depression that was going on in my mind, I was going to have an alcohol problem on top of everything else as well. I didn't want this. For me, again, my motivation is my love of God, my family, and my health. Not addressing my mental well-being is a disservice to all that I love. Addressing it with alcohol certainly doesn't honor anyone.

I've shared many strategies already, but here is what I learned to do as I became aware that my anxiety and depression were being triggered. I needed to stop whatever I was doing and ground myself in my breath, my prayer, and my senses. In addition to my "walking rosary," I learned to practice the counting method. When you feel the anxiety and depression come on, count:

- 5 things you can see;
- 4 things you can hear;
- 3 things you can touch;
- 2 things you can smell;
- 1 thing you can taste.

Take a deep breath with each count. This grounds you in the present and distracts your mind from the spiral of negative thoughts that can overwhelm you.

If you are struggling with the lure of addiction on your journey because of anxiety or depression, please go talk to a professional. Find one that works for you. If the first one gives you the heebie-jeebies, find another. Or talk to a pastoral counselor for support. Or join a support group so that you don't feel alone. You have a ton on your plate right now; the healthiest approach with cancer is dealing with it and getting help. Addiction is just as much of a disease as cancer or other life-threatening issue and you don't want to be battling multiple diseases through the rest of your life. There is no judgment here, just a loving plea to get yourself the help you need and not turn to substances to try to cope.

Big hugs, —*Anna*

Your Story . . .

What are your unhealthy coping mechanisms?

_____

_____

_____

_____

_____

_____

_____

_____

_____

How do you feel about drugs, alcohol, and/or other substances?

_____

_____

_____

_____

_____

_____

_____

_____

_____

Who can you go to for help?

_____

_____

_____

_____

_____

_____

_____

A Year with Cancer

Beat your plowshares into swords, and your pruning hooks into spears; let the weakling say, "I am a warrior." (Joel 3:10)

How I Felt . . .

A year ago today, I got that call from the surgeon that the biopsy of my lymph node was positive for follicular lymphoma. The picture of that moment is seared on my brain. I remember my husband sitting at the bar that overlooked our kitchen as he was working. My children were chattering away upstairs—I remember hearing them. I sat down on the foot of our staircase, and laughed at the surgeon. "You are joking, right? I don't have cancer." We hung up the phone.

Our farm box of veggies had just been delivered. I remember stabbing the box with the kitchen shears trying to open it to put away the vegetables. And I remember putting my head on that box and sobbing. My son came in the kitchen just at that moment. He burst into tears to see me crying. I held him really tight. I couldn't imagine how to have this conversation with my family. I couldn't bear to break the news to my mom. Shock doesn't begin to cover what you feel. My emotions ran the gamut. The experts would say everything I felt during that shocking diagnosis was completely normal. The experts will tell you that everything I've shared and experienced with you so far is normal.

I find no comfort that my experience is normal. You never feel normal when you've been diagnosed with cancer or any other awful disease. And while many talk of "finding the new norm," I am not sure there will ever be a new norm for me. Just like I am never sure that people who go into remission feel they "get rid" of having cancer. I have come to believe that whether I live for forty years with this lymphoma or at some point in the future I go into treatment and then, hopefully, remission, I have been undeniably changed by this experience. In my mind's eye, cancer will always be a part of me. It is making me into who I am today. While I never expected cancer on my journey, it's continuing to make me, me.

My practice of posting on my blog regularly has stalled. There have been a variety of reasons for this lapse. I have been writing—but on other topics not related to my illness. There will be two more books out by me in the New Year: *Christ Walk Kids*[1] and *Sally and the Constellations*.[2] So there are successes to this story.

But I've also been silent because I have found that somewhere along the six- to eleven-month part of this journey, I looked into a mirror and saw a fractured image of myself. I was there, but parts of me were broken. To say I moved on from anger and frustration would be to lie. I *still* get annoyed when I allow myself to think of my cancer. Who has time for cancer? It irritates me on the days it rears its head and says, "Slow down." And being unable to do anything about the cancer is a bit of a kick in the gut. I don't always watch and wait well. God always seems to be trying to teach me the art of patience. I often fail miserably and I don't know that I will ever get over that. Waiting is a part of that whole "new norm" thing that causes me to roll my eyes. Waiting doesn't fit into the worldview of the action hero I want to be when I grow up. Whoever heard of the "Watch and Wait Wonder Woman?" That's just not cool. The new norm forces you to think about your perceptions of yourself.

This new norm really forced me the last several months to stop and focus. I really had to work with my doc on a way to live with cancer and still function, because it was tenuous at times. Those broken bits of me kept trying to fall out. And I found myself needing to apply glue to me. And in a very private way, I needed to do it without blogging.

Glue comes in many shapes, forms, and substances. It came in the form of prayer over the last year—others and my own. We pray as a family every night that God continues to take care of mommy's

---

1. Anna Fitch Courie, *Christ Walk Kids: A 40-Day Journey for Tweens and Teens* (New York: Morehouse Publishing, 2016).

2. Anna Fitch Courie, *Sally and the Constellations* (Charleston, SC: CreateSpace Publishing, 2016).

cancer—and thus far, God continues to show me grace in many ways. Glue comes in the form of friends—those who were willing to listen. Those who were willing to receive random texts about fear and anxiety. Those who were a distraction. Those who treated me like "Anna" so I could figure out how to treat myself like "Anna" again as well. Glue comes from professionals who were patient enough to answer repeated questions of the same thing over and over; were calm when new symptoms cropped up; and were unfailingly reassuring that watching was still the right thing to do. Glue comes in the form of the mundane—the pleasure of walking. The pleasure of doing things with the kids. The pleasure of writing. The pleasure of still having value in the world although I am a broken, semirepaired, cancer-carrying child of God.

When I was receiving this diagnosis, my book *Christ Walk* was being published. I could not imagine that the book would do well. Who wants to learn about living a fit, healthy, and spiritually fulfilled life from a cancer patient? I was so afraid that this diagnosis was the end of my passion for health in the church. I thought God had made a mockery of what I perceived was my calling in life.

But God works in funny ways. My book has gone on to do very well. Church Publishing, Incorporated, tells me I am one of their best sellers. They've graciously decided to pick up my second book, *Christ Walk Kids*. And people want to hear my story of faith, fitness, and health. People desperately want to know they have value in the world; that they are needed, and that they are just as important when they have illness and disease. Illness, cancer, disease—these labels are devaluing to what we think of ourselves. We need to stop this. *Every* single one of us is broken, diseased, or damaged, and we *all* have value in God's creation. I can still be healthy: mind, body, and spirit, even with disease. I really believe this. My cancer is a part of my journey and me, and will continue to be for a long time.

This is where I am now a year later. I am in a good place. I exercise daily, but not always running and training for distance. I pick things that feel good and bring me joy in movement. Each day, I search for the lovely in my life. I am awed by God's grace. When I feel anxious or fearful of the future, I stuff glue in those pieces of me that want to fall out and pass the glue bottle to God to hold it all together. There is much I will never understand. There is much I have little patience for, and when those failings come to get me, I remind myself that I do trust God more than I trust in my limited understanding—and funnily, peace follows.

In two weeks, I go for my annual CT scans. They will pump me full of radiographic material to see if anything lights up in my body as a new or growing tumor. They keep telling me that I'll know when things start to go south. Huh. I still look at them a little crazy when they tell me this. It is so anathema to current medical practice not to treat when detected early. I'm not sure what to ask you to pray for: spontaneous remission (always good); continued status quo (also acceptable); patience with the "new norm" (okay); lots of glue bottles if things go south (eh, it could happen)? I believe in prayer. I'll take whatever you are willing to offer.

So keep walking with me. I am still on this journey and we will continue to find faith, fitness, and health together. I've decided to hold the hand of my cancer and bring it along with us. It's teaching me a thing or two. It might not have been the lessons I was seeking, but it's always teaching me. I hope you are learning something too.

With love, and prayers for another 365-day report, —*Anna*

What I Learned . . .

Living with cancer isn't easy. Living in the aftermath of cancer treatment isn't easy either. But you still have a life, and it is still a very valuable life to God and the world. Whatever place you are in, you have a reason to be here and a purpose within the whole context of your cancer and disease experience.

What you have encountered in sharing my epic adventure with cancer over the course of the last 365 days is an unfolding of the grief experience. Kubler-Ross first described the stages of grief: anger, denial, bargaining, depression, and acceptance.[3] These aren't necessarily stages you go through in a linear progression and you may not experience them at all, but you've seen hallmarks of these stages

---

3. Elizabeth Kubler-Ross, *On Death and Dying* (New York: MacMillan, 1969).

throughout this adventure I've shared with you. I most certainly experienced anger and depression. There were times of bargaining where I thought if only I changed certain behaviors, the cancer would go away. I experienced denial and often asked my doctors if they were sure I had cancer. And I very much wobble between depression and acceptance. But each day, I come closer to accepting my situation and moving on.

You may bounce back and forth through the stages as I did, but eventually you do (or at least I hope you do) get to a point of acceptance. Acceptance doesn't mean that you don't get anxious or worry about your situation ever again: it simply means that you do learn to live with it, finding purpose and even value in the journey you have been given. I believe we find a deeper understanding of God through our grief and suffering. Our faith is often honed to a very precise belief that we are nothing without God, and therefore our cancer and our disease is just what happens to our earthly bodies. Remember, God's message to us through the resurrection of Christ is that all things will be made whole through God. Acceptance is learning that your cancer is just one part of your human journey—you are so much more than a diagnosis. And even if you continue to struggle with your disease, or the aftermath of your disease, I profoundly believe that there is something more to this life and that God consistently promises to be with us.

Grieving is a normal part of this cancer and disease journey. I hope you've found through telling your own story along with mine that you've seen your stages of grief unfold as well. Perhaps you've found your own version of your superhero in sharing my epic adventure with me. Maybe you've discovered that God's grace is your superpower, along with your own cape of invincibility consisting of your friends, family, loved ones, prayer, and peace. All combined to help you fight the good fight with your disease each day. I hope and pray deeply you have come to a stage of acceptance or are on your way there. When we get to acceptance, we see that there is hope, that there is a future, and that there is still so much more God has planned for us. Our lives may be irrevocably changed, but they have taken on new meaning, new direction, or even a newer purpose than where we started. No matter what, those lives are still important to God.

Your Story . . .

What stage of grief do you think you are in now?

_____

_____

_____

_____

_____

_____

_____

_____

What purpose do you see for yourself in this experience?

_____

_____

_____

_____

_____

_____

_____

_____

_____

_____

What do you think God has in store for you?

_____

_____

_____

_____

_____

_____

_____

_____

_____

_____

Forty Things I've Learned Since Turning Forty

Jesus spoke to the people again, saying, "I am the light of the world. Whoever follows me won't walk in darkness but will have the light of life." (John 8:12 CEB)

How I Felt . . .

Yes, I know it is hard to believe, but I hit the 4-0 today. In honor of my birthday, I thought I would try to sum up some big lessons I've learned on the road I am traveling. Enjoy.

40. Food is not the enemy. Our attitude and what we have been taught about food frames our perception about it. Bring joy back to the table and the anxiety that people have about food will be lessened. (Also, eat real food: life is too short for that processed crap. Eat and love real food.)

39. Don't feel guilty about exercise. Exercise to enjoy what you are doing. Exercise to put the body to work for God's work in the world and you will have more motivation to get up each day. No exercise is worth it if it makes you feel less than you are.

38. Learn to love *you*. God made you for a reason.

37. Cured and healed are not the same thing. I am not cured of my disease, but I am very healthy in spite of it. God heals.

36. Stop and watch the butterflies.

35. Enjoy color. I have a bad habit of watching the pavement when I run. I push myself each time to identify colors around me in every season.

34. The Bible tells us multiple times to "*Trust in the Lord.*" This is harder to do than it sounds. Trust in God for the big and the small stuff. I trust in God with my health every single day. I trust in God with my anxiety every single day. When I am overwhelmed, my

trust in God somehow creates the hours I need to get it done. This may be the most important lesson: trust in God in *everything*.

33. There are some years I would rather have a retake in my life: years 12–15, 17, 20–21, 30, and 38–39. These weren't stellar years by my reckoning, but if I stop, I realize I learned a lot during those years. Even in the midst of crisis, learning and love bloom. I cannot regret those years—they've made me who I am.

32. God really does love us and want us to be happy. Love can come out of crappy things.

31. Each moment, month, and year is just a slice out of the overarching scope of our lives. We shouldn't judge the quality of our life by moments. Look at the big picture.

30. However, don't miss the flowers, the trees, or the children for the big picture. God is the only absolute in life. Everything else is just shade and nuance.

29. Parenting is hard. It's the hardest job I have ever had. I am fairly sure my kids will identify many things I did wrong . . . just like I did with my own parents. The good thing is, they get to make their own mistakes trying to get it right.

28. Apologies don't cost anything but my pride.

27. My friends and family are my bedrock—you think I am a strong person? It is only because I am built on the love of my friends and family.

26. I love to travel.

25. I love to read.

24. I love to eat. I have a love affair with food. I love chocolate. Pizza (see my recipe on page 201) is my deathbed food.

23. I love coffee. I love wine. I love to share all these things with friends in fellowship.

22. I *love* my cochlear implants. I am blessed that God gifted people with the brains to create the technology that lets me hear. I love country music. My only regret is that I can no longer sing. Or rather, I can sing, but you wouldn't want to listen. My kids cringe when I belt out tunes. On the upside, I get secret pleasure out of embarrassing them with my rusty pipes.

21. My father taught me about the church. My mother taught me about my faith. These are important distinctions. I don't always agree with the church, but my faith in God never waivers.

20. It seems to me, on both sides of whatever political or theological fence you sit, there are a lot of people that hurl accusations, labels, derogatory comments, and untruths. I wish we would all think a little about what we are saying. You can defend your beliefs without tearing someone down. People rarely fit into the box in which labels put them. It only builds resentment and walls.

19. It's *really* important to understand church history. The Christian faith *is* influenced by history, society, and culture. God may never change, but our understanding of God changes all the time based on the microcosm of our lives.

18. I finally feel comfortable calling myself a writer. I am not sure how I am a nurse *and* a writer, but I am. I am not very sure I am excessively good at either, but where your heart is, there also is your treasure.

17. I'm fairly sure God has a lot more things to teach me. Sometimes this scares me a lot.

16. I've learned to see ministry where I am in life. Sure, I'd love to hop on a plane and be a missionary in Haiti, Africa, or somewhere else, but it's equally important that I see my mission in my local community and as a mother. As a mother, I am raising (hopefully) the next members of the church. The church would die without mothers.

15. I *love* cooking in soup kitchens.

14. My body is no longer twenty years old. I regret not enjoying it when I was that age. The flip side is that I'm getting better about not putting myself down. This is a pretty dang awesome body at forty years. It's got scars and mileage, some stupid mistakes, some great children, and lots of love in it. It may not be much, but I'm proud of what it's done. I'm ok with myself these days (however, I am *not* okay with whiskers—that's just cruel and unusual punishment, and proof that God has a sense of humor).

13. I am cherishing every moment my kids can still curl up in my lap. Every year, I realize they are getting bigger and bigger. It

makes my heart ache a bit. Time moves faster and faster the older you get.

12. I wish I had been less judgmental in my twenties and thirties. I thought I knew it all. I am so sorry for those that had to deal with my opinions. I hope I wasn't too overbearing. And feel free to call me on my comments these days. I am learning to make myself a better person daily, just like you.

11. I love that I have a zest for life. I hope it never goes away. I really do want to go out with a "Woo-Hoo" on my lips and a smile on my face.

10. Life, work, and family balance are crucial to a healthy life. If any of that gets out of balance, things go to pot.

9. It's really important to identify for yourself what the most important things are in your life. These can be your guideposts on where you spend your time. For me, the most important things in my life are God, my family, and my health.

8. You cannot divorce your spirituality from your physical and mental health. It simply isn't possible. If your spirit is sick, your body will suffer as well as your mind.

7. Stress is a killer. I am 99 percent sure my stress level contributed to my cancer diagnosis. I am very good at sweating the small stuff. I've learned it really isn't worth it.

6. Stuff is just stuff. It goes in the small stuff box. Material stuff, career stuff, physical stuff. It's just stuff. It's not going with me to heaven.

5. We don't think enough about heaven. Some people may think it's a given, a foregone conclusion to life. I am not 100 percent sure about that. I continue to study and pray about it, but I do think what we do in this world and how we act toward others is important. How does all that play out in the end? I'll let you know when I get there, but I think we should all think about heaven a lot more.

4. It is okay not to have an answer or an opinion on everything going on in the church. Discernment involves careful study, prayer, conversation, and theological reflection. You would be surprised by the number of things I am unclear about in the church, and I am okay with that. It goes back to the principle of *trust in God*.

3. Work is good for the human body.
2. Miracles happen every day.
1. I am blessed beyond measure and understanding. I have far more than I could want or hope for in my life and I think it directly correlates to *trust in God*.

I love all y'all. Here is to forty more beautiful years of work together. —*Anna*

What I Learned . . .

After all this, I have learned (and believe fiercely) that you and I are more than our cancer and our disease. Our journeys do not end because of a new diagnosis. We learn to take steps differently, but God still expects us to live a journey devoted to God in the middle of disease.

We are superheroes of God in our story. God's grace empowers us to so much more than drugs, surgeries, IVs, side effects, bald heads, and vomit. A life lived in grace is a good one no matter the outcome. Remember, this is not the end of your story.

Your Story . . .

Pick your age:

Write down the things you have learned so far, equal to your numerical age (i.e., just like I did above, forty things I've learned since turning forty):

_____

_____

_____

_____

_____

_____

_____

JENNY'S PIZZA DOUGH

Jenny makes her pizza dough in a bread maker. I make mine in my mixing bowl with the kneading attachment. We've both made it so many times now that although this recipe is what we sort of follow, it also is a little bit in our minds at this point, so we go by memory as well.

INGREDIENTS:

- 1½ cups warm water
- 1 teaspoon sugar
- 1 packet of active dry yeast
- 3½ to 4½ cups flour
- 1 teaspoon salt
- 1 tablespoon olive oil

DIRECTIONS:

1. Put the warm water, sugar, and yeast in a measuring cup or bowl. Let the yeast bloom (it gets fuzzy looking).
2. Put 1½ cups of the flour (I use organic unbleached flour—this makes your pizza healthy) and salt into your mixer with the kneading attachment (or pull out a wooden spoon and some muscle and mix it by hand).
3. Add the yeast and water mixture and mix it until it is smooth.
4. Add the flour slowly 1 cup at a time until the dough comes together in an elastic-type ball (not too sticky). It can take anywhere between 3 to 4½ cups of flour depending on heat, humidity, and all sorts of environmental factors. When the dough is in a ball and not too sticky, you've got it right.
5. Drizzle the dough with the olive oil, cover, and let rise until it doubles in volume. This takes about an hour, but I often make this in the morning and let it sit until I am ready to do something with it.
6. When ready, punch it down and knead it on a floured surface for a bit. Give it some love. Pray over it. Ask God to bless your pizza.

Continued

7. Then cut it in half and roll it out. The recipe makes 2 medium- to large-size pizzas.

8. Put the rolled-out dough on your pizza stone (the *best* way to cook pizza), top with my pizza sauce below, cheese, and what- ever toppings float your boat.

9. Cook at 450 degrees for roughly 15 minutes. It may take a little longer or a little less depending on your oven. I like to make sure the bottom is just brown before pulling it out.

10. *Let it cool!* You will burn your tongue otherwise.

11. Then pray and give thanks that God loves us so much that someone created pizza, and enjoy.

ANNA'S MARINARA SAUCE

INGREDIENTS:

- Tuscan seasoning
- Olive oil
- 1 can crushed tomatoes

DIRECTIONS:

1. Simmer 2 tablespoons olive oil with 1 tablespoon of Tuscan seasoning for about 1 minute.

2. Add in 1 large can of crushed tomatoes.

3. Mix it together and let it hang out on low until you are ready to use. Save the leftovers to dip your grilled cheese sammies in another day.

Thank me later. This really is delicious food. You can make food healthy by using good ingredients and watching your portion sizes. I love pizza. It will always be on some sort of "diet" I follow because, well, it's just good.

Epilogue

As I close this book three-plus years after my diagnosis, I am still watching and waiting with my lymphoma. I still have the disease. It was disappointing to me this last checkup as my tumors have grown a bit. In my mind, I had worked myself up to believe this was going to be the appointment where my doctor told me that I'd gone into spontaneous remission. I think God is still telling me that I need to learn patience. There is growth in learning to pause, watch, and wait. There is learning every day that the only thing I have is trust in God.

As I write this, I am preparing for another military move. The evil, anxious, worrying part of my brain is convinced that I will move across the country and be stuck in a place where my dad dies, my dog dies, my grandfather dies (he is one hundred this year, it could happen), my cancer grows, and I'll be somewhere without friends or family facing treatment and fear over my disease. As you can see, my "what-if" section of my brain is still working strong.

But the grace side of my brain is working strong too. I still hear God whispering, "Trust me." I know that when I have the worried, what-if thoughts, God will see me through. God has brought me thus far; God will continue to be with me no matter where things go.

My life is a blessed life. This does not come from the stance that I am blessed with a house, clothes, food, or things . . . all those things are nice, but I don't feel that God blesses us with stuff. I believe that God blesses us with God. I have come to realize that regardless of what I do or do not have, I have nothing without God. This story is nothing without God. I would have nothing to say to you without God woven through my story.

For me, faith is knowing that all that is important is the love of God. The love of God never waivers—even in the middle of disease, death, and mortality. As you persevere on your journey, perhaps like me, continue to watch, wait, and pray for peace. Whatever lies ahead, you've found that grace of knowing that no matter what, we are loved by God.

With love and blessings to all who have read and shared in my journey.

Thank you, —*Anna*

Acknowledgments

My life is incomplete and my story is without purpose without Treb, Patton, and Merryn. I love you dearly. For my family: thank you for my faith and your love that brought me safe thus far. Margaret, Babcock, Sandra, Simeon, Alice, Caroline, Ellis, the nieces and nephews, Weedo, Sallie, James, Evelyn, Hunter, Stuart, Big Daddy, Gus, Margaret, all the cousins. All the second cousins. All the cousins once removed.

My Groots: Jenny, Louie, Jenn, and Sara. Keep calm. We are Groot. If you get this, text me.

My South Carolina Cancer Posse: Julia, Jim, Ben, Stacy and Richelle, Kasie and Charlie, Paige, and Barbara.

My Kansas Cancer Posse: Katie, Lindsay, Christianne, Heidi, Cristin, Elizabeth, Amanda, Kate, Erin, Stephanie, the JAG wives, Jimmie, Father Michael, the St. Paul's Crew, and the St. Paul's Community Kitchen.

My Virginia Cancer Posse: Patricia, Jill, Matthew, Dave, Katie, Debbie, Leslie, Kerry, Sherri, and Michele.

My military peeps: Sara, Michelle, Andrea, Jason, Sarah, Jackie, Kim, Katie, Jenn, Katie, and Kristin. You've remained my battle buddies. Thank you.

For my work buds: Kym, Carrie, Kelsey, Jo, Renee, and Cindy. HP Rocks. Always.

For my churches near and far: your prayers have been felt. Prayer has power.

Sharon: We are three for three with you as my editor. Can we make it four? Thank you for your wisdom and guidance, and your patience with my excessive use of the word "so," two spaces after a period, and my preference for typing in caps, which you so patiently change to italics. You are soooo appreciated.

Church Publishing: Thank you for taking a special part of me and making it a part of the Church Publishing story. Together, we tell the story of God's work in the world.

As you've seen, no one goes on a journey of illness and disease alone. There is no (absolutely impossible, inconceivable, incapable, improbable) possible way I could have done this on my own. Never gonna happen. I am just not that strong. My superpowers don't come from me. They come from the people that lift me up and continue to drive me to make each step, one more step of faith on this journey. If there was someone I forgot, mea culpa—it was not intentional. Finally, this journey, this book, is not remotely possible without God. Every step, every moment that I cried, "This isn't the story I want," God replied, "Trust me."